Nutritional Management of Cancer Treatment Effects

Nagi B. Kumar

Nutritional Management of Cancer Treatment Effects

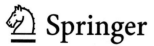 Springer

Nagi B. Kumar, Ph.D
University of South Florida
Heather Oak Place
33647 Tampa Florida
USA
nagi.kumar@moffitt.org

ISBN 978-3-642-27232-5   e-ISBN 978-3-642-27233-2
DOI 10.1007/978-3-642-27233-2
Springer Heidelberg Dordrecht London New York

Library of Congress Control Number: 2012931866

Printed on acid-free paper

Springer is part of Springer Science+Business Media (www.springer.com)

I dedicate this book to the individuals, their families and friends who have been touched by Cancer - for the courage, resiliency and hope that they have demonstrated and most of all, for their willingness to participate in our research studies during the past decades. Their participation has facilitated our understanding and has brought us closer to finding the answers to control, prevent and treat this disease better than we ever did before, with a hope to continue to improve the quality of life of our survivors and their loved ones.

Preface

Although the benefits of novel cancer treatments and approaches are continuing to be well established, many cancer patients are at risk for developing physiological and psychological sequelae of cancer and its treatment that may lead to premature morbidity and mortality. The prevalence of symptoms of cancer and cancer treatment are highly significant issues in clinical oncology. The objective of the book is to present the most current nutritional approaches to mange symptoms of cancer and cancer treatment using an integrated model of pharmacological approaches and non-pharmacological approaches to maximize patient outcomes and improve quality of survival.

Acknowledgement

I acknowledge my mentors, colleagues and my research team at the Moffitt Cancer Center, Tampa, Florida, and my family for their consistent support and encouragement over the years.

Contents

Introduction

The International Agency for Research on Cancer (IARC, World Health Organization) [1] estimated an incidence of 6,617,855 cancers around the world in 2008 with 4,219,626 deaths associated with this disease (IARC 2011). The American Cancer Society estimates that 1,596,670 new cancer cases will be diagnosed in 2011 with half of all men and one third of all women developing cancer in their lifetimes; 571,950 Americans are expected to die of cancer, representing more than 1,500 people a day and accounting for nearly one of every four deaths (ACS) [2], making cancer the second most common cause of death in the USA, exceeded only by heart disease. The National Institutes of Health estimates the total costs of cancer in 2010 to be $263.8 billion: $102.8 billion for direct medical costs (total of all health expenditures), $20.9 billion for indirect morbidity costs (cost of lost productivity due to illness), and $140.1 billion for indirect mortality costs (cost of lost productivity due to premature death) [2].

IARC also estimates that there are 22 million cancer survivors worldwide [1]. In the USA, the 5-year relative survival rate for all cancers diagnosed between 1999 and 2006 is 68%, up from 50% in 1975–1977. The National Cancer Institute estimates that approximately 11.7 million Americans with a history of cancer were alive in January 2007; some of these individuals were cancer free, while others still had evidence of cancer and may have been undergoing treatment.

The significant survival rate that is observed in cancer patient populations reflects the progress made over the past decade in cancer prevention (screening, early detection, lifestyle strategies to prevent cancer) and in cancer treatment. With rapid advances in molecular biology and cancer genetics, better understanding of basic cancer biology, and the development of powerful technologies, cancer therapies have now entered a dynamic era of novel, propitious approaches which target specific tumor sites and are personalized for each individual patient [3]. Under today's treatment paradigm, most cancer patients will successfully be treated with some combination of chemotherapy, surgery, radiation therapy, and/or immunotherapy and survive their disease, as demonstrated in the significant change in the decrease in mortality [1–5]. Increases in life expectancies combined with increases in early detection and improvements in treatment suggest that the number of cancer survivors will continue to increase [1, 2, 4, 5].

N.B. Kumar, *Nutritional Management of Cancer Treatment Effects*,
DOI 10.1007/978-3-642-27233-2_1, © Springer-Verlag Berlin Heidelberg 2012

Despite the improvement in survival, many cancer patients remain at risk of developing physiological and psychological sequelae of cancer and related treatment that can lead to premature morbidity, mortality, and decreased quality of life. In addition to an increased cancer risk (either a recurrence of the cancer for which they were initially treated or an independent development of a second cancer), [6] patients are at risk of adverse long-term (chronic /persistent) or late treatment-related effects, including other comorbid conditions as a result of therapy itself. These conditions may occur months to years after cancer treatment has ended. Additionally, oncology practitioners are realizing that despite the clinical success of therapies, cancer survivors are facing previously unrecognized issues related to survivorship, including functional and psychosocial side effects and practical and economic issues related to adjusting to life after their cancer diagnosis [7]. It is widely reported that the meaning of health and life itself can be altered following a diagnosis of cancer [8–10]. The majority of these effects resulting from disease and treatment are highly prevalent across the cancer continuum and present from a cancer patient's diagnosis and treatment through survivorship and end of life.

As reported subjectively by this patient population, and evaluated objectively in clinical settings, several of these symptoms are disabling, distressing, and persistent and extend in duration or severity beyond the point of compromising normal functioning and quality of life. Examples of the most common symptoms of cancer and cancer treatment include cachexia, anorexia, nausea and vomiting, radiation enteritis, fatigue, constipation, dysphagia, taste and smell alterations, neurocognitive impairment, mucositis, psychological distress, and insomnia. These symptoms are in addition to effects due to other comorbidities, such as hormonal perturbations and anemia, which contribute to impaired function, increased mortality, and a significantly decreased quality of life (Fig. 1.1). Exacerbating the risks of these late effects are the administration of multiagent, intensive, and multimodal therapies or long-term treatment regimens. While these therapies improve survival, they also produce relatively more toxicities and a wide range of treatment-related problems notable for their variability and unpredictability and obscure the delineation of the end of cancer treatment. Significant variability in timing, duration, and acuity of symptoms can be attributed to the complexity of cancer itself (e.g., the type of tumor and stage of disease), the multiple therapies that the patient may receive, the intensity of treatment (e.g., doses of chemotherapy or radiation, the extent of surgery needed), timing, age, and underlying health status of the individual at the time of treatment.

In studies using population-based data from the U.S. National Health Interview Survey, Hewitt and colleagues evaluated the health and disability [11] and burden of illness [12] associated with cancer survivorship, comparing those with self-reported cancer to those without cancer. Results of their study found significant decrements among those with cancer in self-rated health, psychological disability and activities of daily living, and among those less than 65 years, health-related work limitations. Yabroff and colleagues [12] compared self-reported cancer survivors to matched controls without cancer and found poorer outcomes among cancer survivors in self-rated health, a health utility index, and days of lost productivity. Similarly, a study using data from the Australian National Health Survey (NHS) to evaluate the health

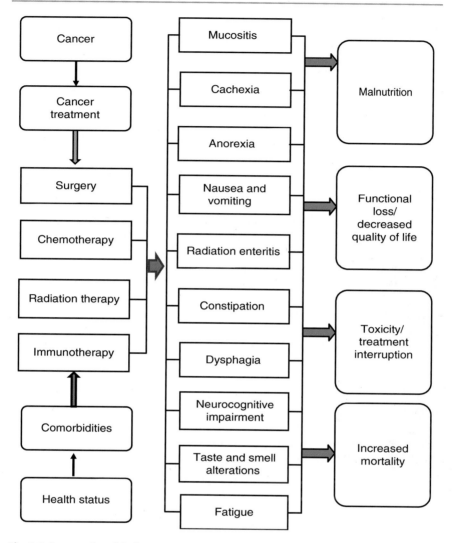

Fig. 1.1 Integrated model of consequences of cancer and cancer treatment

status of longer-term cancer survivors also demonstrated that they have significant decrements in health status and that these are further exacerbated by the presence of comorbid conditions [13].

Despite the significant adverse medical sequelae of cancer and its treatment, the practices relevant to anticipating or managing these symptoms remain poorly characterized, documented, or understood. Currently, an inadequacy remains with regard to our knowledge of the mechanisms underlying these symptoms and co-occurring or symptom clusters, dynamics associated with these closely related and interacting symptoms, the strength of this association and their complex interplay with an individual patient's health status, comorbidities (age, auto immune disorders, osteoporosis, arthritis, anemia, hormonal, or other organ dysfunction) [14], and specific types of cancer [15–21]. Based on this lack in adequate characterization and established management standards, the Institute of Medicine (IOM), Progress Review Group (PRG) documents, and NCI bypass budgets call for research as well as a "survivorship care plan" intended to increase length and quality of life for those diagnosed with and treated for cancer. The guidance reports call for standards for medical follow-up of survivors that include basic standards of care addressing the specific needs of long-term survivors. The IOM Report on cancer survivors diagnosed as adults articulates key areas for research and care delivery, e.g., the development of a formal care plan that integrates, within one document, key treatment relevant variables, exposures, late effect risks, and management/follow-up care needs [1, 2, 4]. At completion of cancer treatment, it is recommended that clinicians provide patients with a summary of treatment delivered and a detailed plan of ongoing care and summarize information critical to the individual's long-term care, such as the cancer diagnosis, treatment, and potential consequences; the timing and content of follow-up visits; tips on maintaining a healthy lifestyle and preventing recurrent or new cancers; legal rights affecting employment and insurance; and the availability of psychological and support services.

With a dynamic environment where novel cancer therapies are continually reaching the bedside, it is critical that symptom characterization, mechanisms, and management strategies be continuously developed in parallel in order to ameliorate new and known effects of these evolving cancers and cancer treatments. Future research should include evaluation of integrated pharmacological and nonpharmacological approaches for the treatment of these symptoms, taking into consideration the underlying mechanisms, moderators, and mediators, as well as other symptom clusters that may confound these symptoms. As research on symptom management continues to evolve, knowledge of the dynamics of symptom interactions and the relationships among commonly observed co-occurring symptoms can lead to the development of appropriate interventions to improve patient outcomes. Treatment and late effects could likely be reduced in the future with the advent of therapies that are tailored to the characteristics of an individual and their cancer. These advances in methods to assess an individual's risk for late effects (e.g., their DNA repair mechanisms related to radiation-induced DNA damage) and to personalize treatments will reduce the symptoms seen in cancer patients on active treatment and cancer survivors, ultimately impacting quality of life [22].

A number of recent reports on cancer survivorship have suggested that cancer, at least those sites with better survival profiles, be managed as chronic conditions [23, 24], with attendant shifts in the health-care system to facilitate transition from acute/oncology settings to primary care and increased attention to key areas of self-management such as lifestyle behaviors known to improve quality of life and function in cancer survivors [25, 26]. Prospective studies that obtain nature (tumor related), prevalence, timing, psychological and physiological mechanisms, and the magnitude of adverse effects in cancer patients throughout the continuum of the cancer treatment and thereafter are important to identify. Integrated interventions, both therapeutic and lifestyle that carry the potential to treat or ameliorate these effects of treatment must be evaluated and implemented. With improved methodological approaches, further research in this area may soon provide clinicians with effective strategies for ameliorating or eliminating these distressing symptoms and enhancing the lives of millions of cancer patients and survivors.

In treating the effects of cancer and cancer treatment, both length and quality of survival are important endpoints [8, 27, 28]. The prevalence of these symptoms is a highly significant issue in clinical oncology due to their high prevalence, deleterious nature, and the lack of insight into the mechanisms underlying most of these symptoms. The objective of the book is to present the most current nutritional approaches to manage symptoms of cancer and cancer treatment, integrated with pharmacological and nonpharmacological approaches, with the ultimate objective of maximizing patient outcomes. In doing so, this text specifically addresses a significant void that exists by providing an integrated methodology that may represent a new avenue for intervention to prevent or manage the most common symptoms in cancer patients that are known to be critical for function, survival, and quality of life. The following chapters guide the field of clinical oncology and are aligned with the goals of the IARC, the Institute of Medicine, and the National Cancer Institute, and may potentially dramatically affect how evidence-based clinical practice may be established and improved over the next decade.

References

1. Ferlay J, Shin HR, Bray F, Forman D, Mathers C, Parkin DM (2010) GLOBOCAN 2008 v1.2, Cancer incidence and mortality worldwide: IARC CancerBase No. 10 [Internet]. International Agency for Research on Cancer, Lyon. Available from: http://globocan.iarc.fr
2. American Cancer Society (2011) Cancer facts & figures, 2nd edn. American Cancer Society, Atlanta
3. Brem S, Kumar NB (2011) Management of treatment-related symptoms in patients with breast cancer. Clin J Oncol Nurs 15(1):63–71
4. Eakin EG, Youlden DR, Baade PD, Lawler SP, Reeves MM, Heyworth JS, Fritschi L (2006) Health status of long-term cancer survivors: results from an Australian population-based sample. Cancer Epidemiol Biomarkers Prev 15(10):1969–1976
5. Howlader N, Noone AM, Krapcho M, Neyman N, Aminou R, Waldron W, Altekruse SF, Kosary CL, Ruhl J, Tatalovich Z, Cho H, Mariotto A, Eisner MP, Lewis DR, Chen HS, Feuer EJ, Cronin KA, Edwards BK (eds) (2011) SEER cancer statistics review, 1975–2008. National Cancer Institute, Bethesda. http://seer.cancer.gov/csr/1975_2008/, based on November 2010 SEER data submission, posted to the SEER web site
6. Parry C, Kent EE, Mariotto AB, Alfano CM, Rowland JH (2011) Cancer survivors: a booming population. Cancer Epidemiol Biomarkers Prev 20(10):1996–2005
7. Gusani NJ, Schubart JR, Wise J, Farace E, Green MJ, Jiang Y, Kimchi ET, Staveley-O'Carroll KF (2009) Cancer survivorship: a new challenge for surgical and medical oncologists. J Gen Intern Med 24(Suppl 2):S456–S458, Review
8. Ganz PA (2009) Survivorship: adult cancer survivors. Prim Care 36(4):721–741, Review
9. Muzzin LJ, Anderson NJ, Figueredo AT, Gudelis SO (1994) The experience of cancer. Soc Sci Med 38(9):1201–1208, Review
10. Vachon CM, Habermann TM, Kurtin PJ, Cerhan JR (2004) Clinical characteristics of familial vs. sporadic non-Hodgkin lymphoma in patients diagnosed at the Mayo Clinic (1986–2000). Leuk Lymphoma 45(5):929–935

11. Hewitt M, Rowland JH, Yancik R (2003) Cancer survivors in the United States: age, health and disability. J Gerontol A Biol Sci Med Sci 58:82–91
12. Yabroff KR, Lawrence SC, Davis WW, Brown ML (2004) Burden of illness in cancer survivors: findings from a population-based national sample. J Natl Cancer Inst 96:1322–1330
13. Eakin EG, Youlden DR, Baade PD, Lawler SP, Reeves MM, Heyworth JS, Fritschi L (2006) Health status of long-term cancer survivors: results from an Australian population-based sample. Cancer Epidemiol Biomarkers Prev 15(10):1969–1976. PMID:17035407
14. Hurter B, Bush NJ (2007) Cancer-related anemia: clinical review and management update. Clin J Oncol Nurs 11:349–359
15. Gedaly-Duff V, Lee KA, Nail L, Nicholson HS, Johnson KP (2006) Pain, sleep disturbance, and fatigue in children with leukemia and their parents: a pilot study. Oncol Nurs Forum 33(3):641–646
16. Fox SW, Lyon DE (2006) Symptom clusters and quality of life in survivors of lung cancer. Oncol Nurs Forum 33(5):931–936
17. Dodd MJ, Miaskowski C, Lee KA (2004) Occurrence of symptom clusters. J Natl Cancer Inst Monogr 32:76–78, Review
18. Kim HJ, McGuire DB, Tulman L, Barsevick AM (2005) Symptom clusters: concept analysis and clinical implications for cancer nursing. Cancer Nurs 28(4):270–282, quiz 283–4. Review
19. Miaskowski C (2006) Symptom clusters: establishing the link between clinical practice and symptom management research. Support Care Cancer 14(8):792–794
20. Fan G, Filipczak L, Chow E (2007) Symptom clusters in cancer patients: a review of the literature. Curr Oncol 14(5):173–179
21. Gleason JF Jr, Case D, Rapp SR, Ip E, Naughton M, Butler JM Jr, McMullen K, Stieber V, Saconn P, Shaw EG (2007) Symptom clusters in patients with newly-diagnosed brain tumors. J Support Oncol 5(9):427–433, 436
22. Gusani NJ, Schubart JR, Wise J, Farace E, Green MJ, Jiang Y, Kimchi ET, Staveley-O'Carroll KF (2009) Cancer survivorship: a new challenge for surgical and medical oncologists. J Gen Intern Med 24(Suppl 2):456–458
23. National Cancer Institute (2006) Facing forward – life after cancer treatment. National Institutes of Health, Bethesda
24. Earle CC (2006) Failing to plan is planning to fail: improving the quality of care with survivorship care plans. J Clin Oncol 24:5112–5116
25. Rowland JH, Hewitt M, Ganz PA (2006) Cancer survivorship: a new challenge in delivering quality cancer care. J Clin Oncol 24:5101–5104
26. Ganz PA, Casillas J, Hahn EE (2008) Ensuring quality care for cancer survivors: implementing the survivorship care plan. Semin Oncol Nurs 24(3):208–217
27. Aziz NM (2007) Cancer survivorship research: state of knowledge, challenges and opportunities. Acta Oncol 46(4):417–432, Review
28. Hewitt M, Greenfield S, Stovall E (2006) From cancer patient to cancer survival: lost in transition. National Academy Press, Washington, DC

Assessment of Malnutrition and Nutritional Therapy Approaches in Cancer Patients

2

2.1 Definition

Malnutrition can be defined as a state of altered nutritional status that is associated with increased risk of adverse clinical events such as complications or death. Nutritional care is fundamental to cancer treatment (Davies M). Malnutrition specific to cancer patient populations has been observed to negatively impact patient's response to therapy; increase the incidence of treatment-related side effects; interrupt serial treatment regimens; extend hospital stay; impair muscle function, performance status, immune function, and quality of life; and ultimately affect survival [1–5]. Depression, fatigue, and malaise also significantly impact on patient well-being. In addition, cancer-related malnutrition is associated with significant health-care-related costs [5, 6]. In a recent study to evaluate the role of malnutrition and mortality in patients undergoing surgery for renal cell carcinoma, Morgan et al. [7] reported that malnutrition is associated with a higher mortality, independent of key clinical and pathological factors. On the other hand, proactive intervention to comprehensively assess and correct malnutrition early has been shown to reduce patient costs and length of hospital stay, improve response to treatment and, most importantly, improve functional status and quality of life in the patient [3]. For example, improvement of nutritional status over time is associated with better survival in ovarian cancer patients [8]. These effects were observed to be independent of age, stage at diagnosis, and prior treatment history and tumor response as determined by CA 125. Others have shown that significantly lower postoperative 30-day mortality after colorectal cancer resection was observed in cases less than 70 years of age, and absence of synchronous liver metastasis, malnutrition, and respiratory and vascular comorbidity were significantly reduced. With continuously evolving treatment modalities and novel agents for the treatment of cancer, it has also become critical to address nutritional care in the entire continuum of cancer (pretreatment, treatment, and posttreatment) to reduce GI toxicities and improve clinical outcomes and to ultimately improve morbidity and mortality in this patient population [8–12].

N.B. Kumar, *Nutritional Management of Cancer Treatment Effects*,
DOI 10.1007/978-3-642-27233-2_2, © Springer-Verlag Berlin Heidelberg 2012

2.2   Prevalence of Malnutrition in Cancer Patients

Malnutrition is the most common comorbidity in cancer patient populations. Studies have demonstrated that anywhere from 30% to 87% of cancer patients are diagnosed with malnutrition [51], with 30–60% of cancer patients diagnosed with protein-calorie malnutrition with higher rates of as much as 80% observed in esophageal cancer patients. The prevalence of malnutrition as high as 67% has been observed on ovarian cancer patients, while only 6% of endometrial cancer patients were malnourished [13, 14]. Others have observed that more than 64% of cancer patients were malnourished, increasing to 81% for patients undergoing palliative care [9, 10]. In clinical observations studies, over 95% of cancer patients indicate one or more symptom involving the gastrointestinal (GI) tract contributing to compromised nutritional status. Malnutrition is thus a frequent manifestation of cancer and a significant contributor of morbidity and mortality.

2.3   Etiology of Malnutrition

The etiology of malnutrition in a cancer patient is multifactorial and can be contributed to several factors: local effects of a tumor, the host response to the tumor, and anticancer therapies resulting in chronic or acute malnutrition. Other causes include reduced food intake (due to systemic effects of the disease, local tumor effects, psychological effects or adverse effects of treatment) and alterations in nutrient metabolism and resting energy expenditure (REE) [5]. Results of inadequate intake or absorption or increased metabolic requirements imposed by disease, including excessive loss of nutrients and drug-nutrient antagonisms, increased demands, inadequate intake, increased losses, relative intake of other nutrients, as well as symptoms of cancer and cancer treatment, can contribute to malnutrition. Figure 2.1 summarizes the multifactorial etiology of malnutrition in cancer.

2.3.1   Tumor-Related Etiology

Nutritional deficits are frequently observed in cancers of the gastrointestinal tract that can physically obstruct nutritional intake or produce metabolic and physiological disturbances that result in poor assimilation or reduction of nutritional intake. Stenosis of the GI tract, dysphagia, and previous surgery may affect the digestive capacity, or an abdominal tumor mass, disturbance of the motility, or repeated (sub) ileus may contribute to nausea and vomiting and therefore to reduced nutrient intake [15]. Pancreatic as well as gastric resections can result in pancreatic exocrine and endocrine insufficiency, creating major nutrition problems such as steatorrhea and hyperglycemia that may impede nutritional intake. Extensive resection of the small bowel can lead to malabsorption, whereas small resections of the bowel usually do not lead to major nutrition problems [16]. Liver cancer patients are confronted with the additional risk of malnutrition because the disease is often associated with hepatitis, liver cirrhosis, and metabolic disturbances [17]. Several agents produced by

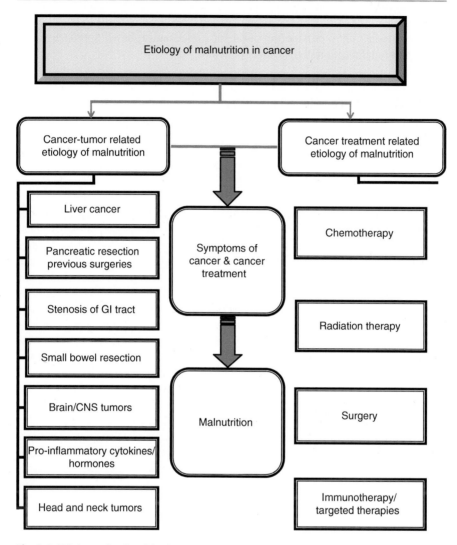

Fig. 2.1 Etiology of malnutrition in cancer

the tumor directly, or systemically in response to the tumor, such as proinflamma-tory cytokines and hormones, have been implicated in the pathogenesis of malnutri-tion and cachexia. A recent ASPEN and ESPEN guidelines group examined the pathophysiology of malnutrition and agreed that an etiology-based approach that incorporates a current understanding of inflammatory response would be most appropriate. The committee proposes the following nomenclature for nutrition diag-nosis in adults in the clinical practice setting. "Starvation-related malnutrition," when there is chronic starvation without inflammation; "chronic disease-related malnutrition," when inflammation is chronic and of mild to moderate degree; and "acute disease or injury-related malnutrition," when inflammation is acute and of severe degree [18]. Although the recommended classification needs to be validated in future studies, they provide the basis for a mechanism-based approach to the treatment of malnutrition in the cancer patients.

2.3.2   Treatment-Related Etiology

Patients with cancer have increased nutritional needs due to hypermetabolism, impaired organ function, increased nutrient loses, and therapy-related symptoms of dysphagia, mucositis, pain, cachexia, anorexia, fatigue, and radiation enteritis, all contributing to malnutrition. In addition, patients with cancer may also have increased requirements for both micro- and macronutrients due to the prolonged period of deficits prior to diagnosis [19]. Intensive therapy for multiple myeloma was significantly associated with decline in nutritional status [20], although these returned to pretherapy levels 6 months posttreatment. Nausea, vomiting, loss of appetite, weight loss, and poor quality of life were all reported by this patient population. Decrease in grip strength and triceps skin fold, as well as decline in hepatic proteins, testosterone, and gonadotropin in intensive treatment of patients with acute myeloid leukemia (AML) have been observed, suggesting a catabolic metabolism leading to impaired nutritional status [20]. Malnutrition is commonly associated to head and neck cancer patients, especially aggravated by radiotherapy or concurrent chemoradiation therapy [21–23]. In a study to characterize the effect of radiotherapy for head and neck cancer and GI cancers on nutritional status, Mahdavi et al. [24] observed that after treatment, the incidence of malnutrition increased significantly in patients in both groups with significant weight loss and decreased energy and protein intake in addition to decreases in serum zinc, copper, and albumin levels. Significantly lower antioxidants and selenium were found in lung cancer patients compared to healthy controls. Those patients with lower functional scores using the Eastern Cooperative Oncology Group (ECOG) performance scales had significantly lower levels of β-carotene and selenium compared to those with higher functional scores [25]. Similarly, we and others have observed lower serum levels of antioxidants lycopene in prostate cancer patients compared to disease-free men [26]. Thus, irrespective of baseline nutritional deficits, cancer patients experience a progressive decline in nutritional symptoms as they go through cancer treatment. Although some cancer patients recover from these nutritional consequences over time, significant variability in individual response to both disease and treatment makes this recovery to baseline nutritional status a complex, unpredictable, and challenging endeavor for the health-care team.

2.4   Assessment of Malnutrition in Cancer Patients

Nutritional care process that encompasses nutritional assessment and therapy of cancer patients in a clinical setting is accomplished in six basic steps: nutritional screening, initial comprehensive nutritional assessment, planning and implementation of nutritional therapy, education of the patient and family, communication with multidisciplinary team and reassessment to monitor response, and change in nutritional status as evaluation of efficacy of therapy. Timely nutritional screening to identify current and potential challenges to maintaining nutrition status and assessment and early nutritional therapy to replenish, improve, and manage exacerbation of symptoms may provide the best opportunity to prevent the debilitating consequence of cancer and cancer treatment. Figure 2.2 below provides a model for an integrated nutritional care process in the cancer continuum.

2.4.1   Nutritional Screening

The goal of screening is to identify patients who present with malnutrition or, due to recent diagnosis, comorbidities, and planned treatment approaches may be at high risk for malnutrition. Validation of these screening tools have been completed utilizing objective markers of malnutrition such as serum hepatic proteins and anthropometrics including body density measurements, weight loss history, and total body potassium. Instruments such as patient-generated subjective global assessment (PG-SGA) [13], SGA [27], and simple screeners using the nutritional risk index or NRS 2000 with more objective variables have been found to be valid for use in cancer patient populations [28]. Other screening tools such as Mini Nutritional Assessment have shown good correlation with laboratory parameters related to inflammation markers such as albumin, CRP, adiponectin, and leptin and were independently associated with survival [29]. In a study of 300 cancer patients to determine whether the Mini Nutritional Assessment (MNA) could effectively rate the nutritional status of patients with liver cancer in Taiwan, Tsai et al. [17] evaluate two modified versions of the MNA in short and long forms. MNA-Taiwan version 1 adopted population-specific anthropometric cut points, whereas version 2 replaced mid-arm and calf circumferences in place of body mass index. Results showed that both versions of the MNA were effective in predicting nutritional status, with nutritional scores correlating well with hemoglobin, serum albumin, C-reactive protein, r-glutamyl transpeptidase, TNM (tumor, node, metastasis) staging, and severity of cirrhosis [17]. Some of the practical variables used in clinical settings for nutritional screening are (a) hepatic proteins (prealbumin <10 mg/dL, albumin <2.1 g/dL, transferrin <100 mg/dL), (b) weight loss compared to percentage of usual weight, (c) body mass index (<20 kg/m^2), (d) lymphocyte counts, and (e) anticipated time to resolution of symptoms that impede nutritional intake (and gastrointestinal function not expected to resolve within 7–10 days or nutritional intake less than 50% of needs >7 days) – all of which form the basis to inform the medical team of the patient's initial nutritional status. Pretreatment weight loss has been documented as a predictor of poor survival, irrespective of type of tumor [30]. Since abnormalities in immune function have been associated with malnutrition, measures of total lymphocyte count may be useful on initial evaluation of the newly diagnosed patient with a solid tumor. However, the application of these parameters during treatment is limited due to the immunosuppressive effects of steroids and

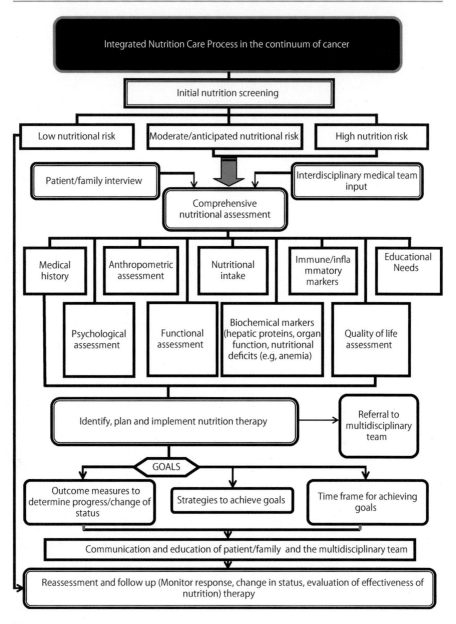

Fig. 2.2 Integrated nutrition care process in the continuum of cancer

many chemotherapy agents. Also, some hematological cancers are known to cause depression of bone marrow function resulting in leukopenia. Combinations of these indicators can stratify patients into low-, moderate-, and high-risk categories for nutrition-related surgical complications [2, 31–33]. Although these specific variables have been consistently shown to correlate to and predictive of malnutrition and poor prognosis, no one individual variable has contributed to identifying a patient at risk for malnutrition. Combinations of these indicators have been used to stratify cancer patients at clinical presentation into no risk, mild, moderate, and severe malnutrition [34–37]. Although a patient is screened initially with the diagnosis of mild or moderate malnutrition, based on the cancer and treatment trajectory, this condition can progress from moderate to severe malnutrition, requiring frequent rescreening and assessment. It is also critical that the initial screening tool must be simple and uncomplicated for application in a clinical setting [38], with readily available objective data [39]. The goal of the nutritional screen originated to identify and prioritize those patients at highest nutritional risk that needed to be evaluated and triaged for nutrition intervention. In most settings, all health professionals including nurses and intake specialists must be trained to screen patients for malnutrition. Whether screening in an acute-care setting or in an ambulatory clinical setting, all newly diagnosed cancer patients are screened on first contact with the health professional. Once patients are identified at high or moderate risk, a comprehensive nutritional assessment follows. Those at mild malnutrition or no risk must be under surveillance for change in condition or treatment. Several tools to screen cancer patients have been developed and validated [13, 40]. Assessment tools have included simple, objective, easily obtainable indicators, while some combine objective and subjective parameters to screen cancer patients.

2.4.2   Nutritional Assessment

The primary aim of assessing a cancer patient comprehensively is to design and implement optimal nutritional therapy, taking into consideration baseline nutritional status, current diagnosis, and comorbidities; planned cancer treatment and anticipated symptoms; and increased nutritional needs. Nutritional assessment is used to guide and inform the planning of nutritional therapy with the goal of improving treatment outcomes, managing symptoms, and improving function and quality of life. A comprehensive assessment of nutritional status is usually based on demographics (specific consideration to age); anthropometric measures; biochemical or laboratory tests; medical history including comorbidities, clinical indicators, and assessment of cancer and cancer-related symptoms; dietary assessment; oral assessment; current and planned medications; psychosocial assessment; swallowing ability; functional assessment including physical activity; and most importantly an assessment of patient and family cultural and religious belief systems. A comprehensive nutritional assessment is performed with objective data available in the patient's medical records and information provided by patients and their families in addition to information gleaned from other members of the multidisciplinary team.

2.4.2.1 Medical History
In addition to current diagnosis and stage of cancer, information regarding the patient's past medical history, presence of complications such as infection or sepsis,

present and past antineoplastic therapy, prior surgeries especially gastrointestinal, treatment and physical manifestations of disease, or nutrient deficits are essential to assessment of nutritional status and development of plan for nutrition therapy. Information on other comorbidities such as diabetes; heart disease; renal, hepatic, or inflammatory bowel disease; and current medications used to treat these illnesses can be useful. Other history of symptoms including toxicities from treatment including mucositis, nausea, vomiting, diarrhea, steatorrhea, constipation, or recent unintentional weight loss; oral or dental disease; or limitations should be obtained from patient or family. Constitutional, dermatological, gastrointestinal (GI), metabolic, and pain symptoms can be obtained using the NCI-CTG Common Toxicity Criteria Checklist

2.4.2.2 Psychosocial History

Social risk factors can also be identified at this time such as smoking history, alcohol or drug use, socioeconomic status [41–43], and availability of social support system. Emergent programs taking into consideration the need for psychosocial support for management of cancer and symptoms have shown to benefit both patients and their family members [44–46]. The need for a support system consisting of family, peers, and friends is a common thread in every culture and has been quantitatively assessed and equated with hope. Factors such as impediments due to personal, family, caregiver, or insurance issues that could interfere with symptom management must be discussed and resolved [47]. On the other hand, emotional suppression and distress through helplessness/hopelessness and stress can increase distress and depression with cancer diagnosis. Information on religious, cultural, and social support systems that can mediate and impact nutritional intake is essential to plan individualized nutritional therapy. Individuals who live alone have been shown to be at risk of having a poor intake [44]. Social deprivation or isolation also increases risk and has been associated with weight loss [45]. Social networks play a role in the maintenance of adequate food intake, and socialization results in increased food intake during a meal. Research has drawn attention to the challenges that patients receiving treatment for head and neck cancers experience, including the physical and emotional impact of diagnosis and treatment, weight loss, challenges related to eating, and strategies used by patients to address nutritional problems. It is clear that patients experience physical, emotional, and social losses associated with a changed meaning of food. Acknowledging the significance of eating problems and the changed meaning of food is required in order to provide patients with the appropriate support, strategies, and interventions to manage with the changes and losses [46]. The goal of psychosocial support is thus to provide tools to manage stress, encourage social interaction during meal times, and proactively educate patients with regard to anticipated symptoms that they may experience while providing strategies to cope with these scenarios. Approaches to education of patient and family, enhanced problem solving skills, stress management, psychosocial support, group support to improve mood and coping response, psychotherapy, and tailored behavioral interventions have shown promise in reducing symptoms of cancer.

2.4.2.3 Anthropometric Data

Body Weight and Body Mass Index

Anthropometric measurements such as patient's height, weight, and body mass index are considered relevant and objective measures of a cancer patient's nutritional status, with few potential errors in measurement in a clinical setting [48, 49]. Body weight and weight history are essential components of the initial nutritional assessment due to the significant impact of weight loss and underweight on morbidity and mortality. Unplanned weight loss occurs more commonly in more aggressive lymphomas, colon and lung cancers. Greatest weight loss is observed in gastric and pancreatic cancer patients [30]. In many forms of cancer, weight loss is an independent predictor of shorter overall survival even prior to chemotherapy, and individuals with weight loss are found to suffer more severe toxicity from chemotherapy [30, 50]. Unintentional weight loss with cancer is found in up to 80% of patients with pancreatic cancer and up to 60% of patients with NSCLC [51, 52]. Current weight is only useful as an indicator of nutritional risk or depletion if it is evaluated in comparison to the patient's usual weight. Weight loss must also be assessed in relation to its duration and whether it is unintentional or intended weight loss. Unintentional weight loss can be expressed as a percentage of usual body weight. Current weight that is 20% below ideal body weight is also an indication of nutritional risk. Similarly, a weight of 20% or less below ideal body weight is also indication of potential nutritional risk. In most cases, measurement of body weight and information regarding recent weight loss are important indicators of the presence of malnutrition upon initial screening and assessment; however, it has serious limitations as an outcome measure or monitoring tool since weight is a dynamic variable and is confounded by hydration and use of medications such as corticosteroids. The relevance of rapid and unplanned weight loss (10% of usual body weight in the past 6 months or 5% weight loss in the past 3 months) has been observed consistently to be associated with poor prognosis [30] and thus is an excellent indicator for screening cancer patients for nutritional risk. It is recommended that weight and weight change be assessed in combination with other parameters. Table 2.1 provides the formula used to calculate percent change from usual body weight.

In addition to weight loss, decreasing body mass index (18.5 kg/m^2) has continued to be informative for nutritional assessment of a cancer patient in clinical practice as an indicator of malnutrition [14, 30]. Patients undergoing nephrectomy for localized renal tumors with a BMI of less than 23–25 kg/m^2 have worse outcomes compared to those patients with a BMI >25 kg/m^2 [50, 51], demonstrating that BMI continues to be an important prognostic marker in cancer. Pretreatment body weight has also been shown to be a risk factor for locoregional failure in patients receiving

Table 2.1 Calculation of percent change from usual body weight

$$\% \text{ Weight change} = \frac{\text{Usual weight} - \text{Present weight}}{\text{Usual weight}} \times 100$$

Table 2.2 Body mass index (BMI) calculations and categories

$$BMI = \frac{Mass\,(lb) \times 703}{\left(Height\,(in)\right)^2}$$

Underweight = <18.5
Normal weight = 18.5–24.9
Overweight = 25–29.9
Obesity = BMI of 30 or greater

concurrent chemoradiation therapy for head and neck cancer [23]. Anorexia and weight loss are associated with increased mortality [4]. Studies showing inconsistencies in the relationship between BMI and malnutrition can be attributed to criteria used to determine normal versus obese or undernutrition ranges for BMI. For example, Marin Caro et al. [3] used <20 kg/m² for their definition of malnutrition, while others used up to 25 kg/m² to define malnutrition. Other parameters such as skinfold and circumference measurements and bioelectrical impedance technology have been used in clinical settings to measure lean body mass as well as body fat distribution. However, these methods suffer from errors due to measurement, unless performed by well-trained clinical staff and do not provide meaningful data of efficacy on nutritional therapy. Table 2.2 provides methods for calculating BMI and the categories to estimate under weight to obesity.

Body Composition

Although body weight, unplanned weight loss, and weight as a parameter as it relates to body mass index are valid measures to evaluate malnutrition, weight as an indicator to response to treatment has serious limitations since it is a dynamic variable and confounded by hydration and use of medications such as corticosteroids. Body composition measurements, both total lean body mass (LBM) changes and total bone mineral density (BMD), are relatively better markers that can be applied in order to tailor nutritional treatment to patients' individual requirements [52] as well as to monitor progress in a clinical setting. At present, body composition (BC) is rarely measured in the clinical setting because it is thought to be too unmanageable and time-consuming and burdensome to the patient. Skeletal muscle function is a central determinant of functional capacity in humans. Loss of muscle as seen in cancer patients results in poor function and decreased survival rate following critical illness [53]. Muscle size is therefore considered an important marker of functional status in studies of sarcopenia/cachexia [54–56]. Measurements of body composition combined with physical assessment for signs of obvious muscle wasting may help to identify significant losses in somatic protein stores; however, a more objective and sensitive measure of protein nutriture is the biochemical assessment of visceral protein stores. Using new technologies, the estimation of fat, lean body mass, and body fluids that are significant in the management of nutrition therapies in oncology has improved.

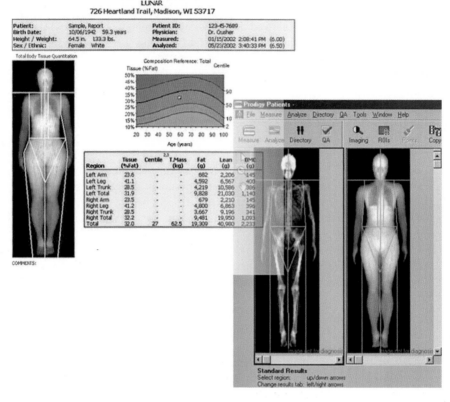

Fig. 2.3 Sample report of body composition as measured by DXA

Dual-Energy X-Ray Absorptiometry (DXA)

Figure 2.3 Sample report of body composition as measured by DXA (Body Composition Center, 77 Birch St., Suite A, Redwood City, CA 94062) has been used to measure human body composition on a high-speed fan-beam scanner. High- and low-energy attenuation pairs, produced by the various combinations of fat mass and fat-free mass in the human body, were compared to attenuation values produced by standard materials (aluminum and acrylic). These standards were measured in various combinations to construct calibration curves for fat and fat-free mass. Primary calibration of the aluminum/acrylic combinations was achieved by direct comparison to the dual energy attenuation produced by stearic acid and pure water. Whole body examinations were accomplished using three 45-s longitudinal passes of the fan beam. These passes were acquired and assembled to create a giant, isocentric fan beam with a single center of focus. In vivo precision was 0.009 g/cm^2 for bone mineral density (BMD) and 425 g for fat mass and fat-free mass (s.d.) [55]. DXA technology is now considered the most valid measure used to assess both total lean body mass (LBM) changes and total bone mineral density (BMD) in a clinical setting without increasing the burden to the cancer patient. Total bone mineral density (BMD) can also be followed as an indirect measure of muscle and patient activity. Total LBM is sometimes called total fat-free mass (FFM) depending upon specific DXA manufacturer. Total lean body mass changes can be calculated with total LBM values taken directly from most current DXA compared to total LBM from baseline DXA. DXA instruments use an X-ray source that generates or is split into two energies to measure bone mineral mass and soft tissue from which fat and fat-free mass are estimated. The exam is quick (1–2 min), precise (0.5–1%), and noninvasive. DXA scanners have the precision required to detect changes in muscle mass as small as 5%. Radiation exposure from DXA scans is minimal. The National Council of Radiation Protection and Measurements (NCRP) has recommended that the annual effective dose limit for infrequent exposure of the general population is 5,000 μSv and that an annual effective dose of 10 μSv be considered a negligible individual dose. The effective dose of a dual-energy X-ray absorptiometry whole body scan on an adult is 2.1 μSv

(a) *MRI of Thigh Muscle*

To obtain accurate measures of change in skeletal and fat mass with nutritional therapy, other direct measure of thigh muscle volume (TMV) may be obtained by MRI scan [56]. However, this is not always a practical option at this time as it not only increases patient burden but also the economic burden to the cancer patient. Subjects will be imaged using an MRI scanner (Siemens) at 1.5 T and a Q-body coil. Caution will be taken to ensure minimal patient motion during scanning (e.g., by placing folded pads/sheets under the legs) and using same positioning used for all subsequent scans. After a rapid survey scan, thigh images will be acquired using a 3D fast-gradient echo Dixon technique sequence (VIBE-Dixon) to cover the entire thigh (knee to hip). The total sequence time will be approximately 25 s. This sequence is superior for intramuscular fat quantitation. The 3D sequences yield automated separate fat images and images of water signal (almost all of which is in skeletal muscle), as well as combined (in-phase T1-weighted) and combined opposed phase images (Fig. 2.4). Muscle and fat compartments will be segmented. Muscle volume will be determined from the segmented calculation and will be made of (a) volume of subcutaneous fat and fat between muscle groups, (b) intramuscular fat volume, and (c) muscle volume. Muscle mass in kilograms will be determined by multiplying muscle volume by density. A density value of 1.0597 g/cm^3 as described in literature from unfixed rabbit and canine muscle tissue will be used for this calculation. Similarly, intermuscle fat content and subcutaneous adipose tissue will be obtained in kilograms by multiplying fat volume by the density of adipose tissue (0.9196 g/mL). Our primary endpoint will be defined by TMV based on MRI [56]. In addition to TMV, MRI will also allow exploratory outcomes (e.g., T2 and ADC) to assess metabolic impact of $N - 3$ FA on skeletal muscle and adipose tissue in the upper leg. This assessment can be related to the metabolic and functional abnormalities of the skeletal muscle in muscle wasting. The MRI pulse sequence used will allow for lipid quantification in the thigh muscle region

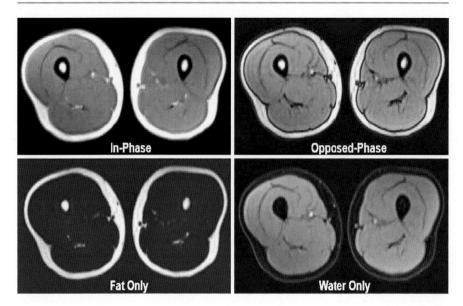

Fig. 2.4 Segmentation of fat and water images of the thigh using a single whole volume 3D gradient echo sequence

(i.e., subcutaneous adipose and intermuscular fat content or intermuscle adipose tissue) Fig. 2.4.

2.4.2.4   Measurements of Function and Strength

(a) *Handgrip Strength Dynamometry Assessment*

Figure 2.5 shows a sample of the Jamar dynamometers used to measure grip strength in a clinical setting. Muscle strength has been shown to be positively associated to muscle mass but negatively associated with inflammatory activity. Handgrip strength is also correlated with serum albumin levels [27]. A validated tool commonly used to assess handgrip strength is the Jamar dynamometer, which is a fast, reliable, and easy-to-perform device commonly used by our team to measure improvements in functional strength [57]. The Jamar dynamometer has a lower percent coefficient of variation and is thus a more precise device than other handgrip dynamometers (Fig. 2.5).

(b) *Functional Markers*

Evaluation of patient's functional status and barriers to obtaining adequate nutrients are also necessary. A physical exam combined with personal interview should include the evaluation of functional status such as the ability to chew and swallow, dental or oral problems causing odynophagia or dysphagia, signs of muscle wasting or anasarca, presence of edema, presence of skin or mouth lesion, and ability to perform instrumental activities of daily living (IADLs) such as cooking, shopping, and feeding self. It is critical to assess activities of daily living, physical activity, exercise, sleep, and ability to work and perform other functional roles. Limitations in the activities of daily living have been

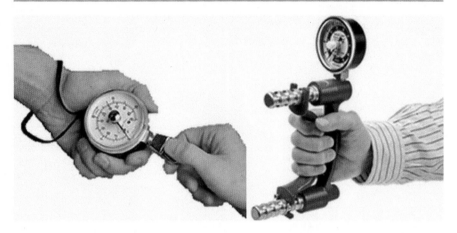

Fig. 2.5 Jamar dymamometers

identified secondary to and as a cause of weight loss in cancer patients. Cancer and other chronic diseases pose difficulties specifically for the cancer patient receiving treatment and the elderly in carrying out activities of daily living. A loss of postural and locomotive muscle mass has been observed within 7 days of inactivity [58]. The Karnofsky Performance Scale Index allows patients to be classified as to their functional impairment. This has been used to compare effectiveness of different therapies and to assess the prognosis in individual patients and has been validated in cancer patient populations [59].

2.4.2.5 Nutritional Intake

A vital component in the assessment of a patient's nutritional status is a detailed diet history and the collection of information regarding the patients eating behavior. This is extremely important in order to identify factors which may result in diminished nutrient intake. Nutritional intake is best assessed by conducting random weekly, 2 weekdays + 1 weekend day, 24-h dietary recalls (gold standard for collecting dietary data) using a five-step multipass procedure [32, 33] (which has been found to assess mean energy intake within 10% of actual intake). Food portion visuals should be provided to the patient to assist with documenting portions of food consumed [44, 60]. Nutritional history should include habitual diet and any change in diet pattern, frequency of meals or snacks, quantity of food at meals, self-imposed food restrictions, use of supplements, and other complementary therapies and vitamin/mineral use. Other symptom-related assessment must include ability to chew or swallow, specific intolerance to texture or type of food, presence of mechanical obstruction, poor dentition or pain with swallowing, recent or prolonged food or smell aversions, taste changes, early satiety, nausea or vomiting, pain, fatigue, appetite loss, and food allergies or intolerance. Questions should be open-ended to allow for accurate recall of diet history. After diet history is obtained, current nutrient intake should be compared to predicted requirements to determine adequacy of intake and need for intervention. Several nutritional analysis software are available today which range from free to the more the frequently updated University of Minnesota Nutrition Data System for Research (NDSR) version database for analysis of nutrient composition.

2.4.2.6 Biochemical Markers

(a) *An Objective Evaluation of Organ Function Can Be Determined Using Standard Comprehensive Metabolic Profile (CMP) and Complete Blood Count (CBC)*
   Complete Blood Count (CBC): The CMP is performed using electronic cell sizing sorting cytometry/microscopy are recommended at baseline and periodically. Tests performed as part of the CBC panel include the following: WBC, RBC, HgB, HCT, MCV, MCH, MCHC, RDW, PLT, MPV, absolute neutrophils, absolute bands, absolute lymphs, absolute monocytes, absolute eosinophils, and absolute basophils.
   Comprehensive Metabolic Panel, Direct: The CMP is performed using spectrophotometry, ion selective electrode (ISE), and hexokinase. Tests performed as part of the CMP panel will include the following: albumin, total bilirubin, alkaline phosphatase, AST, ALT, total protein, calcium, serum glucose, creatinine, urea nitrogen (BUN), BUN-to-creatinine ratio, sodium, potassium, chloride, and carbon dioxide.

(b) *Protein Status (Serum Albumin, Prealbumin, and Transferrin)*
   Serum hepatic protein (albumin, transferrin, and prealbumin) levels have historically been linked to nutritional status. Nutritional status and protein intake are the significant correlates with serum hepatic protein levels. Evidence has consistently suggested that serum hepatic protein levels correlate with morbidity and mortality and thus are useful indicators of severity of illness. Although serum hepatic proteins do not measure nutritional repletion (with the exception of prealbumin), it has been shown to be useful in identifying those who are the most likely to develop malnutrition, even if well nourished prior to onset of illness [61]. Serum proteins provide indirect information about visceral protein levels, indicating less hepatic synthesis which is usually a consequence of intake deficits. In cancer patients who are provided nutrition therapy including protein-sparing diets supplemented with proteins, an increase in serum hepatic proteins could signify an anabolic response. With half-lives of prealbumin (2–3 days) and serum transferrin (8 days) being relatively much shorter compared to serum albumin (15–20 days), changes in response to nutritional therapy can be observed within days of repletion [62]. Serum prealbumin and transferrin are thus considered relatively more sensitive parameters of the efficacy on nutrition interventions.
   Serum albumin is the most validated as a prognostic index and readily available biochemical parameter used to assess protein status. However, its relatively long half-life (14–20 days) makes it slow to respond to dietary interventions. Since the intervention period is 12 weeks, we have selected this to measure change in visceral protein stores. Perioperative serum albumin has also been observed to predict prognosis and survival in colorectal cancer patients undergoing surgical treatment [63]. In a comprehensive review of epidemiological data investigating

the prognostic value of serum pretreatment albumin levels and survival in a heterogenous group of cancers, Gupta and Lis [8] demonstrated the this was an excellent prognostic marker and may be used to better define baseline nutritional risk in cancer patients. Marin Caro et al. [3] observed a significant association between patients with low serum albumin levels and nutritional intake.

Prealbumin changes to short-term interventions are best indicated by prealbumin since it has a 2-day half-life versus albumin, making it a good indicator for early monitoring. Prealbumin is also unaffected by hydration status and, together with transferrin, predictive of changes in serum albumin [62, 64]. Prealbumin levels may be reduced with hepatic dysfunction, acute catabolic stress, sepsis, surgery, trauma, or severe enteritis or ulcers which may result from cancer treatment or progression of disease versus inadequate intake.

Transferrin is a serum beta globulin protein synthesized primarily in the liver, but unlike albumin it is located intravascularly as a transporter of iron, has a shorter half-life (8–10 days), and responds more rapidly to changes in protein status. Although transferrin levels are affected by iron status, serum transferrin, either singly or as part of a multiparameter index, is the *strongest predictor of cancer patient mortality and morbidity* [62, 64, 65]. Serum transferrin receptor is a marker of severe iron deficiency only when iron stores are exhausted. Clinical studies indicate that serum transferrin is less affected by inflammation [65]. The limitation of using transferrin as an indicator of nutritional status in cancer patients is that serum levels will decrease in chronic infections, acute catabolic states, surgery, and with renal impairment.

It may be important to recognize the challenge that patients with a syndrome like cachexia or with multiple, confounding symptom clusters may have inconsistencies in hepatic protein levels. Other potential confounding factors include stage of disease and impact of prospective concurrent anticancer therapies including surgery, chemotherapy, and radiation therapy. There is substantial evidence of the correlation between serum hepatic proteins and inflammation, making these the most relevant biomarkers in CC. Serum transferrin, prealbumin, and albumin have been observed as intermediate endpoint biomarkers and independently associated with worse outcome in cachexia [66, 67]. Measurements of body composition combined with more objective and sensitive measure of protein nutriture is ideal for the biochemical assessment of intravascular and visceral protein stores. Over 70% of patients of both genders with advanced cancer receiving palliative care have been shown to consistently have below normal serum hepatic protein levels [30]. Plasma levels of proteins (prealbumin, albumin, and transferrin) have been consistently used as indicators of protein-calorie malnutrition in the general population [62–70].

2.4.2.7 Immune and Inflammatory Markers

Unlike anorexia, in CC, there is a range of metabolic responses triggered by inflammatory and immunological responses. It is believed that the putative mediators of CC are cytokines, and increased expression of tumor necrosis factor and interleukin-6 has been observed in patients with CC. Cytokines will be measured in a panel including IL-1, IL-4, IL-6, IL-8, IL-10, GM-CSF, IFN-γ, TNF-α, and CRP (BioRad-Bioplex). All of these biomarkers have been shown to increase with disease, aging, and cytotoxic agents. Though we realize these intermediate endpoint biomarkers of cytokines cannot be reliably interpreted, as over 70% of the subjects as observed in our preliminary studies were on active treatment with cytotoxic agents, these variables are important to determine as they may provide useful information and contribute to the better understanding of the mechanistic process.

With our knowledge of the basis for some of symptoms such as cachexia observed in cancer, other novel markers of inflammation such as elevated C-reactive proteins and systemic inflammation–based scores such as Glasgow prognostic score, neutrophil-to-lymphocyte ratio, and platelet-to-lymphocyte ratio are being evaluated for use with cancer patients [71]. In addition to identifying patients at risk, these inflammation-based scores can potentially provide therapeutic targets in future intervention trials for the treatment of nutritional decline.

2.4.2.8   Quality of Life

Nutritional related symptoms such as cachexia, anorexia, weight loss, fatigue, cognitive impairment, and gastrointestinal manifestations such as mucositis and diarrhea are not only reflective of nutritional status but, in most cases, also reflective of social isolation and nonprogressive or declining functional status, ultimately impacting quality of life. The evaluation of nutritional status should include an assessment of quality of life in order to optimize nutritional treatment for patients' individual requirements. Because of the potentially clinically relevant impact of nutritional intervention on quality of life, nutritional care should be included in any antineoplastic strategy [72]. Other factors such as depression and distress have also been correlated to poor nutritional intake and compromise nutritional status in the cancer patient [73]. The Rand Short Form (SF)-36 [74] (Medical Outcomes Study SF36) has been used extensively with both general, high-risk, and cancer populations and has available norms for mail and telephone versions and comparisons between group and individual scores. Scores are calculated and transformed to a 0–100 scale, with higher scores indicating increased health status. Reliability of the SF-36 scales was measured by Cronbach α coefficient, and the results ranged from 0.78 in general health perceptions to 0.91 in the physical functioning domain.

2.5   Nutrition Therapy

Once the nutritional needs have been assessed, the best mode of nutritional delivery must be determined in consultation with the multidisciplinary team, utilizing the expertise of clinical nutritionist and clinical pharmacists. Determinants for options of supportive nutrition in cancer patients include presence or absence of functional GI tract; treatment plans – surgery, hormonal therapy, radiation therapy, chemotherapy, or biological response modifier therapy; degree of baseline deficit; quality of life and prognosis; and cost effectiveness/utility [75]. The choice of nutritional support is dependent on the degree of function of the gastrointestinal tract, access, patient comfort and motivation, type of therapy, anticipated disease course, duration of therapy, anticipated toxicities [76], and, most importantly, the choice of the patient. The availability of caregivers, patient's performance status, and financial resources should also be considered. In spite of the clear understanding of the effectiveness of nutritional therapy on intermediate markers of nutrition status [77], the ultimate effect on proven clinical outcomes such as morbidity, mortality, quality of life, tolerance to therapy, and cancer outcomes are all still limited [78]. Similarly, there is a clear correlation between degree of malnutrition and increased risk of perioperative complications in cancer patients undergoing surgery, although the beneficial effects of NST in perioperative patients have been difficult to demonstrate consistently [79]. This can be attributed to the complex effects of not only malignancies but also the continuously evolving treatment modalities with novel and targeted agents on the host's physiological, psychological, and metabolic milieu. In addition, these inconsistencies may be in part, due to methodological problems with trials performed in this setting, including the use of suboptimal feeding regimens and the inclusion of well-nourished patients unlikely to benefit from nutritional support regimens [79]. With our understanding of the metabolic and physiological mechanisms involved in the development of cancer and cancer-treatment related consequences, nutrition therapy for the cancer patient has now evolved to be an integrated, multimodality therapy that includes both pharmacological and nonpharmacological approaches that need to be individualized for specific patient populations. Nutritional support, addressing the specific needs of this patient group, is required to help improve prognosis and reduce the consequences of cancer-associated nutritional decline [5]. Nutritional intervention or therapy should be considered as a supportive measure within the global oncology strategy [72]. In curative oncology care, it contributes to reduced postoperative infection rate, better control of cancer-related symptoms, shortened length of hospital stay, and improved tolerance to treatment. In palliative care, the nutritional intervention focuses on controlling symptoms, thus improving quality of life [72]. If feasible, pretreatment nutritional therapy should be considered. Although earlier studies did not show the benefit of pretreatment nutritional support prior to head and neck radiation therapy [80], more recent studies have demonstrated benefit. Additionally, nutritional interventions adapted to diets modified based on side effects using oral route, combination of oral and tube feedings as with tube feeding only all resulted in improvement in increase in caloric and protein intake [21], demonstrating the benefits of nutritional therapy. Intensive nutrition interventions targeted specifically for head and neck cancer patients receiving radiation therapy improved intake of calories and proteins compared to standard interventions using nutritional education [81]. Furthermore, administration of the supplemented diet before and after surgery seemed to be the best strategy to reduce complications and length of hospital stay [82].

2.5.1   Estimation of Nutritional Needs

2.5.1.1 Calories

It is well accepted that many malignancies exert a metabolic effect on the host; however, the difficulty lies in predicting to what degree metabolic rate is affected due to the great variability in individual response as well as type of cancer and combination of therapies. Studies have measured the basal energy expenditure in a variety of cancer

Table 2.3 Calculating energy requirements

Basal energy expenditure (BEE)

For females: $55(9.6 \times \text{wt in kg}) + (1.7 \times \text{ht in cm}) - (4.7 \times \text{age})$

For males: $66.5(13.7 \times \text{wt in kg}) + (5 \times \text{ht in cm}) - (6.8 \times \text{age})$

For weight maintenance needs: $\text{BEE} \times 1.15 - 1.3$

For weight anabolism needs: $\text{BEE} \times 1.5$

Harris and Benedict [90]

patients. Cancer patients with pancreatic tumors, solid tumors, and liver carcinomas have been observed to be hypermetabolic [83–85]; however, other studies have not demonstrated a similar pattern in lung, colon, esophageal, and metastatic liver cancers [60, 86, 87]. Although others have demonstrated no differences in basal metabolic rate (BMR) between cancer patients and controls, the decrease in energy expenditure that is normally seen in starvation and weight loss in healthy men and women could not be demonstrated in weight-losing gastric or colorectal cancer patients [60]. Squamous cell carcinoma of the head and neck is associated with significant weight loss prior to, during, and after cancer diagnosis and treatment. A meta-analysis of effectiveness of nutritional intervention using appetite stimulants, dietary counseling, and prophylactic enteral tube feeding to meet compromised nutritional needs in patients receiving radiation and/or chemotherapy support the use of these proactive interventions to optimize nutrition in this population [88]. However, more randomized clinical trials are needed in this area. Caloric and protein supplementation has been shown to improve clinical outcomes in general populations, specifically in cancer patient populations too. Anorexia and weight loss are associated with increased mortality [4]. Oral supplementation is a simple, noninvasive option to increase nutritional intake in patients who are unable to meet nutritional requirements despite counseling [19] and modification of intake as per tolerance and has shown.

The best and most accurate method of determining calorie expenditure is by measuring metabolic rate via direct or indirect calorimetry under a variety of conditions. However, these methods are limited by the expense and availability of the necessary equipment and the added inconvenience of performing addition diagnostic testing on the already stressed and anxious patient. Another simpler method for calculating expected metabolic rate is with a formula developed by Harris and Benedict [89] (Table 2.3). This equation, used in combination with accepted activity and stress factors, is widely used for calculating basal energy expenditure in hospitalized patients. This method takes into account the patient's gender, height, weight, and age, factors known to influence metabolic rate. The accuracy of this equation has been verified in validation studies comparing actual measurements and predicted values of healthy individuals with a mean difference of only 4% [89].

The calculations of predicted total energy expenditure (TEE) are derived using the Harris-Benedict equation multiplied by an activity factor or a stress factor (Table 2.4). These factors are based on data collected by Long et al. [91] measuring the metabolic

Table 2.4 Activity and stress factors for calculating total energy expenditure

Activity level	
Bedrest	1.2
Low activity	1.3
Moderate activity	1.5–1.75
Highly active	2.0
Injury factors:	
Minor surgery	1.1
Major surgery	1.3
Mild infection	1.2
Moderate infection	1.2–1.4
Sepsis	1.4–1.8
Skeletal trauma	1.2–1.4
Skeletal or head trauma (treated with steroids)	1.6–1.8

Source: From Long [89]

response to injury and illness. In order to determine an estimate of energy requirements, it is critical to obtain information regarding the patient's nutritional status, treatment, and any additional metabolic stresses as identified in the nutritional assessment. To determine calorie needs in the absence of surgery or infection, as is often the case with cancer patients, a factor of 1.15×BEE can be used for weight maintenance or 1.5×BEE, for repletion and anabolism [92] The average caloric deficit in weight-losing patients observed by us and other teams is approximately 250–400 kcal/day with significant variations based on stage and severity of disease. In most clinical settings, these deficits in nutritional intake have been compensated by providing caloric and protein supplementation with a goal of meeting nutritional needs of the individual patient. The average supplementation of 1 cal/mL supplements have not shown to improve nutritional status of patients on chemotherapy [93, 94]. However, recent studies using a more calorie-dense (1.5 kcal/mL) and higher protein supplementation have suggested that at least weight stabilization can be achieved [95], although improvements in lean body mass has not been observed in these studies. Our preliminary studies have also demonstrated that high-calorie and high-protein supplemental (calorie- and protein-dense) feedings result in substitution of regular meals and thus a reduction of caloric and protein intake in this patient population who experience early satiety as a symptom cluster with anorexia or cancer cachexia. It is important to take into consideration that these guidelines were established several decades ago and continue to be used for lack of alternate evidence-based guidelines. Because these calculations are an estimate and not based on actual measurement of caloric expenditure, the best indicator of adequacy is the patient's response to the nutrition regimen. Monitoring of patient progress and adjustments of calorie goals as needed are essential parts or the nutrition care plan.

2.5.1.2 Protein

Injury and illness are known to produce marked losses of protein as indicated by increases in urinary nitrogen excretion [89]. Acceleration of protein turnover and derangements in protein metabolism have also been seen in cancer patients [96]. Protein-calorie deficits have been shown to contribute to malnutrition in esophageal cancer patients. Provision of exogenous energy and protein has been shown to invoke an anabolic response as indicated by an increase in serum prealbumin and transferrin level in this patient population [62]. In contrast to simple starvation where the body attempts to spare protein, the opposite is true under conditions of metabolic stress such as the cancer process itself or combined with antineoplastic therapy. The most accurate method of determining protein requirements in a hypermetabolic patient is based on urinary nitrogen loss; however, this is impractical in most settings due to the labor intensity involved in collecting 24-h urine specimens and fecal specimens for total nitrogen output in addition to accurately calculating protein intake. The only setting in which this might be feasible is in critical care. The estimated protein requirement is determined based on the degree of protein depletion and the metabolic stress factors. For the well-nourished, mildly stressed individual, the protein needs may only be 0.8–1.0 g/kg IBW; however, with mild to moderate depletion combined with metabolic stress, 1.5–2.0 g/kg IBW may be required to achieve positive nitrogen balance and protein repletion. Another method of estimating protein requirements is by calculating the ratio of nitrogen to nonprotein calories. It is recommended to provide 1 g nitrogen (protein in grams divided by 6.25) per 120–150 nonprotein calories for anabolism in the moderately to severely malnourished or stressed patient [97, 98]. As with estimating calorie requirements, the best indicator of whether protein needs are being met is with monitoring and reassessment for weight gain and nitrogen retention in the malnourished patient and weight maintenance and nitrogen equilibrium in the well-nourished patient [99]. Initially, the pathophysiology of CC had two principle components – a failure of food intake and a systemic hypermetabolism/hypercatabolism syndrome. Additionally, diets adequate in calories from fats and carbohydrates were required in "protein-sparing" quantities for muscle anabolism [100]. Protein intake must also be sufficient for wound repair, resistance to infection, and synthesis of enzymes and plasma proteins [101, 102]. Supplementation with glutamine, arginine, and branched-chain amino acids appears to support improvement in reducing complications and improving treatment outcomes [103]. Future clinical trials should evaluate the impact of multimodal interventions using, in addition to nutrients and appetite stimulants, immune modulatory nutrients for the treatment of malnutrition in well-powered clinical trials. Guidelines for estimating protein requirements are provided in Table 2.5. However, as with total calories, these calculations are an estimate and not based on actual measurement of protein expenditure in cancer patient populations. Thus, the best indicator of adequacy is the patient's response to the nutrition regimen. Monitoring of patient progress and adjustments of protein intake goals as needed are essential parts or the nutrition care plan.

2.5.1.3 Fats/Lipids

There are no recommended dietary allowances for lipids and carbohydrates in cancer patient populations.

Table 2.5 Calculating protein requirements

For calculating protein needs : Divide IBW by 2.2 = kg of IBW

For protein maintenance : Multiply $0.8 - 1.4 \times$ kg of IBW

For protein anabolism : Multiply $1.5 \times$ kg of IBW

2.5.1.4 Vitamins and Minerals

The need for vitamins and minerals is increased in this patient population. Oxidative stress and inflammation contribute to several organ toxicities, including neurotoxicities, after common cancer chemotherapy regimens. Doxorubicin and other platinum-based therapies have been documented to cause the generation of free radicals and the induction of oxidative stress, associated with cellular injury [104]. The debate continues as to the safety of antioxidant use *during* chemotherapy to reduce oxidative stress, other than a multivitamin-mineral supplement that meets the current USRDA. Increased doses higher than the USRDA may not be recommended based on the safety and nutrient-cytotoxic agent interaction concerns, if administered during active therapy. In September 2005, studies were published [105, 106] warning against the concurrent use of antioxidants with cytotoxic therapies. Supplementing with antioxidants and anti-inflammatory agents posttreatment may serve to "rescue" tissues from the effects of the oxidative damage, in addition to replenishing depleted status of these critical nutrients and reversing oxidative damage. However, these theories have not been tested in well-powered trials, in clinical trials targeting cancer patients.

2.5.1.5 Determining Hydration

Daily fluid replacement is essential, specifically in chronically or acutely ill patients who are on diuretics, laxatives, or other therapeutic regimens for cancer treatment. In addition, dehydration is commonly observed in the elderly as they have reduced thirst sensation and diminished water conservation by the kidneys. Nutritionally related symptoms as a result of cancer treatment such as diarrhea, inability to swallow liquids, or fever may also increase requirements contributing to clinical dehydration. Recurrent urinary tract infections have been documented in hospitalized elderly women. A minimum schedule of 30–35 mL fluid/kg of body weight or a minimum of 1,500 mL a day is recommended.

2.6   Route of Nutrition Intervention

2.6.1   Oral Intake

The preferred method of nutrition intervention, the least expensive and least invasive, is a standard or modified diet plus oral supplementation [107]. Several options of commercial and homemade recipes are recommended as tolerated and/or preferred by the patient. Several pharmacological and nonpharmacological strategies to improve appetite and nutritional intake and prevent early satiety are developed with individual patients. However, if patients are unable to consume sufficient protein and calories for greater than 7–10 days with continued decline in nutritional status as indicated by serum hepatic proteins, weight loss, and anthropometrics, alternate means of support via enteral support or total parenteral nutrition (TPN) may be indicated. Table 2.4 provides general guidelines/criteria for selection of route of feeding.

2.6.2   Enteral Nutrition

Enteral nutrition involves the nonvolitional delivery of nutrients by tube into the gastrointestinal tract. Patients who cannot, should not, or will not eat adequately, in whom the benefits of improved nutrition outweigh the risk, and have a functional gastrointestinal tract are candidates for enteral tube feedings [108]. Enteral feeding provided through a tube, catheter, or stoma delivers nutrients distal to the oral cavity (Fig. 2.6). The chosen route for enteral feedings depends on the patient's clinical status, risk for aspiration, and anticipated duration of tube feeding. Short-term feedings (less than 3–4 weeks) usually are administered via nasogastric, nasoduodenal, or nasojejunal tubes. The nasoduodenal and nasojejunal (postpyloric) routes are preferable to the nasogastric route if the patient is at risk for aspiration. A decision to perform a tube enterostomy (esophagostomy, gastrostomy, jejunostomy) is usually made for long-term feedings (>3–4 weeks). Jejunostomy is the preferred approach when the patient is at risk for aspiration or is unable to consume adequate calories due to uncontrolled nausea or vomiting. If patient is critically ill, timely, early nutritional intervention using the enteral route may be beneficial. If oral intake is not feasible, early enteral nutrition may be instituted, especially in head and neck cancer patients [19, 109]. If enteral nutrition is insufficient or fails to alter nutritional status, parenteral nutritional therapy may be considered, taking into consideration the often-reduced demand for exogenous substrates, especially in the critically ill patient [110]. The impact of timing of PEG tube placement on clinical endpoints in patients undergoing concurrent chemoradiation therapy showed a significant clinical benefit from early placement for nutritional supplementation [111]. However, the effect of prophylactic GT placement on acute and long-term outcomes in patients treated with definitive chemoradiotherapy for head and neck cancer is still not certain, with recent reports demonstrating a higher rate of late esophageal toxicity and need for weighing the benefits to risk in this patient population [112]. In the ASPEN guidelines for surgical cancer patients, it is recommended that EN should not be used routinely in patients undergoing major cancer surgery. However, it is recommended that perioperative EN may be beneficial in moderately or severely malnourished patients if administered for 7–14 days preoperatively, but the potential benefits of EN must be weighed against the potential risks of the EN itself and of delaying surgical procedures [79].

Although concerns about PEG feeding have been documented, specific risk factors have been examined. Factors such as cirrhosis and radiation therapy were predictors of infection. Post-PEG bleeding and other complications were found to be a rare event in a large population-based study. Even in patients taking concurrent anticoagulants, no elevated risk was observed with PEG feedings [113]. Jejunostomy tubes (JT) which are usually placed at time of esophagectomy have also been

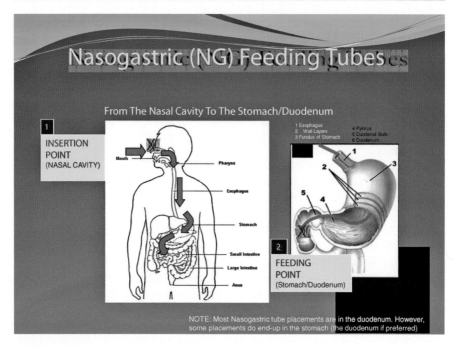

Fig. 2.6 Insertion and feeding points for nasogastric feeding tubes

associated with low morbidity. Although no major contraindications were observed, the only absolute indication for JT placement after esophagectomy was a BMI <18.5 kg/m^2 or based on the surgeon's judgment [114]. More recently, several novel methodologies to insert PEGs for long-term feeding of cancer patient populations has received attention. The safety of pull-type and introducer-type insertion of PEG have been evaluated, and the introducer PEG procedure for long-term tube feeding has been found to produce significantly higher complications and mortality rates in patients with head/neck or esophageal malignancies treated with chemotherapy and radiation therapy compared to pull-type PEG placement [115, 116]. Techniques for PEG placement using the T-fastener gastropexy technique in head and neck cancer patients and esophageal cancer patients also resulted in lower overall complication rate compared to the pull method [117]. Enteral nutrition has been shown to reduce infectious complications and mortality compared to parenteral nutrition [118]. Although enteral nutrition is generally considered safe, gastrointestinal, metabolic, and respiratory complications have been documented [79]. Inappropriate formula advancement or feeding interruptions may result in underfeeding. Gastrointestinal intolerance is often due to improper methods of feeding, such as bolus delivery into the small intestine. The most common problems associated with enteral feedings can be minimized or prevented through proper formula preparation and equipment selection, controlled administration, and monitoring. A reduced incidence of metabolic abnormalities and other improved outcomes of enteral nutrition have been demonstrated when patients are managed by a multidisciplinary team. Figure 2.6 below provides examples of placement of nasogastric tube feedings (Table 2.6).

Table 2.6 General guidelines/criteria for selection of route of feeding

Criteria for enteral feeding via oral route.	Criteria for enteral feeding via tube feeding	Indications for parenteral nutrition	Ethically acceptable guidelines for nutritional support in end-stage disease
(a) If the gastrointestinal tract is working- use this.	If patient's condition is not anticipated to resolve in <7 days, consider enteral tube feeding	In patient where enteral feeding is not feasible and the gastrointestinal problems are anticipated to persist – consider parenteral feeding if benefits outweigh other risks:	In cancer patients not receiving curative antineoplastic therapy/end-stage disease.
(b) Evaluate risk for dysphagia, aspiration, nausea, vomiting, diarrhea, gastric motility or abdominal pain while eating.	(a) Nutritional intake below 50% of needs	(a) If problems with GI tract function is anticipated	(a) Nutritional support – viewed as a palliative measure
	(b) Functioning gastrointestinal tract	(b) Severely malnourished	(b) The goal is to support hydration
(c) Absent above symptoms or if above symptoms are anticipated to resolve in <7 days	(i) Nasogastric (NG) feeding (insertion point: nasal cavity, feeding point: stomach/duodenum)	(c) GI problems will persist >7–10 days	(c) IV route for hydration may also serve as a route for delivering necessary medications
(d) Consider oral intake.	(ii) Percutaneous endoscopic gastrostomy (PEG): does not require general anesthesia	(d) Nutritional needs not met–(<50%) over 7–10 days	(d) Decision must be made based on patients desire. Family preferences should be taken into account
	(iii) PEG-J: jejunal extension in patients at risk for aspiration	(e) Not at risk for sepsis or multiple, resistant infections	(e) Informed decision based on stage of cancer and prognosis
		(f) Unsuccessful enteral feedings	(f) Anticipated consequences of not receiving hydration or nutrition should be communicated to patient and family
		(g) Aggressive malignancy and persistent obstruction – functioning GI tract – consider total parenteral nutrition	(g) Risks involved in administering support: fluid overload, infection, malabsorption
		(h) Monitor patient for	(h) Allow patients to eat for enjoyment
		(i) Serum glucose >300 mg/dL	(i) Quality of life is key
		(ii) Serum phosphorous <2 mg/dL	(j) Educate family on nutritional care for the patient based on patient's wishes.
		(iii) BUN >100 mg/dL	(k) Patient will be unable to tolerate if intake is planned to meet increased needs.
		(iv) Serum potassium >5.7 or <3.0 mEq/L	(l) Provide emotional support consulting with spiritual counselor, palliative care services when available.
		(v) Catheter-related infection	
		(vi) Malfunction of catheters due to clotted or clogged ports	
		Wean to enteral as soon as patient consumes 50% of calories and protein based on need.	

(continued)

Table 2.6 (continued)

Contraindications for enteral feeding using the gastrointestinal tract	Contraindications for enteral tube feeding using the gastrointestinal tract	Contraindications for parenteral feeding
(a) If patient is hemodynamically unstable	(a) If patient is hemodynamically unstable	(a) End stage disease
(b) Malabsorption	(b) Malabsorption	(b) Multiple organ failure
(c) Short-bowel syndrome	(c) Short-bowel syndrome	(c) Sepsis
(d) Pseudo obstruction	(d) Pseudo obstruction	(d) Resistant infections
(e) Gastrointestinal fistula	(e) Gastrointestinal fistula	(e) Nutritional support – viewed as a palliative measure
(f) Mesenteric ischemia – interruption in blood flow to all or part of the small intestine or the right colon radiation enteritis	(f) Mesenteric ischemia – interruption in blood flow to all or part of the small intestine or the right colon radiation enteritis.	(f) The goal is to support hydration
(g) Paralytic ileus – either by a physical obstruction of the lumen such as a growing tumor, or by a loss of normal peristaltic function	(g) Paralytic ileus – either by a physical obstruction of the lumen such as a growing tumor, or by a loss of normal peristaltic function	(g) Decision must be made based on patients desire.
		(h) Family preferences should be taken into account. Informed decision based on stage of cancer and prognosis

2.6.3   Parenteral Nutrition

In patients where enteral nutrition is not feasible nor tolerated, parenteral nutrition offers the possibility of increasing or ensuring nutrient intake [78]. The ESPEN guidelines [119] on enteral nutrition in oncology recommends that several of the indications for parenteral nutrition are similar to those for enteral nutrition (weight loss or reduction in food intake for more than 7–10 days), but only those who, for whatever reason, cannot be fed orally or enterally are candidates to receive parenteral nutrition. Other groups where short-term parenteral nutrition is recommended are in patients with CC using a high fat-to-glucose ratio may be advised because these patients maintain a high capacity to metabolize fats and in patients with acute gastrointestinal complications from chemotherapy and radiotherapy. Long-term (home) parenteral nutrition has been found to be critical in patients with subacute/chronic radiation enteropathy. Other patient populations that have shown to benefit from home PN are incurable cancer patients who are hypophagic/(sub)obstructed patients (if there is an acceptable performance status) if they are expected to die from starvation/undernutrition prior to tumor spread [119]. In a study to evaluate the effects of TPN and EN on biochemical and clinical outcomes in pancreatic cancer patients who underwent pancreaticoduodenectomy (PD), Liu et al. [120] observed that although there were no preoperative differences between the groups, significant differences in liver and kidney function parameters were observed with incidence of pancreatic fistulas and hemorrhages significantly greater in the TPN group compared to the EN group. Although the specific criteria for using TPN instead of PN in the first place are not indicated and the sample size of the target population was small, these studies demonstrate that EN is a better choice if the gut is functioning versus TPN in this patient population [120]. Others have examined if early preoperative enteral nutrition improved postoperative course, since most patients post-PD have symptoms of nausea, diarrhea, and abdominal distention presenting challenges to initiate PN. In a pilot trial to examine both EN and EN plus TPN in this target group, the rate of discontinuance was significantly greater in the EN group compared to the EN plus TPN group, with no differences in the infection rate between the two groups [121]. The ESPEN [119] guidelines recommend that perioperative parenteral nutrition only be used in malnourished patients if enteral nutrition is not feasible. In nonsurgical, well-nourished oncologic patients, routine parenteral nutrition is not recommended, since it has not offered any advantage and is associated with increased morbidity. A benefit, however, is reported in patients undergoing hematopoietic stem cell transplantation [119]. The benefit of administering TPN as means of support or for repletion of nutritional status continues to remain controversial due to the lack documentation for a favorable impact of TPN on response to therapy or survival. The decision to use TPN as an adjunct to therapy remains a matter of clinical judgment. However, malnourished patients unable to tolerate enteral feedings with a clear response or potential response to antineoplastic treatment are usually considered candidates for parenteral support, taking into consideration problems and challenges identified in patient populations with organ failure, circulatory disorders, and effects of other therapies used and tumor effects.

2.7   Reassessment and Follow-up Nutritional Care

Improved management of malnutrition with nutritional therapy may require a multimodal intervention by multidisciplinary teams using a comprehensive and integrated approach. Initial screening and knowledge of treatment trajectory of the cancer patient should guide a plan for reassessment of the cancer patient at regularly planned intervals. Subjective and objective data on progress and response to nutritional therapy may be assessed using the indicators used in the comprehensive nutritional assessment. Newly developed symptoms resulting from treatment or progression of disease may require additional monitoring or revision of nutritional therapy. Nutritional reassessment is also indicated in those patients initially identified at low or no risk for malnutrition. Criteria for reassessment in this group is indicated when treatment symptoms are anticipated or develop; a deficiency in nutritional intake is observed compared to assessed requirements; patient exhibits nutritional symptoms such as nausea, vomiting, and diarrhea; or patient is on serial treatment regimens that have been shown to increase nutritional risk. Reassessment/reevaluation for monitoring and evaluation of nutritional therapy must include monitoring of clinical, functional, dietary, and behavioral outcomes that were identified by the comprehensive nutritional assessment.

2.8   Patient and Family Communication/Education

The goals of nutritional therapy, the outcome measures planned, and strategies to achieve these goals, as well a time frame within which these goals can be achieved, must be communicated both to the patient as well as the interdisciplinary medical team throughout the continuum of cancer care. Patient education may include information about the results of nutritional assessment, planned nutritional therapy and patient's role in planning this therapy, symptoms that can be anticipated based on treatment regimen, and strategies to manage symptoms. Patient and family education, proactively, has been the single most important component of managing nutrition therapy in cancer patients. Patients must be educated on reporting symptoms and not take for granted that these symptoms are a part of cancer treatment. Approaches to education of patient and family, enhanced problem solving skills, stress management, psychosocial support, peer group support to improve mood and coping response, psychotherapy, and tailored behavioral interventions have shown promise in reducing symptoms of cancer.

2.9   Communication with Interdisciplinary Team

Ongoing communication/education as to the rationale of nutritional therapy must be communicated to all members of the health-care team including the attending physician, social worker, speech therapist, physical therapist, dietitian, and nursing staff, and the patient's family or caregiver is essential in developing and implementing the best possible care plan for the patient. Physician-nurse communication has been identified as one of the main obstacles to progress in patient safety. Breakdowns in communication between physicians, nurses, and members of the health-care team often result in errors, many of which are preventable [122]. Clear and complete communication between health-care providers is a prerequisite for safe patient management [123]. These studies have continued to support the development of structured communication interventions to improve quality of nurse-physician communication. Errors in dose of chemotherapy, medications, and other treatment are preventable if communication is structured, timely, and thorough. When referral is made to dental health, radiology, nutritionists, or other health professionals for pretreatment, specific information about patient's diagnosis, anticipated start date and restrictions to medications or therapeutic procedures, and contact information for further questions must be provided by the lead medical oncologist to maximize the effectiveness of service provided by other team members. With outstanding communication devices and systems in place, timely communication between team members should not present a challenge.

2.10   Future Directions

It is clear that patients with cancer and those who receive treatment for cancer are at a nutritional risk throughout the continuum of cancer. Nutritional screening, assessment, support, and reassessment should be considered a valuable measure within the overall oncology strategy. Despite extensive research in the field of clinical nutrition, examining the value of nutritional interventions in specific cancers and treatments, definite guidelines to base rational nutritional assessment and support in cancer patients are still debated. This may be attributed to a dynamic environment in oncology, where novel agents and treatment modalities–chemotherapeutic agents, radiation therapy, chemoradiation, immune therapies, and targeted therapies – have flooded the practice of clinical oncology. Although the focus of clinical oncologists continue to be in the treatment of cancers and improving morbidity and mortality in the cancer patient, they rely upon the expertise and partnership of their multidisciplinary teams to provide supportive care to their patients. Future research testing effectiveness of cancer treatment approaches should also include in parallel, an integrated evaluation of safety and effectiveness of supportive care approaches to manage symptoms and comorbidities. The results of these studies can inform the practice of nutritional and other supportive care that can significantly impact treatment outcomes and quality of survival in the cancer patient. The following chapters comprehensively examine some of the most common symptoms of cancer and treatments which have an implication on nutrition status and examine their significance, prevalence, etiology, current treatment strategies, and guidelines for management in a clinical setting using an integrated, multidisciplinary approach.

References

1. Davies M (2005) Nutritional screening and assessment in cancer-associated malnutrition. Eur J Oncol Nurs 9(suppl 2):S64–S73
2. Leandro-Merhi VA, de Aquino JL, Sales Chagas JF (2011) Nutrition status and risk factors associated with length of hospital stay for surgical patients. JPEN J Parenter Enteral Nutr 35:241–248
3. Marin Caro MM, Gomez Candela C, Castillo Rabaneda R, Lourenco Nogueira T, Garcia Huerta M, Loria Kohen V et al (2008) Nutritional risk evaluation and establishment of nutritional support in oncology patients according to the protocol of the Spanish Nutrition and Cancer Group. Nutr Hosp 23(5):458–468
4. Morley JE (2009) Calories and cachexia. Curr Opin Clin Nutr Metab Care 12(6):607–610
5. Van Cutsem E, Arends J (2005) The causes and consequences of cancer-associated malnutrition. Eur J Oncol Nurs 9(Suppl 2):S51–S63
6. Panis Y, Maggiori L, Caranhac G, Bretagnol F, Vicaut E (2011) Mortality after colorectal cancer surgery: a French survey of more than 84,000 patients. Ann Surg 254(5):738–744
7. Morgan TM, Tang D, Stratton KL, Barocas DA, Anderson CB, Gregg JR et al (2011) Preoperative nutritional status is an important predictor of survival in patients undergoing surgery for renal cell carcinoma. Eur Urol 59(6):923–928, PMCID: 3085569
8. Gupta D, Lis CG (2010) Pretreatment serum albumin as a predictor of cancer survival: a systematic review of the epidemiological literature. Nutr J 9:69, PMCID: 3019132
9. Paccagnella A, Morassutti I, Rosti G (2011) Nutritional intervention for improving treatment tolerance in cancer patients. Curr Opin Oncol 23(4):322–330
10. Kumar NB, Kazi A, Smith T, Crocker T, Yu D, Reich RR, Reddy K, Hastings S, Exterman M, Balducci L, Dalton K, Bepler G (2010) Cancer cachexia: traditional therapies and novel molecular mechanism-based approaches to treatment. Curr Treat Options Oncol 11(3–4): 107–117, Review
11. Baldwin C (2011) Nutritional support for malnourished patients with cancer. Curr Opin Support Palliat Care 5(1):29–36
12. Demoor-Goldschmidt C, Raynard B (2009) How can we integrate nutritional support in medical oncology? Bull Cancer 96(6):665–675
13. Laky B, Janda M, Bauer J, Vavra C, Cleghorn G, Obermair A (2007) Malnutrition among gynaecological cancer patients. Eur J Clin Nutr 61(5):642–646
14. Sarhill N, Mahmoud FA, Christie R, Tahir A (2003) Assessment of nutritional status and fluid deficits in advanced cancer. Am J Hosp Palliat Care 20(6):465–473
15. Ockenga J, Valentini L (2005) Review article: anorexia and cachexia in gastrointestinal cancer. Aliment Pharmacol Ther 22(7):583–594, Review
16. Capra S, Ferguson M, Ried K (2001) Cancer: impact of nutrition intervention outcome–nutrition issues for patients. Nutrition 17:769–772
17. Tsai AC, Hsu WC, Chan SC, Chang TL (2011) Usefulness of the mini nutritional assessment in predicting the nutritional status of patients with liver cancer in Taiwan. Nutr Cancer 63(3):334–341
18. Jensen GL, Mirtallo J, Compher C, Dhaliwal R, Forbes A, Grijalba RF et al (2010) Adult starvation and disease-related malnutrition: a proposal for etiology-based diagnosis in the clinical practice setting from the International Consensus Guideline Committee. Clin Nutr 29(2):151–153
19. Kruizenga HM, Wierdsma NJ, van Bokhorst MA, de van der Schueren, Haollander HJ, Jonkers-Schuitema CF, van der Heijden E, Melis GC, van Staveren WA (2003) Screening of nutritional status in The Netherlands. Clin Nutr 22(2):147–152
20. Iversen PO, Ukrainchenko E, Afanasyev B, Hulbekkmo K, Choukah A, Gulbrandsen N et al (2008) Impaired nutritional status during intensive chemotherapy in Russian and Norwegian cohorts with acute myeloid leukemia. Leuk Lymphoma 49(10):1916–1924

21. Goncalves Dias MC, de Fatima Nunes Marucci M, Nadalin W, Waitzberg DL (2005) Nutritional intervention improves the caloric and proteic ingestion of head and neck cancer patients under radiotherapy. Nutr Hosp 20(5):320–325

22. Epstein JB, Huhmann MB (2011) Dietary and nutritional needs of patients undergoing therapy for head and neck cancer. J Am Dent Assoc 142(10):1163–1167

23. Platek ME, Reid ME, Wilding GE, Jaggernauth W, Rigual NR, Hicks WL Jr et al (2011) Pretreatment nutritional status and locoregional failure of patients with head and neck cancer undergoing definitive concurrent chemoradiation therapy. Head Neck 33(11):1561–1568

24. Mahdavi R, Faramarzi E, Mohammad-Zadeh M, Ghaeammaghami J, Jabbari MV (2007) Consequences of radiotherapy on nutritional status, dietary intake, serum zinc and copper levels in patients with gastrointestinal tract and head and neck cancer. Saudi Med J 28(3):435–440

25. Klarod K, Hongsprabhas P, Khampitak T, Wirasorn K, Kiertiburanakul S, Tangrassameeprasert R et al (2011) Serum antioxidant levels and nutritional status in early and advanced stage lung cancer patients. Nutrition 27(11–12):1156–1160

26. Kumar NB, Besterman-Dahan K, Kang L, Pow-Sang J, Xu P, Allen K, Riccardi D, Krischer JP (2008) Results of a randomized clinical trial of the action of several doses of lycopene in localized prostate cancer: administration prior to radical prostatectomy. Clin Med Urol 1:1–14

27. Pham NV, Cox-Reijven PL, Wodzig WK, Greve JW, Soeters PB (2007) SGA and measures for muscle mass and strength in surgical Vietnamese patients. Nutrition 23(4):283–291

28. Ryu SW, Kim IH (2010) Comparison of different nutritional assessments in detecting malnutrition among gastric cancer patients. World J Gastroenterol 16(26):3310–3317, PMCID: 2900724

29. Gioulbasanis I, Georgoulias P, Vlachostergios PJ, Baracos V, Ghosh S, Giannousi Z et al (2011) Mini nutritional assessment (MNA) and biochemical markers of cachexia in metastatic lung cancer patients: interrelations and associations with prognosis. Lung Cancer 74:516–20

30. Dewys WD, Begg C, Lavin PT, Band PR, Bennett JM, Bertino JR, Cohen MH, Douglass HO Jr, Engstrom PF, Ezdinli EZ, Horton J, Johnson GJ, Moertel CG, Oken MM, Perlia C, Rosenbaum C, Silverstein MN, Skeel RT, Sponzo RW, Tormey DC (1980) Prognostic effect of weight loss prior to chemotherapy in cancer patients. Eastern Cooperative Oncology Group. Am J Med 69(4):491–497

31. Franch-Arcas G (2001) The meaning of hypoalbuminaemia in clinical practice. Clin Nutr 20(3):265–269, Review

32. Kanda M, Fujii T, Kodera Y, Nagai S, Takeda S, Nakao A (2011) Nutritional predictors of postoperative outcome in pancreatic cancer. Br J Surg 98(2):268–274

33. Brugler L, Stankovic AK, Schlefer M, Bernstein L (2005) A simplified nutrition screen for hospitalized patients using readily available laboratory and patient information. Nutrition 21(6):650–658

34. Smith RC, Ledgard JP, Doig G, Chesher D, Smith SF (2009) An effective automated nutrition screen for hospitalized patients. Nutrition 25(3):309–315, Epub 2008 Nov 28

35. Santarpia L, Contaldo F, Pasanisi F (2011) Nutritional screening and early treatment of malnutrition in cancer patients. J Cachexia Sarcopenia Muscle 2:27–35

36. Huhmann MB, Cunningham RS (2005) Importance of nutritional screening in treatment of cancer-related weight loss. Lancet Oncol 6(5):334–343, Review

37. Gavazzi C, Colatruglio S, Sironi A, Mazzaferro V, Miceli R (2011) Importance of early nutritional screening in patients with gastric cancer. Br J Nutr 17:1–6

38. Nitenberg G (2000) Nutritional support in sepsis: still skeptical? Curr Opin Crit Care 6(4):253–266

39. Huhmann MB, August DA (2008) Review of American Society for Parenteral and Enteral Nutrition (ASPEN) Clinical Guidelines for Nutrition Support in Cancer Patients: nutrition screening and assessment. Nutr Clin Pract 23(2):182–188

40. Kim JY, Wie GA, Cho YA, Kim SY, Kim SM, Son KH, Park SJ, Nam BH, Joung H (2011) Development and validation of a nutrition screening tool for hospitalized cancer patients. Clin Nutr 30:724–9

41. Conway DI, McMahon AD, Smith K, Black R, Robertson G, Devine J, McKinney PA (2010) Components of socioeconomic risk associated with head and neck cancer: a population-based case–control study in Scotland. Br J Oral Maxillofac Surg 48(1):11–17
42. Fontana V, Decensi A, Orengo MA, Parodi S, Torrisi R, Puntoni R (1998) Socioeconomic status and survival of gastric cancer patients. Eur J Cancer 34(4):537–542
43. Kuwahara A, Takachi R, Tsubono Y, Sasazuki S, Inoue M, Tsugane S, JPHC Study Group (2010) Socioeconomic status and gastric cancer survival in Japan. Gastric Cancer 13(4):222–230
44. Ramic E, Pranjic N, Batic-Mujanovic O, Karic E, Alibasic E, Alic A (2011) The effect of loneliness on malnutrition in elderly population. Med Arh 65(2):92–95
45. Hopkinson JB (2010) The emotional aspects of cancer anorexia. Curr Opin Support Palliat Care 4(4):254–258, Review
46. McQuestion M, Fitch M, Howell D (2011) The changed meaning of food: physical, social and emotional loss for patients having received radiation treatment for head and neck cancer. Eur J Oncol Nurs 15(2):145–151
47. Townsend D, Accurso-Massana C, Lechman C, Duder S, Chasen M (2010) Cancer nutrition rehabilitation program: the role of social work. Curr Oncol 17(6):12–17
48. Bollag D, Genton L, Pichard C (2000) Assessment of nutritional status. Ann Med Interne (Paris) 151(7):575–583
49. Gregg JR, Cookson MS, Phillips S, Salem S, Chang SS, Clark PE, Davis R, Stimson CJ Jr, Aghazadeh M, Smith JA Jr, Barocas DA (2011) Effect of preoperative nutritional deficiency on mortality after radical cystectomy for bladder cancer. J Urol 185(1):90–96, Epub 2010 Nov 12
50. Daly JM, Redmond HP, Gallagher H (1992) Perioperative nutrition in cancer patients. JPEN J Parenter Enteral Nutr 16(suppl 6):100S–105S, Review
51. Ross PJ, Ashley S, Norton A, Priest K, Waters JS, Eisen T, Smith IE, O'Brien ME (2004) Do patients with weight loss have a worse outcome when undergoing chemotherapy for lung cancers? Br J Cancer 90(10):1905–1911
52. Ferrucci LM, Bell D, Thornton J, Black G, McCorkle R, Heimburger DC, Saif MW (2011) Nutritional status of patients with locally advanced pancreatic cancer: a pilot study. Support Care Cancer 19(11):1729–1734
53. Lee CE, McArdle A, Griffiths RD (2007) The role of hormones, cytokines and heat shock proteins during age-related muscle loss. Clin Nutr 26(5):524–534, Epub 2007 Jun 21
54. Evans WJ (2010) Skeletal muscle loss: cachexia, sarcopenia, and inactivity. Am J Clin Nutr 91(4):1123S–1127S, Epub 2010 Feb 17
55. Kelly TL, Berger N, Richardson TL (1998) DXA body composition: theory and practice. Appl Radiat Isot 49(5–6):511–513
56. Gray C, MacGillivray TJ, Eeley C et al (2010) Magnetic resonance imaging with k-means clustering objectively measures whole muscle volume compartment in sarcopenia/cancer cachexia. Clin Nutr 30(1):106–111
57. Trutschnigg B, Kilgour RD, Reinglas J et al (2008) Precision and reliability of strength. (Jamar vs. Biodex handgrip) and body composition (dual-energy x-ray absorptiometry vs bioimpedance analysis) measurements in advanced cancer patients. Appl Physiol Nutr Metab 33:1232–1239
58. Al-Majid S, McCarthy DO (2001) Cancer-induced fatigue and skeletal muscle wasting: the role of exercise. Biol Res Nurs 2(3):186–197
59. Schag CC, Heinrich RL, Ganz PA (1984) Karnofsky performance status revisited: reliability, validity, and guidelines. J Clin Oncol 2:187–193
60. Fredrix EW, Soeters PB, Rouflart MJ, von Meyenfeldt MF, Saris WH (1991) Resting energy expenditure in patients with newly detected gastric and colorectal cancers. Am J Clin Nutr 53:1318–1322
61. Fuhrman MP, Charney P, Mueller CM (2004) Hepatic proteins and nutrition assessment. J Am Diet Assoc 104(8):1258–1264

62. Guerra LT, Rosa AR, Romani RF, Gurski RR, Schirmer CC, Kruel CD (2009) Serum transferrin and serum prealbumin as markers of response to nutritional support in patients with esophageal cancer. Nutr Hosp 24(2):241–242, PMID: 19593499
63. Sun LC, Chu KS, Cheng SC, Lu CY, Kuo CH, Hsieh JS et al (2009) Preoperative serum carcinoembryonic antigen, albumin and age are supplementary to UICC staging systems in predicting survival for colorectal cancer patients undergoing surgical treatment. BMC Cancer 9:288, PMCID: 2745428
64. Neyra NR, Hakim RM, Shyr Y, Ikizler TA (2000) Serum transferrin and serum prealbumin are early predictors of serum albumin in chronic hemodialysis patients. J Ren Nutr 10(4):184–190
65. Beguin Y (2003) Soluble transferrin receptor for the evaluation of erythropoiesis and iron status. Clin Chim Acta 329:9–22
66. Kemik O, Kemik AS, Begenik H, Erdur FM, Emre H, Sumer A, Purisa S, Tuzun S, Kotan C (2011) The relationship among acute-phase response proteins, cytokines, and hormones in various gastrointestinal cancer types patients with cachectic. Hum Exp Toxicol
67. Barber MD, Fearon KC, Tisdale MJ, McMillan DC, Ross JA (2001) Effect of a fish oil-enriched nutritional supplement on metabolic mediators in patients with pancreatic CC. Nutr Cancer 40(2):118–124
68. Anthony D, Reynolds T, Russell L (2000) An investigation into the use of serum albumin in pressure sore prediction. J Adv Nurs 32(2):359–365
69. Cano NJ (2002) Metabolism and clinical interest of serum transthyretin (prealbumin) in dialysis patients. Clin Chem Lab Med 40(12):1313–1319
70. Dequanter D, Lothaire P (2011) Serum albumin concentration and surgical site identify surgical risk for major post-operative complications in advanced head and neck patients. B-ENT 7(3):181–183
71. McMillan DC (2009) Systemic inflammation, nutritional status and survival in patients with cancer. Curr Opin Clin Nutr Metab Care 12(3):223–226
72. Marin Caro MM, Laviano A, Pichard C (2007) Impact of nutrition on quality of life during cancer. Curr Opin Clin Nutr Metab Care 10(4):480–487
73. Daudt HM, Cosby C, Dennis DL, Payeur N, Nurullah R (2011) Nutritional and psychosocial status of colorectal cancer patients referred to an outpatient oncology clinic. Support Care Cancer
74. Fouladiun M, Körner U, Gunnebo L, Sixt-Ammilon P, Bosaeus I, Lundholm K (2007) Daily physical-rest activities in relation to nutritional state, metabolism, and quality of life in cancer patients with progressive cachexia. Clin Cancer Res 13(21):6379–6385
75. Robuck JT, Fleetwood JB (1992) Nutrition support of the patient with cancer. Focus Crit Care 19:129–130, 132–134, 136–138
76. Goldstein MK, Fuller JD (1994) Intensity of treatment in malnutrition. The ethical considerations. Prim Care 21(1):191–206, Review
77. Bozzetti F (2002) Rationale and indications for preoperative feeding of malnourished surgical cancer patients. Nutrition 18(11–12):953–959, Review
78. Bozzetti F (2011) Nutritional support in oncologic patients: where we are and where we are going. Clin Nutr 30:714–717
79. Huhmann MB, August DA (2009) Nutrition support in surgical oncology. Nutr Clin Pract 24(4):520–526, Review
80. Rabinovitch R, Grant B, Berkey BA, Raben D, Ang KK, Fu KK et al (2006) Impact of nutrition support on treatment outcome in patients with locally advanced head and neck squamous cell cancer treated with definitive radiotherapy: a secondary analysis of RTOG trial 90–03. Head Neck 28(4):287–296
81. Isenring EA, Bauer JD, Capra S (2007) Nutrition support using the American Dietetic Association medical nutrition therapy protocol for radiation oncology patients improves dietary intake compared with standard practice. J Am Diet Assoc 107(3):404–412

82. Andreoli A, De Lorenzo A, Cadeddu F, Iacopino L, Grande M (2011) New trends in nutritional status assessment of cancer patients. Eur Rev Med Pharmacol Sci 15(5):469–480

83. Falconer JS, Fearon KC, Plester CE, Ross JA, Carter DC (1994) Cytokines, the acute-phase response, and resting energy expenditure in cachectic patients with pancreatic cancer. Ann Surg 219:325–331

84. Hyltander A, Korner U, Lundholm KG (1993) Evaluation of mechanisms behind elevated energy in cancer patients with solid tumours. Eur J Clin Invest 23:46–52

85. Merli M, Riggio O, Servi R, Zullo A, DeSantis A, Attili AF, Capocaccia L (1992) Increased energy expenditure in cirrhotic patients with hepatocellular carcinoma. Nutrition 8:321–325

86. Nixon DW, Kutner M, Heymsfield S, Foltz AT, Carty C, Seitz S, Casper K, Evans WK, Jeejeebhoy KN, Daly JM et al (1988) Resting energy expenditure in lung and colon cancer. Metabolism 37:1059–1064

87. Thomson SR, Hirshberg A, Haffejee AA, Huizinga WK (1990) Resting metabolic rate of esophageal carcinoma patients: a model for energy expenditure measurement in a homogenous cancer population. J Parenter Enteral Nutr 14:119–121

88. Garg S, Yoo J, Winquist E (2010) Nutritional support for head and neck cancer patients receiving radiotherapy: a systematic review. Support Care Cancer 18(6):667–677

89. Long CL (1984) Nutritional assessment of the critically ill patient. In: Wright RA, Heymsfield SB (eds) Nutritional assessment. Blackell Scientific Publications, Boston, p 168

90. Harris JA, Benedict FG (1919) Biometric studies of basal metabolism in man. Carnegie Institute, Washington, DC, Publ. No. 279

91. Long CL, Schaffel N, Geiger JW, Schiller WR, Blakemore WS (1979) Metabolic response to injury and illness: estimation of energy and protein needs from indirect calorimetry and nitrogen balance. JPEN 3:452–456

92. Dempsey DT, Mullen JL (1985) Macronutrient requirements in the malnourished cancer patient. Cancer 55:290–294

93. Charney P (2008) Nutrition screening vs nutrition assessment: how do they differ? Nutr Clin Pract 23(4):366–372

94. Bozetti F (1987) Nutritional assessment from the perspective of a clinician. JPEN 11:115S–121S

95. Huffman GB (2002) Evaluating and treating unintentional weight loss in the elderly. Am Fam Physician 65(4):640–650

96. Shike M, Brennan M (1989) Nutritional support. In: DeVita VT, Hellman S, Rosenberg SA (eds) Cancer: principles and practice of oncology, 3rd edn. J.B. Lippincott, Philadelphia, pp 2029–2044

97. Long CL, Schaffel N, Geiger JW, Schiller WR, Blakemore WS (1979) Metabolic response to injury and illness: estimation of energy and protein needs from indirect calorimetry and nitrogen balance. JPEN J Parenter Enteral Nutr 3:452–456

98. Dempsey DT, Mullen JL (1985) Macronutrient requirements in the malnourished cancer patient. Cancer 55:290–294

99. Charney P (2008) Nutrition screening vs nutrition assessment: how do they differ? Nutr Clin Pract 23(4):366–372

100. Bosaeus I (2008) Nutritional support in multimodal therapy for CC. Support Care Cancer 16(5):447–451, Epub 2008 Jan 15. PMID: 18196284

101. Morley JE (2002) Pathophysiology of anorexia. Clin Geriatr Med 18(4):661–673, v. Review. PMID: 12608495

102. Morley JE (2003) Anorexia and weight loss in older persons. J Gerontol A Biol Sci Med Sci 58(2):131–137

103. Blackburn GL, Moldawer LL, Usui S, Bothe A Jr, O'Keefe SJ, Bistrian BR (1979) Branched chain amino acid administration and metabolism during starvation, injury, and infection. Surgery 86(2):307–315

104. Whitney KA, Lysaker PH, Steiner AR, Hook JN, Estes DD, Hanna NH (2008) Is "chemobrain" a transient state? A prospective pilot study among persons with non-small cell lung cancer. J Support Oncol 6(7):313–321

105. D'Andrea GM (2005) Use of antioxidants during chemotherapy and radiotherapy should be avoided. CA Cancer J Clin 55:319–321
106. Parker-Pope T (2005) Cancer and vitamins: patients urged to avoid supplements during treatment. Wall St J D:1
107. Mercandante S (1996) Nutrition in cancer patients. Support Care Cancer 4:10–20
108. Teitelbaum D, Guenter P, Howell WH, Kochevar ME, Roth J, Seidner DL (2005) Definition of terms, style, and conventions used in A.S.P.E.N. guidelines and standards. Nutr Clin Pract 20(2):281–285
109. Antoun S, Merad M, Raynard B, Ruffie P (2006) Malnutrition in cancer patients. Rev Prat 56(18):2025–2029
110. Kreymann KG (2008) Early nutrition support in critical care: a European perspective. Curr Opin Clin Nutr Metab Care 11(2):156–159
111. Rutter CE, Yovino S, Taylor R, Wolf J, Cullen KJ, Ord R et al (2011) Impact of early percutaneous endoscopic gastrostomy tube placement on nutritional status and hospitalization in patients with head and neck cancer receiving definitive chemoradiation therapy. Head Neck 33(10):1441–1447
112. Chen AM, Li BQ, Lau DH, Farwell DG, Luu Q, Stuart K et al (2010) Evaluating the role of prophylactic gastrostomy tube placement prior to definitive chemoradiotherapy for head and neck cancer. Int J Radiat Oncol Biol Phys 78(4):1026–1032
113. Richter-Schrag HJ, Richter S, Ruthmann O, Olschewski M, Hopt UT, Fischer A (2011) Risk factors and complications following percutaneous endoscopic gastrostomy: a case series of 1041 patients. Can J Gastroenterol 25(4):201–206, PMCID: 3088695
114. Fenton JR, Bergeron EJ, Coello M, Welsh RJ, Chmielewski GW (2011) Feeding jejunostomy tubes placed during esophagectomy: are they necessary? Ann Thorac Surg 92(2):504–511; discussion 11–12
115. Van Dyck E, Macken EJ, Roth B, Pelckmans PA, Moreels TG (2011) Safety of pull-type and introducer percutaneous endoscopic gastrostomy tubes in oncology patients: a retrospective analysis. BMC Gastroenterol 11:23, PMCID: 3068968
116. Grant DG, Bradley PT, Pothier DD, Bailey D, Caldera S, Baldwin DL et al (2009) Complications following gastrostomy tube insertion in patients with head and neck cancer: a prospective multi-institution study, systematic review and meta-analysis. Clin Otolaryngol 34(2):103–112
117. Chadha KS, Thatikonda C, Schiff M, Nava H, Sitrin MD (2010) Outcomes of percutaneous endoscopic gastrostomy tube placement using a T-fastener gastropexy device in head and neck and esophageal cancer patients. Nutr Clin Pract 25(6):658–662
118. Petrov MS, Whelan K (2010) Comparison of complications attributable to enteral and parenteral nutrition in predicted severe acute pancreatitis: a systematic review and meta-analysis. Br J Nutr 103(9):1287–1295
119. Bozzetti F, Arends J, Lundholm K, Micklewright A, Zurcher G, Muscaritoli M (2009) ESPEN guidelines on parenteral nutrition: non-surgical oncology. Clin Nutr 28(4):445–454
120. Liu C, Du Z, Lou C, Wu C, Yuan Q, Wang J et al (2011) Enteral nutrition is superior to total parenteral nutrition for pancreatic cancer patients who underwent pancreaticoduodenectomy. Asia Pac J Clin Nutr 20(2):154–160
121. Nagata S, Fukuzawa K, Iwashita Y, Kabashima A, Kinoshita T, Wakasugi K et al (2009) Comparison of enteral nutrition with combined enteral and parenteral nutrition in post-pancreaticoduodenectomy patients: a pilot study. Nutr J 8:24, PMCID: 2703645
122. Manojlovich M (2010) Nurse/physician communication through a sensemaking lens: shifting the paradigm to improve patient safety. Med Care 48(11):941–946, Review
123. Tjia J, Mazor KM, Field T, Meterko V, Spenard A, Gurwitz JH (2009) Nurse-physician communication in the long-term care setting: perceived barriers and impact on patient safety. J Patient Saf 5(3):145–152

Cancer Anorexia (CA)

3

Core Messages

Anorexia can be defined as a lack of appetite or loss of desire to eat resulting in the involuntary decline in food intake contributing to malnutrition. Although cancer cachexia and cancer anorexia have been used synonymously in research literature, there are distinct differences between the two symptoms observed in cancer patient populations. In cancer anorexia, without cachexia, metabolism is almost normal, and nutritional deficits and symptom management can be achieved. If a patient with cancer anorexia continues to develop or demonstrate persistent metabolic disturbances, it is likely that this patient is cachectic and should be screened, staged, and treated for cancer cachexia with anorexia.

It is estimated that greater than 50% of cancer patients may suffer from cancer anorexia involving cancer-induced or treatment-related anorexia. This condition may be higher in advanced cancer patient and patients with pancreatic, head and neck, and gastrointestinal cancers. Myeloablative conditioning regimens commonly lead to prolonged anorexia and poor oral intake.

The pathogenesis of anorexia, like cancer cachexia, is complex and multifactorial, with three potential explanatory models existing with regard to the etiology of cancer anorexia.

Anorexia or reduction of nutritional intake has been reported to be tumor-related as well as treatment-related. Stenosis of the GI tract, dysphagia, previous surgery or an abdominal tumor, and pancreatic as well as gastric resections can lead to anorexia. Anorexia may be worsened by the side effects of treatment such as alterations in taste sensation and decreased taste and smell of food as a result of chemotherapy and radiation therapy, especially in patients treated for head and neck cancers. Anorexia can also result from a learned aversion to food because of treatment-related symptoms such as nausea, vomiting, or diarrhea. Symptoms of constipation, poor GI motility, and malabsorption can also contribute to early satiety and reduced food intake.

N.B. Kumar, *Nutritional Management of Cancer Treatment Effects*,
DOI 10.1007/978-3-642-27233-2_3, © Springer-Verlag Berlin Heidelberg 2012

Others have associated anorexia to perturbations of the physiological regulation of eating behavior at the hypothalamic level. This model is characterized by the release of endogenous transmitter substances or products of tumors leading to anorexia and cancer cachexia. Regulation of appetite is altered in cancer patients because of the central effects of cytokines or tumor peptides.

The third model takes into account the social and psychological etiology of cancer anorexia and has attributed depression and distress due to disease diagnosis and the burden to them and their families during treatment to be major contributor. Dementia and mood disorders have also been observed to contribute to loss of appetite or inadequate intake. Lack of support, social deprivation, or isolation also increases risk and has been associated with weight loss.

Irrespective of the etiology, cancer anorexia can contribute to malnutrition and poor clinical outcomes in cancer patients, in addition to contributing to distress in both the patient and care takers. Recent studies have also shown that advanced malnutrition resulting from anorexia is much more difficult to treat in the elderly than in younger adults, and the consequences of failure to correct malnutrition delay recovery and have a significant impact on functional dependence and quality of life. Similar to cancer cachexia, cancer anorexia continues to be an important problem in clinical oncology.

3.1 Definition/Description

Anorexia can be defined as a lack of appetite or loss of desire to eat resulting in the involuntary decline in food intake contributing to malnutrition [1, 2]. Although cancer cachexia (CC) and cancer anorexia have been used synonymously in research literature, there are distinct differences between the two symptoms observed in cancer patient populations. Anorexia, although often present in cancer cachexia, is insufficient to account for the metabolic abnormalities and wasting of skeletal muscles observed in cachexia. CC is a pathological syndrome where loss of muscle (skeletal and visceral) and fat occurs, manifested in the cardinal feature of emaciation, weakness affecting functional status, impaired immune system, and metabolic dysfunction [3–8]. On the other hand, massive depletion of skeletal muscle does not occur during anorexia, unless cancer anorexia is not identified and treated. In addition, cachexia can occur without anorexia [8]. Anorexia clearly contributes to weight loss and malnutrition in the cancer patient population and complicates treatment course and poor outcomes in cancer patients, especially if identified at the time of cancer diagnosis. Systematic reviews of the evidence of symptom management of cancer-related anorexia and cachexia indicate that nutritional repletion does not result in improved nutritional status, tumor response, survival, or quality of life [9] in cancer cachexia. In addition, nutritional supplementation does not replace loss of lean body mass [8, 9] in cancer cachexia. On the other hand, cancer anorexia, in most cases, is specifically reversible with nutritional support and treatment of contributing etiology. Appetite loss alone is not usually distressing to patients as it is to patient families [10]. However, anorexia coupled with hypermetabolic state of malignancy that leads to rapid and dramatic changes in body composition and weight can be psychologically damaging to patients and their families [9], in addition to contributing substantially to malnutrition. Data consistently indicate that this degree of malnutrition reduces responsiveness to chemotherapy and radiation therapy, increases perioperative morbidity in cancer patients, worsens their quality of life, and indeed diminishes survival [11, 12].

3.2 Prevalence

It is estimated that greater than 50% of cancer patients may suffer from cancer anorexia involving cancer-induced or treatment-related anorexia. This condition may be higher in advanced cancer patient and patients with pancreatic and gastrointestinal cancers [1–9, 13]. Studies have shown that patients with gastrointestinal malignancies as a result of anorexia have a higher prevalence of weight loss before surgery and during the first postoperative months with an additional 10% unplanned weight loss reported in this population [14–18]. Similarly, higher prevalence of anorexia is observed in patients with head and neck cancers [19, 20]. Over 85% of pancreatic cancer patients experience anorexia. Myeloablative conditioning regimens commonly lead to prolonged anorexia and poor oral intake. Over 92% significantly reduced caloric intake [21]. Anorexia may occur early in the disease or later, if the cancer grows or spreads. Some patients already have anorexia when they are diagnosed with cancer. Almost all patients who have advanced cancer will have anorexia. Anorexia is the most common cause of malnutrition in cancer patients. Dewys et al. [22] reported that a weight loss of >5% prior to chemotherapy [23] may be a defining point for the poor response to therapy, interruption of serial treatment, and survival. Recent studies have also shown that anorexia, similar to CC, is much more difficult to treat in the elderly than in younger adults, and the consequences of failure to correct malnutrition delay recovery and have a significant impact on functional dependence and quality of life in this patient population [24]. Recent studies have also shown that advanced malnutrition resulting from anorexia is much more difficult to treat in the elderly than in younger adults, and the consequences of failure to correct malnutrition delay recovery and have a significant impact on functional dependence and quality of life [7, 8, 25]. Similar to cancer cachexia, cancer anorexia continues to be an important problem in clinical oncology.

3.3   Etiology and Potential Mechanisms

The pathogenesis of anorexia, like cancer cachexia, is complex and multifactorial, with three potential explanatory models existing with regard to the etiology of cancer anorexia.

3.3.1   Tumor- and Treatment-Related Etiology of Anorexia

Anorexia or reduction of nutritional intake has been reported to be tumor-related as well as treatment-related. Stenosis of the GI tract, dysphagia, and previous surgery may affect the digestive capacity, or an abdominal tumor mass disturbance of the motility or repeated (sub) ileus may contribute to nausea and vomiting and therefore to reduced nutrient intake [26]. Pancreatic as well as gastric resections can result in pancreatic exocrine and endocrine insufficiency, creating major nutrition problems such as steatorrhea and hyperglycemia that may impede nutritional intake. Extensive resection of the small bowel can lead to malabsorption, whereas small resections of the bowel usually do not lead to major nutrition problems [27]. Anorexia may be worsened by the side effects of treatment such as alterations in taste sensation and decreased taste and smell of food as a result of chemotherapy and radiation therapy, especially in patients treated for head and neck cancers. Anorexia can also result from a learned aversion to food because of treatment-related symptoms such as nausea, vomiting, or diarrhea. Symptoms of constipation, poor GI motility, and malabsorption can also contribute to early satiety and reduced food intake. Physical limitations due to a head and neck tumor may limit or impair swallowing ability or dysphagia caused by treatment-related factors such as radiation or surgery may limit intake of foods [19, 28, 29]. Pain due to stomatitis, dyspnea, or delirium may also contribute to symptoms of anorexia. Central and peripheral mechanisms may be involved in the genesis of early satiety contributing to anorexia [30]. These would include central sensory-specific satiety, food aversions, diurnal changes in intake, gastric motility and accommodation, and as gastrointestinal hormones. Early satiety, increased brain tryptophan, dysfunctional hypothalamic membrane adenylate cyclase [9]. Hospitalization, surgery, radiation, and chemotherapy can also lower appetite and decrease food intake [31].

3.3.2   Perturbations of the Physiological Regulation of Eating Behavior as Etiology of Anorexia

Others have associated anorexia to perturbations of the physiological regulation of eating behavior at the hypothalamic level [2, 32]. This model is characterized by the release of endogenous transmitter substances or products of tumors leading to anorexia and cancer cachexia. Regulation of appetite is altered in cancer patients because of the central effects of cytokines or tumor peptides. Energy intake is controlled by the hypothalamus, where peripheral signals on energy intake (e.g., ghrelin, CCK) and adiposity status (e.g., insulin, leptin) are signaled. In the hypothalamus, particularly in the arcuate nucleus, this information is transduced into behavioral responses [32]. In cancer-free populations, peripheral signals are integrated by the hypothalamus to modulate energy intake. However, in cancer patients, increased cytokine expression in the brain prevents the hypothalamus from responding appropriately to these peripheral signals. Anorexigenic systems are persistently activated, inhibiting prophagic pathways [33]. Hypothalamic monoaminergic neurotransmission has been reported to contribute to these effects [34]. Because of their central role in energy homeostasis, a number of studies have also investigated the role of the prophagic (orexigenic) signal neuropeptide Y (NPY) in the pathogenesis of cancer anorexia. In weight-loss conditions, NPY is important in stimulating hunger and hyperphagia. Leptin and insulin are capable of blocking NPY production, and, vice versa, increased NPY decreases leptin and insulin production. Next to orexigenic also anorexigenic signals are involved in energy homeostasis. The hypothalamic anorexigenic neuropeptides melanocortin, CFR, and α-MSH, which is a product of proopiomelanocortin, have a role in normal control of food intake. α-MSH induces anorexia by activating the receptors MC3R and MC4R, which are both expressed in the hypothalamus and other brain regions. The inability of the hypothalamus to respond appropriately to consistent peripheral signals in cancer anorexia seems to be related to the central effect of cytokines [35]. Barrett et al. [36] recently demonstrated that peptides containing leptin sequences 1–33 r 61–90 are taken up by the rat brain and recently examined if these affect food intake and body weight in mature rats. They conclude that peptides 1–33 and 61–90 indeed acted as leptin antagonists significantly stimulating food intake and body weight increases. In animal studies, a negative correlation was observed between cerebrospinal fluid IL-1α and a tumor-bearing rat model [37], and intrahypothalamic microinjections of IL-1 receptor antagonist (IL-1ra) were associated with improvement in food intake in sarcoma-bearing rats [38]. In other studies in prostate tumor–bearing mouse models, upregulation of IL-1β mRNA in their brain regions was associated to development of anorexia. Treatment-related anorexia has been widely reported where cancer chemotherapeutic drugs have been demonstrated to increase proinflammatory cytokines and anorexia. Malone et al. observed a significant elevation of plasma cytokines that affect appetite (IL-2, IL-6, TNFα) and associated anorexia in patients undergoing myeloablative conditioning regimens. Etoposide (VP16) administration increased serum IL-6 in healthy mice and induced anorexia, loss of body weight, and decreased hemoglobin levels and voluntary wheel-running activity [39]. Although the role of cytokines in cancer anorexia is elegantly demonstrated in preclinical models, these correlations have been inconsistent in clinical trials [40]. These inconsistencies in translating the preclinical evidence to clinical trials may be potentially attributed to a lack of clear distinction made in patient selection in these trials—targeting those with cancer anorexia or cancer cachexia with anorexia. With recent advances in this distinction in the diagnosis, future studies targeting these specific populations may provide more succinct and valid data on the association of cytokines to anorexia.

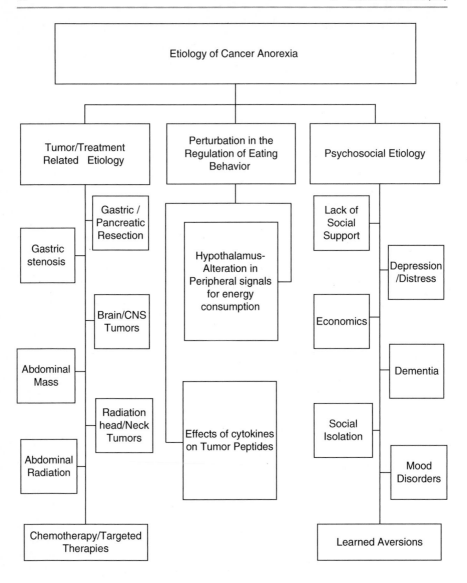

3.3.3   Psychosocial Etiology of Anorexia

The third model takes into account the social and psychological etiology of cancer anorexia and has attributed depression and distress due to disease diagnosis and the burden to them and their families during treatment to be major contributor [8, 41–45]. Dementia and mood disorders have also been observed to contribute to loss of appetite or inadequate intake [42]. Psychosocial support for management of cancer and symptoms has shown to benefit for both patients and their family members [41, 46–48]. The need for a support system consisting of family, peers, and friends is a common thread in every culture and has been quantitatively assessed and equated with hope. Factors such as impediments due to personal, family, caregiver, or insurance issues that could interfere with symptom management must be discussed and resolved [46]. On the other hand, emotional suppression and distress through helplessness/hopelessness and stress can increase distress and depression with cancer diagnosis. Individuals who live alone have been shown to be at risk of having a poor intake [47]. Social deprivation or isolation also increases risk and has been associated with weight loss [41]. Social networks play a role in the maintenance of adequate food intake, and socialization results in increased food intake during a meal. Research has drawn attention to the challenges that patients receiving treatment for head and neck cancers experience, including the physical and emotional impact of diagnosis and treatment, weight loss, challenges related to eating, and strategies used by patients to address nutritional problems. It is clear that patients experience physical, emotional, and social losses associated with a changed meaning of food. Acknowledging the significance of eating problems and the changed meaning of food is required in order to provide patients with the appropriate support, strategies, and interventions to manage with the changes and losses [48]. The goal of psychosocial support is thus to provide tools to manage stress, encourage social interaction during meal times, and proactively educate patients with regard to anticipated symptoms that they may experience, while providing strategies to cope with these scenarios. Approaches to education of patient and family, enhanced problem-solving skills, stress management, psychosocial support, group support to improve mood and coping response, psychotherapy, and tailored behavioral interventions have shown promise in reducing symptoms of cancer.

More recently, measurement of the quality of symptom management and end-of-life care has received significant attention as this could help provide a basis for improving supportive care for advanced cancer patients, where psychosocial issues are critical to quality of life of patients as well as caregivers. In a pilot evaluation of a comprehensive set of 92 supportive oncology quality indicators, Cancer Quality-ASSIST, including outpatient and hospital indicators for symptoms commonly related to cancer and its treatment and information and care planning, the authors successfully identified 41 that were feasible, reliable, and valid to be used for patients with advanced cancer in these settings. This set of indicators shows promise for describing key supportive care processes in advanced cancer [45].

3.4   Current Therapies for Cancer Anorexia

Over the years, anorexia, reduced food intake [8, 25] leading to malnutrition and consequences of malnutrition, has been well recognized and documented in cancer patients at diagnosis, during treatment as well as posttreatment and recovery period. It has also been clear that reversal of anorexia can impact patient's quality of life and functional status facilitating improvements in treatment outcomes. Although the pathogenesis of anorexia is multifactorial, the etiology for the large part has demonstrated four key principles, based upon which it is feasible to develop and implement a therapeutic approach to treating cancer patients with anorexia. In cancer anorexia, without cachexia, metabolism is almost normal, and nutritional deficits and symptom management can be achieved. If a patient with cancer anorexia continues to develop or demonstrate persistent metabolic disturbances, it is likely that these patients are cachectic and should be screened, staged, and treated for cancer cachexia with anorexia.

3.4.1   Timing of Diagnosis and Intervention

The first principle is that timing of intervention may be critical as anorexia is identified at diagnosis, worsens in some populations during treatment, and has residual effects posttreatment. In advanced cancer patients, anorexia may be recognized as an initial symptom of the development of cancer cachexia syndrome. The second principle is to screen and comprehensively assess all symptoms at admission. Once symptoms are identified, treating underlying causes when benefits exceed risk and prioritizing treatments is critical [49] since it is now recognized that multiple symptom clusters occur with anorexia [50, 51]. Thirdly, since cancer patients are hypermetabolic and their anorexia is exacerbated with increased caloric needs, the optimal nutritional approach should also be multifaceted combining a nutrition counseling, nutritional intervention, and drug therapy to improve appetite, taking into consideration other symptom clusters that are identified in these patients [49, 52–54] that may have implications in providing nutritional support. Some of the major factors that may impact nutrition interventions are tumor and treatment location that will impact route of feeding, cancer pain requiring preparing the patient prior to feedings/mealtimes, or dysphagia that will impact consistency of food intake or route of feeding. Studies report that optimum dietary intervention and reversal of anorexia can be achieved if interventions are specifically targeted to alleviate symptoms contributing to anorexia and meet increased dietary needs of macro- and micronutrients, providing an appetite stimulant to ensure that nutritional intake is sufficient to stabilize and enhance nutritional status. With the emerging data on the pathogenic mechanism and role of cytokines and tumor-derived factors in cancer anorexia, supplementing diets with those nutrient-derived substances that target the inflammatory pathways has demonstrated some success in early clinical trials [2, 36, 52–55]. More recently, in a phase II dose titration study of thalidomide, also an immune modulatory agent was used to treat cancer-associated anorexia. Davis et al. [30] treated 35 subjects with 50 mg PO thalidomide for 14 days and observed that this agent reduced multiple symptoms associated with cancer anorexia and improved quality of life. Last, but not least, studies have demonstrated that it may be important to identify social and psychological etiology of anorexia and provide psychosocial support for patients with cancer anorexia. These interventions have demonstrated benefit to both the patient and their caregivers [41, 42, 56].

3.4.2   Nutrition Supplementation

The average caloric deficit in weight-losing patients observed by us and other teams is approximately 250–400 kcal/day, although significant variations can exist among patients with severe illness and later stage disease. In most clinical setting, these deficits in nutritional intake have been compensated by providing calorie and protein supplementation with a goal of meeting nutritional needs of the individual patient. The average supplementation of 1 cal/ml supplements has not shown to improve nutritional status of patients on chemotherapy [20, 57]. However, recent studies using a more calorie dense (1.5 kcal/ml) and protein supplementation have suggested that at least weight stabilization can be achieved [6], although improvements in lean body mass have not been observed in these studies. Our preliminary studies have also demonstrated that high-calorie and high-protein supplemental (calorie/protein dense) feedings result in substitution of regular meals and thus a reduction of caloric and protein intake in this patient population who experience early satiety as a symptom cluster with anorexia. However, since these patients are hypermetabolic and have irregular feeding patterns, enhancing appetite using appetite stimulants, it may be important to make available to them a variety of dense high-calorie and high-protein supplements to prevent intake deficits and, at a minimum, stabilize weight loss. Supplementation with omega-3 fatty acids stabilized weight and offered benefits verifiable with improvements in biochemical markers of protein status, functional and clinical markers [1, 53]. Supplementation with glutamine, arginine, and branched chain amino acids appears to support improvement in reducing complications and improving treatment outcomes [53]. However, although these early studies appear promising, there is a significant need for well-powered, randomized clinical trials to confirm these early provocative results.

3.4.3   Appetite Stimulants and Other Pharmacotherapies to Treat Anorexia

To ensure adequate intake, other approaches have included providing appetite stimulants such as progestogens, cannabinoids, corticosteroids, and antidepressants in addition to nutritional supplementation. The most common agent used to enhance patient appetite is orexigenic agents such as megestrol acetate (MA) which acts by reducing cytokine production. In a meta-analysis by Berenstein and Ortiz [58], the effectiveness, efficacy, and safety of megestrol acetate for the treatment of anorexia in cancer was evaluated. This analysis showed a benefit of megestrol compared with placebo, particularly with respect to appetite improvement and weight gain in cancer patients. In another meta-analysis by Lesniak et al. [59], they observed that although megestrol reduced symptoms of anorexia, there were no improvements in survival. In a study of elderly patient, similar results were observed with megestrol. However, treated elderly patients reported significantly greater improvement in appetite, enjoyment in life, and well-being [60]. MA also decreased the rate of protein degradation in incubated isolated skeletal muscles. Real-time PCR analysis revealed that MA treatment resulted in a decrease in ubiquitin, E2, and atrogin-1 mRNA content in muscles, therefore suggesting that the main antiproteolytic action of the drug may be based on an inhibition of the ATP-ubiquitin-dependent proteolytic system [61]. The drug also improved appetite, weight loss, total physical activity, and grip force. With the exception of a few small studies, these studies have been of poor quality using heterogeneous populations of subjects and have not collected valid and reliable data on markers of protein status nor have they observed any meaningful gain in lean body mass. In addition, megestrol acetate is also associated with a reduction in steroid hormones which results in decline in muscle mass and an increase in fat mass [1, 8, 10, 62–67]. Addition of olanzapine (Zyprexa) to megestrol was associated to improved appetite and weight gain in advanced cancer patients [67]. Although optimum dose of 800 mg/day of megestrol acetate provided the best evidence for improved appetite and weight gain, doses as low as 80–160 mg a day were also beneficial [65]. Other common agents include dronabinol, a cannabis derivative, demonstrated to enhance appetite and mood in cancer patients [10, 62–64]. In a small open-label study, doses ranging from 7.5 to 15 mg of dronabinol a day improved appetite and were tolerated well [68]. However, at a lower dose of 5 mg/day used in a multicenter, randomized clinical trial, no improvement in appetite was observed [69]. In a pilot retrospective chart review [70] of 156 patients diagnosed and treated for cancer anorexia, we evaluated the prevalence, type, and effectiveness of appetite stimulants used at our Cancer Center. We observed this patient population for a 12-week period. All subjects in the study were provided with high protein and calorie supplementation in addition to their regular diets to meet their nutritional needs. The most common appetite stimulants used in this patient population were cannabinoids (50%), steroids (24%), and megestrol (26%). Our studies showed no improvement in serum albumin or skeletal proteins with supplementation and appetite stimulants. In contrast, serum albumin levels decreased in all groups receiving progestogens (2.9–2.8 mg/dl), cannabinoids (3.4–3.3 mg/dl), and corticosteroids (3.0–2.5 mg/dl). No improvement in immune markers (WBC count) was observed. We observed no significant changes in weight, with the exception of an increase in weight in subjects on cannabinoids. We attributed this increase in weight, in the absence of improvements in visceral and skeletal proteins, to alterations in hydration status, inflammation, and edema. Weight is thus not considered a valid marker in these advanced cancer patients on treatment. Over 33% of these subjects were diagnosed with lung cancer, and all were on active treatment for cancer [10]. In a large randomized trial, megestrol at a dose of 800 mg/day was observed to be superior to dronabinol for treating anorexia [71]. In addition, the pharmacokinetics of this agent in cancer patients on treatment has never been examined. In addition, mood alterations secondary to drug can be confused with dementia, especially in subjects who have never used cannabinoids in the past. More recently, antidepressants such as Remeron have been used to treat depression, which may be a major reversible contributor of weight loss in patients with anorexia attributed to distress due to diagnosis and the burden of treatment and consequences. A growing body of evidence is emerging with other novel compounds such as ghrelin, a peptide hormone secreted in the stomach, as well as parathyroid hormone–related proteins as appetite stimulators in animal models with promising results to be considered for future evaluation for the treatment of anorexia.

3.4.4 Increase Lean Body Mass with Physical Activity

Other strategies include increasing physical activity, aerobic and anaerobic, as a nonpharmacological means to improve muscle and bone mass [72–75] similar to those recommended for cancer cachexia. In spite of a number of cancer patients reporting fatigue, there is some preliminary evidence that at least some cancer patients are willing and able to tolerate physical activity interventions, with some patients demonstrating improvement in select supportive care outcomes postintervention with physical activity interventions [76]. Since energy expenditure in anorexia is frequently increased while energy intake is decreased, physical activity interventions should be initiated with caution and attention paid to achieving optimal energy balance. Relaxation, hypnosis, and short-term psychotherapy have some benefits with regard to treatment of anorexia [56]. However, methodologically rigorous future clinical trials in a substantial number of cancer patients using valid outcome markers are required to advance this area of research. More recently, multimodal approaches combining physical activity along with traditional approaches to treat both anorexia and cancer cachexia suggest potential improvement in overall improvement in physical function and quality of life [56, 73–77]. Future large scale studies will be required to confirm these initial results.

3.5 Guidelines for Treatment

Currently, there are no standard agents or therapies established to treat the symptom cluster associated to CA. The following guidelines are considered best practice standards. Improved management of CA may require a *multimodal approach by multi-disciplinary teams*. Approach to treatment includes proactive screening guidelines for early detection, ongoing and comprehensive symptom assessment and treatment. Treatment should include nutritional intervention supported by pharmacotherapy, psycho social intervention and physical activity. A monitoring schedule must be established and patients should be monitored closely for change of status and assessment of response to treatment.

3.5.1 Nutrition Guidelines

Nutritional assessment must be performed within 24 h of admission of the patient by a registered dietitian/nutritionist.

The goals for nutritional support in a cancer patient on active treatment may be as follows:

- To slow down the wasting process by reducing anorexia (ensuring adequate nutritional intake and appetite stimulants)
- Attenuating the systemic inflammation
- Attenuating skeletal muscle catabolism or stimulating the muscle protein anabolism (n – 3 fatty acid supplementation)
- Prevent or reverse nutrient deficiencies
- Help patients better tolerate treatments
- Minimize nutrition-related side effects and complications
- Maintain strength and energy
- Protect immune function, decreasing the risk of infection
- Aid in recovery and healing
- Maximize quality of life
- Take into consideration patient wishes
- Common symptom clusters in patients with anorexia:
  - Cachexia
  - Constipation(laxatives, stool softeners, prokinetics based on etiology)
  - Oral pain (lidocaine swishes/Oragel)
  - Nausea and vomiting
  - Early satiety (adopt suggestions provided below)
  - Hypermetabolism
  - Inventory nutritional symptoms and treat consistently integrating both pharmacological and nonpharmacological approaches
1. Screen patient within 24 h of admission. This order for nutritional screening can be a standard order for all cancer patient admissions to avoid delay in timing of screening.
2. In addition to standard nutritional assessment parameters described in Chap. 2, assess all symptoms: gastrointestinal tract: taste alterations, smell alterations, dysphagia, dyspnea, other pain, early satiety, dry mouth, too much saliva production, anorexia, diarrhea, constipation, nausea, vomiting, dehydration, and fatigue; psychosocial: family/caregiver support, depression, and activities of daily living (ADL).
3. Assess current nutritional status and estimate caloric, protein and multivitamin/mineral needs. There are no specific guidelines that have been evaluated in the cancer patient population. The recommendations provided here are usual standards of care that is provided in this patient population based on best practice standards as follows.
4. Provide adequate nutrition by including "calorie" and "protein" booster education material and nutritional supplements to ensure intake of proteins (recommended 0.8 g–1.0 g/kg/day). Provide dense caloric supplements up to 400 cal/day containing 1.5 kcal/ml. If intake is insufficient in protein intake, supplement with modular protein supplements, adding this to favorite beverage (http://www.nestle-nutrition.com/Products/Default.aspx; http://abbottnutrition.com/). The choice of nutritional supplements can be based in the personal choice of the patient, patient needs, and tolerance to product as well as other comorbidities.

5. Include a standard multivitamin mineral supplementation to prevent any further deficits and meet increased needs.

6. Assess adequacy of intake and provide an appetite stimulant (megestrol acetate 800 mg/day or alternate) if patient has cancer anorexia to ensure adequate intake and prevent further weight loss.

7. Provide each patient with nutritional guidelines to ensure adequate intake of calories and proteins and a list of suggested high-calorie and high-protein nutritional supplements to choose from, taking into consideration taste alterations, early satiety, nausea, and vomiting that are common symptoms observed in this patient population.

8. Recommend prescription for standardized omega-3 fatty acid supplement if benefits outweigh risks.

9. Other tips to enhance nutritional intake:
   - Meal and snack times need to be planned to occur at regular intervals and not in response to the hunger mechanism, which may be absent or altered.
   - Snacks of high caloric and protein density must be planned between meals, such as high-calorie puddings, shakes, high-calorie and protein drink supplements, sandwiches, avocados, and nuts.
   - Plans must be made for special circumstances. If meals need to be missed or delayed due to a test or therapy, snacks or a meal must be planned for consumption after the event/test.
   - High-calorie and protein-dense foods may be essential. Choose high-calorie foods, such as avocados, nuts, pudding, cream soups, cooked cereals, and vegetables with added butter or margarine. Use extra olive oil in salads.
   - Season foods with exotic flavors, fresh herbs, and spices that stimulate appetite. Unless contraindicated, use salt and sweetening as desired.
   - Consider the role of smell, texture, and eye appeal to help stimulate the desire to eat, such as the smell of fresh bread baking or a colorful fruit cup.
   - Use garnishes on foods to increase the visual "eye" appeal.
   - Fresh fruits and vegetables may be more appealing than canned or frozen ones.
   - Experiment with different food textures as crunchy, creamy, and crispy foods.
   - When shopping, recommend choosing foods that are beautiful, colorful, fresh, and full-flavored.
   - If the patient is unable to tolerate red meats, recommend including other protein sources in the diet such as poultry, fish, milk, eggs, bean and legumes, peanut butter, and other nut butters.
   - Some patient may be able to take advantage of a diurnal variation in appetite, usually an increased appetite in the morning.
   - Remove dietary restrictions if possible.
   - Ensure regular oral check up/fastidious oral care.
   - Recommend scheduled times to drink fluids.

10. Alter consistency of foods as needed, based on ability to chew and swallow.

11. Selection of route of feeding may be informed based on general guidelines and criteria provided in Table 2.7 of Chap. 2.

3.5.2 Pharmacotherapy

Assessment must be performed within 24 h of admission of the patient by a clinical pharmacist closely working with the registered dietitian.

Appetite Stimulants: Current therapies used to improve appetite and to reduce breakdown of muscle proteins (proteolysis):
* *Corticosteroids*
  – Dexamethasone (Decadron®)
  – Methylprednisolone (Solu-Medrol®)
  – Prednisone (Deltasone®)
* *Orexigenic agents*
  – Megestrol acetate (Megace®)
* *Anabolic steroids*
  – Medroxyprogesterone acetate (Provera®, Depo-Provera®)
* *Antiemetic*
  – Dronabinol (Marinol®)
* *Antidepressants*
  Proteasome inhibitors: (Experimental therapies)
* *Omega-3 fatty acids*
  – Lovaza (GSK)

3.5.3 Speech Therapist

Refer for video fluoroscopic assessment for dysphagia and obtain recommendation for alterations in consistency to prevent aspiration if needed.

3.5.4 Physical Activity

Since fatigue and poor nutritional status are classic symptoms of CA, patients should proactively receive a comprehensive assessment of physical status by a licensed physical therapist and therapy initiated within 24 h of assessment.

Markers and Instruments for Patient Monitoring and Assessment of Response to Treatment by the Interdisciplinary Medical Team:
1. *Anthropometric measurements* such as participant's height, weight, and body mass index can be performed at admission and at regular intervals established by the medical team.
2. *Body composition by DXA scan:* DXA should be used to assess both total lean body mass (LBM), fat mass (FM), and total bone mineral density (BMD). Total bone mineral density (BMD) is a valid indirect measure of skeletal muscle and patient activity. Total LBM is sometimes called total fat-free mass (FFM) depending upon specific DXA manufacturer. DXA instruments use an X-ray source that generates or is split into two energies to measure bone mineral mass and soft tissue from which fat and fat-free mass are estimated. The exam is

quick (1–2 min), precise (0.5–1%), and noninvasive. DXA scanners have the precision required to detect changes in muscle mass as small as 5%. Radiation exposure from DXA scans is minimal. The National Council on Radiation Protection and Measurements (NCRP) has recommended the annual effective dose limit for infrequent exposure of the general population is 5,000 μSv and that an annual effective dose of 10 μSv be considered a negligible individual dose. The effective dose of a dual-energy X-ray absorptiometry whole body scan on an adult is 2.1 μSv. Studies have shown that quality assurance is an important issue in the use of DXA scans to determine body composition including lean body mass and bone mineral density. DXA instrument manufacturer and model should remain consistent, and their calibration should be monitored throughout treatment. Use of a standardized scan acquisition protocol and appropriate and unchanging scan acquisition and analysis software is essential to achieve consist results.

3. *Dietary intake* must be assessed at baseline and periodical intervals by conducting random weekly, 2-week days +1 weekend day 24-h dietary recalls (gold standard for collecting dietary data) using a five-step multipass procedure (which has been found to assess mean energy intake within 10% of actual intake) and using the frequently updated University of Minnesota Nutrition Data System-Research version (NDS-R) database for analysis of nutrient composition. Food portion visuals can be provided to patients to estimate portion sizes of foods while monitoring intake.

4. *Symptom log* may be completed daily and collected from patients on a monthly basis. Based on these symptoms, all anticipated and unanticipated, grades of constitutional, dermatological, gastrointestinal (GI), metabolic, and pain symptoms can be continuously monitored including those symptoms affecting nutritional intake and utilization.

5. *Monthly* CMP and CBC should be monitored to assess electrolytes and organ function.

6. *Functional markers* (*Karnofsky performance score*): Evaluation of patients' functional status and barriers to obtaining adequate nutrients is also necessary. A physical exam combined with personal interview should include the evaluation of functional status such as the ability to chew and swallow, dental or oral problems causing odynophagia or dysphagia, signs of muscle wasting or anasarca, presence of edema, presence of skin or mouth lesion, and ability to perform instrumental activities of daily living (IADLs) such as cooking, shopping, and self-feeding. It is critical to assess activities of daily living, physical activity, exercise, sleep, and ability to work and perform other functional roles. Limitations in the activities of daily living have been identified secondary to and as a cause of weight loss in cancer patients. Cancer and other chronic diseases pose difficulties specifically for the cancer patient receiving treatment and the elderly in carrying out activities of daily living. A loss of postural and locomotive muscle mass has been observed within 7 days of inactivity. The Karnofsky Performance Scale Index allows patients to be classified as to their functional impairment. This has been used to compare effectiveness of

different therapies and to assess the prognosis in individual patients and has been validated in cancer patient populations. This has been used to compare effectiveness of different therapies and to assess the prognosis in individual patients and has been validated in cancer patient populations.

7. *Godin Leisure-Time Exercise Questionnaire* weekly to monitor physical activity.

8. *Handgrip Strength Dynamometry Assessment*: A validated tool commonly used to assess handgrip strength is the Jamar dynamometer, which is a fast, reliable, and easy-to-perform device commonly used by our team to measure improvements in functional strength. The Jamar dynamometer has a lower percent coefficient of variation and is thus a more precise device than other handgrip dynamometers.

9. *Biochemical markers of protein status (serum albumin and transferrin)*: Assessment of protein status is critical in the identification and treatment of abnormalities in protein metabolism. There is substantial evidence of the correlation between serum hepatic proteins and inflammation, making these the most relevant biomarkers in CC. Serum transferrin, prealbumin, and albumin have been observed as intermediate endpoint biomarkers and independently associated with worse outcome in cachexia [20]. Measurements of body composition combined with more objective and sensitive measure of protein nutriture are ideal for the biochemical assessment of intravascular and visceral protein stores. We have thus included the three major valid intermediate endpoint biomarkers (IEBs) that represent intravascular and visceral protein pools—transferrin, prealbumin, and albumin—as the biochemical indicators of protein status. Although transferrin levels are affected by iron status, serum transferrin, either singly or as part of a multiparameter index, is the strongest predictor of cancer patient morbidity and mortality [97–99].

10. *Immune and inflammatory markers*: Unlike anorexia of aging, in CC, there is a range of metabolic responses triggered by inflammatory and immunological responses. It is believed that the putative mediators of CC are cytokines, and increased expression of tumor necrosis factor and interleukin-6 has been observed in patients with CC. Cytokines will be measured in a panel including IL-1, IL-4, IL-6, IL-8, IL-10, GM-CSF, IFN-κ, TNFα, and CRP (BioRad-Bioplex). All of these biomarkers have been shown to increase with disease, aging, and cytotoxic agents. Though we realize these intermediate endpoint biomarkers of cytokines cannot be reliably interpreted, as over 70% of the subjects as observed in our studies were on active treatment with cytotoxic agents, these variables are important to determine, as they may provide useful information and contribute to the better understanding of the mechanistic process.

11. *Quality of life*: Should be measured at baseline and monthly using the Rand Short Form (SF)-36 (Medical Outcomes Study SF-36) [78]. The SF-36 has been used extensively with both general, high-risk, and cancer populations and

has available norms for mail and telephone versions and comparisons between group and individual scores. Scores are calculated and transformed to a 0–100 scale, with higher scores indicating increased health status. Reliability of the SF-36 scales was measured by Cronbach α coefficient, and the results ranged from 0.78 in general health perceptions to 0.91 in the physical functioning domain.

3.5.5 Follow-up

Patients must be seen by the multidisciplinary team on a regularly scheduled basis to monitor progress and to review compliance to intervention including diet intake adequacy, symptom logs, change in concomitant medications, and any other issues related to treatment. Improved management of malnutrition with nutritional therapy may require a multimodal intervention by multidisciplinary teams using a comprehensive and integrated approach. Initial screening and knowledge of treatment trajectory of the cancer patient should guide a plan for reassessment of the cancer patient at regularly planned intervals. Subjective and objective data on progress and response to nutritional therapy may be assessed using the indicators used in the comprehensive nutritional assessment. Newly developed symptoms resulting from treatment or progression of disease may require additional monitoring or revision of nutritional therapy. Reassessment/reevaluation for monitoring and evaluation of nutritional therapy must include monitoring of clinical, functional, dietary, and behavioral outcomes that were identified by the comprehensive nutritional assessment.

3.6 Future Directions

Early referral to supportive care services and coordination of interdisciplinary care are essential to support patients with CA. Randomized clinical trials with appetite stimulants and supplementation with proteins and calories are current strategies to improve intake and produce stabilization in weight loss in most cancer patients on treatment. Supplementation with omega-3 fatty acids stabilized weight and offered benefits verifiable with improvements in biochemical markers of protein status and functional and clinical markers. Supplementation with glutamine, arginine, and branched chain amino acids appears to support improvement in reducing complications and treatment outcomes. Strategies to enhance appetite, intake of nutrients, and lean body mass including synergistic effects with physical activity interventions have a scientific rationale and merit further evaluation. However, although these early studies appear promising, there is a significant need for well-powered, randomized clinical trials to confirm these provocative observations using meaningful, valid markers demonstrating reversal or cancer anorexia and other symptom clusters seen in this patient population.

Summary for the Clinician

Due to the multifactorial etiology of cancer anorexia, there is no single standard of therapy established to treat the symptoms of anorexia in cancer patients.

Diagnosis and management of anorexia requires timely and careful screening using detailed history and clinical examination by integrated, multidisciplinary teams consisting of treating oncologists (surgeons, radiation oncologists, and medical oncologists), clinical pharmacist, psychosocial worker, physical therapist, and dietitian.

The first principle is that timing of intervention may be critical as anorexia is identified at diagnosis, worsens in some populations during treatment, and has residual effects posttreatment. In advanced cancer patients, anorexia may be recognized as an initial symptom of the development of cancer cachexia syndrome.

The second principle is to screen and comprehensively assess all symptoms at admission. Once symptoms are identified, treating underlying causes when benefits exceed risk and prioritizing treatments is critical, since it is now recognized that multiple symptom clusters occur with anorexia.

Thirdly, since cancer patients are hypermetabolic and their anorexia is exacerbated with increased caloric needs, the optimal nutritional approach should also be multifaceted combining a nutrition counseling, nutritional intervention, and drug therapy to improve appetite, taking into consideration other symptom clusters that are identified in these patients that may have implications in providing nutritional support. Intervention must be proactive and based on ongoing evaluations to monitor patient's change in status based on disease stage, response to treatment, and treatment outcomes as well as use of concomitant medications. Strategies to increase physical activity, aerobic and anaerobic, are recommended as a nonpharmacological means to improve muscle and bone mass.

Last, but not least, studies have demonstrated that it may be important to identify social and psychological etiology of anorexia and provide psychosocial support for patients with cancer anorexia. These interventions have demonstrated benefit to both the patient and their caregivers.

Supplementation with omega-3 fatty acids stabilized weight and offered benefits verifiable with improvements in biochemical markers of protein status and functional and clinical markers. Supplementation with glutamine, arginine, and branched chain amino acids appears to support improvement in reducing complications and treatment outcomes. Strategies to enhance appetite, intake of nutrients, and lean body mass including synergistic effects with physical activity interventions have a scientific rationale and merit further evaluation. However, although these early studies appear promising, there is a significant need for well-powered, randomized clinical trials to confirm these provocative observations using meaningful, valid markers demonstrating reversal or cancer anorexia and other symptom clusters seen in this patient population.

References

1. Kumar NB, Kazi A, Smith T, Crocker T, Yu D, Reich RR, Reddy K, Hastings S, Exterman M, Balducci L, Dalton K, Bepler G (2010) Cancer cachexia: traditional therapies and novel molecular mechanism-based approaches to treatment. Curr Treat Options Oncol 11(3–4):107–117, Review

2. Gupta SC, Kim JH, Kannappan R, Reuter S, Dougherty PM, Aggarwal BB (2011) Role of nuclear factor κB-mediated inflammatory pathways in cancer-related symptoms and their regulation by nutritional agents. Exp Biol Med (Maywood) 236(6):658–671, Epub 2011 May 12. Review

3. Tisdale MJ (2008) Catabolic mediators of cancer cachexia. Curr Opin Support Palliat Care 2(4):256–261, PMID: 19069310

4. Deans C, Wigmore SJ (2005) Systemic inflammation, cachexia and prognosis in patients with cancer. Curr Opin Clin Nutr Metab Care 8(3):265–269, PMID: 15809528

5. Tisdale MJ (2001) Loss of skeletal muscle in cancer: biochemical mechanisms. Front Biosci 6:164–174, PMID: 11171557

6. Fearon KC, Von Meyenfeldt MF, Moses AG, Van Geenen R, Roy A, Gouma DJ, Giacosa A, Van Gossum A, Bauer J, Barber MD, Aaronson NK, Voss AC, Tisdale MJ (2003) Effect of a protein and energy dense N-3 fatty acid enriched oral supplement on loss of weight and lean tissue in cancer cachexia: a randomised double blind trial. Gut 52(10):1479–1486, PMCID: PMC1773823

7. Tisdale MJ (1999) Wasting in cancer. J Nutr 129(1S Suppl):243S–246S, Review. PMID: 9915907

8. Morley JE (2002) Pathophysiology of anorexia. Clin Geriatr Med 18(4):661–673, v. Review. PMID: 12608495

9. Shoemaker LK, Estfan B, Induru R, Walsh TD (2011) Symptom management: an important part of cancer care. Cleve Clin J Med 78(1):25–34

10. Von Roenn JH (1994) Randomized trials of megestrol acetate for AIDS-associated anorexia and cachexia. Oncology 51(Suppl 1):19–24

11. Khalid U, Spiro A, Baldwin C, Sharma B, McGough C, Norman AR, Eisen T, O'Brien ME, Cunningham D, Andreyev HJ (2007) Symptoms and weight loss in patients with gastrointestinal and lung cancer at presentation. Support Care Cancer 15(1):39–46

12. Van Cutsem E, Arends J (2005) The causes and consequences of cancer-associated malnutrition. Eur J Oncol Nurs 9(Suppl 2):S51–S63

13. Schmitz KH, Holtzman J, Courneya KS, Mâsse LC, Duval S, Kane R (2005) Controlled physical activity trials in cancer survivors: a systematic review and meta-analysis. Cancer Epidemiol Biomarkers Prev 14:1588–1595

14. Copland L, Liedman B, Rothenberg E, Bosaeus I (2007) Effects of nutritional support long time after total gastrectomy. Clin Nutr 26:605–613

15. Braga M, Molinari M, Zuliani W, Foppa L, Gianotti L, Radaelli G, Cristallo M, Di Carlo V (1996) Surgical treatment of gastric adenocarcinoma: impact on survival and quality of life. A prospective ten year study. Hepatogastroenterology 43:187–193

16. Hyltander A, Bosaeus I, Svedlund J, Liedman B, Hugosson I, Wallengren O, Olsson U, Johnsson E, Kostic S, Henningsson A et al (2005) Supportive nutrition on recovery of metabolism, nutritional state, health-related quality of life, and exercise capacity after major surgery: a randomized study. Clin Gastroenterol Hepatol 3:466–474

17. Liedman B, Andersson H, Berglund B, Bosaeus I, Hugosson I, Olbe L, Lundell L (1996) Food intake after gastrectomy for gastric carcinoma: the role of a gastric reservoir. Br J Surg 83:1138–1143

18. Takahashi S, Maeta M, Mizusawa K, Kaneko T, Naka T, Ashida K, Tsujitani S, Kaibara N (1998) Long-term postoperative analysis of nutritional status after limited gastrectomy for early gastric cancer. Hepatogastroenterology 45:889–894

19. García-Peris P, Parón L, Velasco C, de la Cuerda C, Camblor M, Bretón I, Herencia H, Verdaguer J, Navarro C, Clave P (2007) Long-term prevalence of oropharyngeal dysphagia in head and neck cancer patients: impact on quality of life. Clin Nutr 26(6):710–717, Epub 2007 Oct 22

20. Couch M, Lai V, Cannon T, Guttridge D, Zanation A, George J, Hayes DN, Zeisel S, Shores C (2007) Cancer cachexia syndrome in head and neck cancer patients: part I. Diagnosis, impact on quality of life and survival, and treatment. Head Neck 29(4):401–411, PMID: 17285641

21. Malone FR, Leisenring WM, Storer BE, Lawler R, Stern JM, Aker SN, Bouvier ME, Martin PJ, Batchelder AL, Schoch HG, McDonald GB (2007) Prolonged anorexia and elevated plasma cytokine levels following myeloablative allogeneic hematopoietic cell transplant. Bone Marrow Transplant 40(8):765–772, Epub 2007 Aug 13

22. Dewys WD, Begg C, Lavin PT, Band PR, Bennett JM, Bertino JR, Cohen MH, Douglass HO Jr, Engstrom PF, Ezdinli EZ, Horton J, Johnson GJ, Moertel CG, Oken MM, Perlina C, Rosenbaum C, Silverstein MN, Skeel RT, Sponzo RW, Tormey DC (1980) Prognostic effect of weight loss prior to chemotherapy in cancer patients. Eastern Cooperative Oncology Group. Am J Med 69:491–497, PMID: 7424938

23. Ross PJ, Ashley S, Norton A, Priest K, Waters JS, Eisen T, Smith IE, O'Brien ME (2004) Do patients with weight loss have a worse outcome when undergoing chemotherapy for lung cancers? Br J Cancer 90:1905–1911

24. Vallas B, Lauque S, Andrieu S, Nurhashemi F, Folland Y, Baumgartner R, Garry P (2001) Nutrition assessment in the elderly. Curr Opin Clin Nutr Metab Care 4(1):5–8

25. Morley JE (2003) Anorexia and weight loss in older persons. J Gerontol A Biol Sci Med Sci 58(2):131–137

26. Ockenga J, Valentini L (2005) Review article: anorexia and cachexia in gastrointestinal cancer. Aliment Pharmacol Ther 22(7):583–594, Review

27. Capra S, Ferguson M, Ried K (2001) Cancer: impact of nutrition intervention outcome–nutrition issues for patients. Nutrition 17:769–772

28. Sink J, Kademani D (2011) Maxillofacial oncology at the University of Minnesota: treating the epidemic of oral cancer. Northwest Dent 90(3):13–16, 38

29. Arias F, Manterola A, Domínguez MA, Martínez E, Villafranca E, Romero P, Vera R (2004) Acute dysphagia of oncological origin. Therapeutic management. An Sist Sanit Navar 27(Suppl 3):109–115

30. Davis MP, Walsh D, Lagman R, Yavuzsen T (2006) Early satiety in cancer patients: a common and important but underrecognized symptom. Support Care Cancer 14(7):693–698, Epub 2006 Apr 20. Review

31. Ryu SW, Kim IH (2010) Comparison of different nutritional assessments in detecting malnutrition among gastric cancer patients. World J Gastroenterol 16(26):3310–3317

32. Schwartz MW, Woods SC, Porte D Jr, Seeley RJ, Baskin DG (2000) Central nervous system control of food intake. Nature 404:661–671

33. Plata-Salaman CR (1996) Anorexia during acute and chronic disease. Nutrition 12:69–78

34. Laviano A, Meguid MM, Rossi-Fanelli F (2003) Cancer anorexia: clinical implications, pathogenesis, and therapeutic strategies. Lancet Oncol 4:686–694

35. Mantovani G, Macciò A, Esu S, Lai P, Santona MC, Massa E, Dessì D, Melis G, Del Giacco S (1997) Medroxyprogesterone acetate reduces the production of cytokines and serotonin involved in anorexia/cachexia and emesis by peripheral blood mononuclear cells of cancer patients. Biochem Soc Trans 25(2):296S

36. Barrett GL, Naim T, Trieu J (2011) Leptin-derived peptides that stimulate food intake and increase body weight following peripheral administration. Regul Pept 170(1–3):24–30, Epub 2011 May 24

37. Opara EI, Laviano A, Meguid MM, Yang ZJ (1995) Correlation between food intake and CSF IL-1 alpha in anorectic tumor bearing rats. Neuroreport 6:750–752

38. Laviano A, Gleason JR, Meguid MM, Yang ZJ, Cangiano C, Rossi Fanelli F (2000) Effects of intra-VMN mianserin and IL-1ra on meal number in anorectic tumor-bearing rats. J Invest Med 48:40–48

39. Wood LJ, Nail LM, Perrin NA, Elsea CR, Fischer A, Druker BJ (2006) The cancer chemotherapy drug etoposide (VP-16) induces proinflammatory cytokine production and sickness

behavior-like symptoms in a mouse model of cancer chemotherapy-related symptoms. Biol Res Nurs 8:157–169

40. Wang W, Lonnroth C, Svanberg E, Lundholm K (2001) Cytokine and cyclooxygenase-2 protein in brain areas of tumor-bearing mice with prostanoid-related anorexia. Cancer Res 61:4707–4715

41. Hopkinson JB (2010) The emotional aspects of cancer anorexia. Curr Opin Support Palliat Care 4(4):254–258, Review

42. Hopkinson JB, Brown JC, Okamoto I, Addington-Hall JM (2012) The effectiveness of patient-family carer (couple) intervention for the management of symptoms and other health-related problems in people affected by cancer: a systematic literature search and narrative review. J Pain Symptom Manage 43(1):111–142, Epub 2011 Jun 30

43. Thomas DR (2009) Anorexia: aetiology, epidemiology and management in older people. Drugs Aging 26(7):557–570

44. Fearon K, Strasser F, Anker SD, Bosaeus I, Bruera E, Fainsinger RL, Jatoi A, Loprinzi C, MacDonald N, Mantovani G, Davis M, Muscaritoli M, Ottery F, Radbruch L, Ravasco P, Walsh D, Wilcock A, Kaasa S, Baracos VE (2011) Definition and classification of cancer cachexia: an international consensus. Lancet Oncol 12(5):489–495, Epub 2011 Feb 4. Review

45. Dy SM, Lorenz KA, O'Neill SM, Asch SM, Walling AM, Tisnado D, Antonio AL, Malin JL (2010) Cancer Quality-ASSIST supportive oncology quality indicator set: feasibility, reliability, and validity testing. Cancer 116(13):3267–3275

46. Townsend D, Accurso-Massana C, Lechman C, Duder S, Chasen M (2010) Cancer nutrition rehabilitation program: the role of social work. Curr Oncol 17(6):12–17

47. Ramic E, Pranjic N, Batic-Mujanovic O, Karic E, Alibasic E, Alic A (2011) The effect of loneliness on malnutrition in elderly population. Med Arh 65(2):92–95

48. McQuestion M, Fitch M, Howell D (2011) The changed meaning of food: physical, social and emotional loss for patients having received radiation treatment for head and neck cancer. Eur J Oncol Nurs 15(2):145–151

49. Snyder CF, Garrett-Mayer E, Blackford AL, Brahmer JR, Carducci MA, Pili R, Stearns V, Wolff AC, Dy SM, Wu AW (2009) Concordance of cancer patients' function, symptoms, and supportive care needs. Qual Life Res 18(8):991–998, Epub 2009 Aug 6

50. Jiménez A, Madero R, Alonso A, Martínez-Marín V, Vilches Y, Martínez B, Feliu M, Díaz L, Espinosa E, Feliu J (2011) Symptom clusters in advanced cancer. J Pain Symptom Manage 42(1):24–31, Epub 2011 Mar 12

51. Kirkova J, Aktas A, Walsh D, Davis MP (2011) Cancer symptom clusters: clinical and research methodology. J Palliat Med 14(10):1149–1166, Epub 2011 Aug 23

52. Laviano A, Seelaender M, Sanchez-Lara K, Gioulbasanis I, Molfino A, Rossi Fanelli F (2011) Beyond anorexia -cachexia. Nutrition and modulation of cancer patients' metabolism: supplementary, complementary or alternative anti-neoplastic therapy? Eur J Pharmacol 668(Suppl 1):S87–S90, Epub 2011 Jul 27

53. Paccagnella A, Morassutti I, Rosti G (2011) Nutritional intervention for improving treatment tolerance in cancer patients. Curr Opin Oncol 23(4):322–330

54. Del Fabbro E, Hui D, Dalal S, Dev R, Noorhuddin Z, Bruera E (2011) Clinical outcomes and contributors to weight loss in a cancer cachexia clinic. J Palliat Med 14(9):1004–1008 [Epub ahead of print]

55. Baker A, Wooten LA, Malloy M (2011) Nutritional considerations after gastrectomy and esophagectomy for malignancy. Curr Treat Options Oncol 12(1):85–95, Review. Erratum in: Curr Treat Options Oncol. 2011 Mar;12(1):109

56. Inui A (2005) Recent development in research and management of cancer anorexia-cachexia syndrome. Gan To Kagaku Ryoho 32(6):743–749, Review

57. Ovesen L, Allingstrup L, Hannibal J, Mortensen EL, Hansen OP (1993) Effect of dietary counseling on food intake, body weight, response rate, survival, and quality of life in cancer patients undergoing chemotherapy: a prospective, randomized study. J Clin Oncol 11:2043–2049, PMID: 8410128

58. Berenstein EG, Ortiz Z (2005) Megestrol acetate for the treatment of anorexia-cachexia syndrome. Cochrane Database Syst Rev (2):CD004310

59. Leśniak W, Bała M, Jaeschke R, Krzakowski M (2008) Effects of megestrol acetate in patients with cancer anorexia-cachexia syndrome–a systematic review and meta-analysis. Pol Arch Med Wewn 118(11):636–644
60. Yeh SS, Lovitt S, Schuster MW (2009) Usage of megestrol acetate in the treatment of anorexia-cachexia syndrome in the elderly. J Nutr Health Aging 13(5):448–454
61. Busquets S, Serpe R, Sirisi S, Toledo M, Coutinho J, Martínez R, Orpí M, López-Soriano FJ, Argilés JM (2010) Megestrol acetate: its impact on muscle protein metabolism supports its use in cancer cachexia. Clin Nutr 29(6):733–737
62. Desport JC, Gory-Dalabaere G, Blanc-Vincent MP, Bachmann P, Béal J, Benamouzig R, Colomb V, Kere D, Melchior JC, Nitenberg G, Raynard B, Schneider S, Senesse P, FNCLCC (2003) Standards, options and recommendations for the use of appetite stimulants in oncology (2000). Br J Cancer 89(Suppl 1):S98–S100, PMID: 12915909
63. Karcic E, Philpot C, Morley JE (2002) Treating malnutrition with megestrol acetate: literature review and review of our experience. J Nutr Health Aging 6(3):191–200, Review. PMID: 12152625
64. Morley JE (2002) Orexigenic and anabolic agents. Clin Geriatr Med 18(4):853–866, Review. PMID: 12608509
65. Donnelly S, Walsh TD (1995) Low-dose megestrol acetate for appetite stimulation in advanced cancer. J Pain Symptom Manage 10:182–183
66. Mulligan K, Zackin R, Von Roenn JH et al (2007) ACTG 313 study team. Testosterone supplementation of megestrol therapy does not enhance lean tissue accrual in men with human immunodeficiency virus-associated weight loss: a randomized, double-blind, placebo-controlled, multicenter trial. J Clin Endocrinol Metab 92:563–570, Abstract
67. Navari RM, Brenner MC (2010) Treatment of cancer-related anorexia with olanzapine and megestrol acetate: a randomized trial. Support Care Cancer 18:951–956
68. Walsh D, Kirkova J, Davis MP (2005) The efficacy and tolerability of long-term use of dronabinol in cancer-related anorexia: a case series. J Pain Symptom Manage 30:493–495
69. Cannabis-In-Cachexia-Study-Group, Strasser F, Luftner D, Possinger K et al (2006) Comparison of orally administered cannabis extract and delta-9-tetrahydrocannabinol in treating patients with cancer-related anorexia-cachexia syndrome: a multicenter, phase III, randomized, double-blind, placebo-controlled clinical trial from the Cannabis-In-Cachexia-Study-Group. J Clin Oncol 24:3394–3400
70. Kumar NB, Hopkins K (2007) A retrospective study of Nutritional supplementation and appetite stimulants in the treatment of cancer cachexia. Abstract. In: Proceedings of research day, Moffitt Cancer Center, Tampa, Fl, USA 2007
71. Jatoi A, Windschitl HE, Loprinzi CL et al (2002) Dronabinol versus megestrol acetate versus combination therapy for cancer-associated anorexia: a North Central Cancer Treatment Group study. J Clin Oncol 20:567–573
72. Fearon KC (2008) Cancer cachexia: developing multimodal therapy for a multidimensional problem. Eur J Cancer 44(8):1124–1132, Epub 2008 Mar 28. PMID: 183475115
73. Walsh D, Nelson KA, Mahmoud FA (2003) Established and potential therapeutic applications of cannabinoids in oncology. Support Care Cancer 11(3):137–143, Epub 2002 Aug 21. Review. PMID: 12618922
74. Al-Majid S, Waters H (2008) The biological mechanisms of cancer-related skeletal muscle wasting: the role of progressive resistance exercise. Biol Res Nurs 10(1):7–20
75. Al-Majid S, McCarthy DO (2001) Cancer-induced fatigue and skeletal muscle wasting: the role of exercise. Biol Res Nurs 2(3):186–197
76. Lowe SS (2011) Physical activity and palliative cancer care. Recent Results Cancer Res 186:349–365
77. Penna F, Busquets S, Pin F, Toledo M, Baccino FM, López-Soriano FJ, Costelli P, Argilés JM (2011) Combined approach to counteract experimental cancer cachexia: eicosapentaenoic acid and training exercise. J Cachex Sarcopenia Muscle 2(2):95–104, Epub 2011 May 11
78. Garratt AM, Ruta DA, Abdalla MI, Buckingham JK, Russell IT (1993) The SF36 health survey questionnaire: an outcome measure suitable for routine use within the NHS? BMJ 306(6890):1440–1444

Cancer Cachexia (CC)

4

Core Messages

Cancer cachexia (CC) is a pathological loss of striated muscle (skeletal and cardiac) and fat stores, manifesting in the cardinal features of emaciation, weakness affecting functional status, impaired immune system, metabolic dysfunction, and poor quality of life.

More recently, staging guidelines for CC have been proposed, following the spectrum of initial unplanned weight loss (precachexia) progressing through degrees of severity (four stages) to the point where the cancer patient is depleted of both muscle and fat and immunocompromised and will likely die from complications.

The complex syndrome of cancer cachexia (CC) is present in 50–80% and a major contributor to the morbidity and mortality of cancer patients.

Multiple approaches, including experimental, preclinical, and early human clinical trials, have been employed to dissect the complex effectors of the CC syndrome.

Although synonymously included or noted in association with cancer anorexia, it is now clear that CC is much more complex relative to cancer anorexia and that it is mediated or modulated by a highly complex interplay of multiple biologic pathways, which are not fully understood.

It is reported that patient weight loss of >5% prior to chemotherapy may be a defining point for poor response, interruption of serial treatment, and survival.

Experimental and clinical studies have demonstrated that cachexia is mediated or modulated by a highly complex interplay of multiple biologic pathways, including pathological levels of proinflammatory cytokines, neuroendocrine hormones, positive and negative growth factors, transcription factors (NF-κB), lipolytic and proteolytic enzymes, and other signaling pathways.

N.B. Kumar, *Nutritional Management of Cancer Treatment Effects*,
DOI 10.1007/978-3-642-27233-2_4, © Springer-Verlag Berlin Heidelberg 2012

Although previous definitions and thus prevalence were based on weight loss associated with this syndrome, a more contemporary characterization of the cachectic state should include loss of skeletal mass, reduced food intake, and systemic inflammation, all of which may be more meaningful in terms of altered clinical outcomes.

4.1   Definition

The complex syndrome of cancer cachexia (CC) is a major contributor to the morbidity and mortality of cancer patients [1–5]. CC is a pathological loss of striated muscle (skeletal and cardiac) and fat stores, manifesting in the cardinal features of emaciation, weakness affecting functional status, impaired immune system, metabolic dysfunction, and poor quality of life [1–9]. More recently, staging guidelines for CC have been proposed [10, 11], following the spectrum of initial unplanned weight loss (precachexia) progressing through degrees of severity (four stages) to the point where the cancer patient is depleted of both muscle and fat and immunocompromised and will likely die from complications [12, 13]. Dewys et al. [14] reported that patient weight loss of >5% prior to chemotherapy, including those with lung cancer [15], may be a defining point for poor response, interruption of serial treatment, and survival. In the elderly, advanced malnutrition is much more difficult to treat or reverse contributing to a significant impact on functional dependence and quality of life [5, 15, 16] CC continues to be a critical problem in clinical oncology.

4.2   Prevalence

Due to multiple clinical symptom presentation and lack of an "all-inclusive" definition for this syndrome, it is difficult to estimate the true prevalence of cachexia. It is estimated that CC occurs in 50–80% of cancer patients and serves as an independent predictor of shorter survival, increased risk of treatment failure, and toxicity [1–5]. With our knowledge of the multidimensional nature of this syndrome, it is important that we do not account for the prevalence of CC, merely based on loss of weight observed in this population. Although previous definitions and thus prevalence were based on weight loss associated with this syndrome, a more contemporary characterization of the cachectic state should include loss of skeletal mass, reduced food intake, and systemic inflammation, all of which may be more meaningful in terms of altered clinical outcomes.

4.3   Etiology of Cancer Cachexia

Multiple approaches, including experimental, preclinical, and early human clinical trials, have been employed to dissect the complex effectors of the CC syndrome. Although synonymously always included or noted in association with cancer anorexia, it is now clear that CC is much more complex relative to cancer anorexia and that it is mediated or modulated by a highly complex interplay of multiple biologic pathways, which are not fully understood. It is also clear that these various experimental methods need to be linked together in order to interpret outcomes in the context of human physiology and pathology [17].

4.3.1   Potential Molecular Mechanisms of CC

Although the etiopathogenesis of CC is not fully understood, experimental and clinical studies have demonstrated that cachexia is mediated or modulated by a highly complex interplay of multiple biologic pathways, including pathological levels of proinflammatory cytokines (IL-1, IL-6, IFNγ, and TNFα) [18–23], neuroendocrine hormones [5, 24], positive and negative growth factors (IGFs, PIF, myostatin) [2, 6, 25–27], transcription factors (NF-κB, STATs) [28–33], lipolytic and proteolytic enzymes (adipose triglyceride lipase, caspases, proteasome subunits) [10, 34–36], and other signaling pathways. Loss of skeletal muscle in CC is the result of imbalance between protein synthesis and degradation [37]. The ubiquitin proteasome pathway accounts for the majority of skeletal muscle degradation in CC and is stimulated by several proinflammatory cytokines including TNFα, Il-6, IFNγ, and the PIF [6, 26, 27]. NF-κB which is an important regulator of skeletal muscle proteasome expression and protein degradation is upregulated in CC [13, 28, 30–33, 36, 38–40] increasing the rate of myosin heavy chain and telethonin degradation, compromising sarcomere integrity [41]. Pathologic levels of proinflammatory cytokines [18–23, 38] are associated with muscle wasting, exerted through inhibition of myosin expression and myogenic differentiation and stimulation of apoptosis [21–23]. Several investigators have suggested that actomyosin, actin, and myosin are specifically targeted for proteasome degradation in CC. Thus, both myosin synthesis and degeneration are affected in cachexia. Activation of apoptosis via Bax or caspases precedes myofibrillar protein breakdown during muscle wasting in CC [42–44].

The role of TNFα, IL-1, and IL-6 in CC development has been evaluated and confirmed in several studies [14, 18–20, 45, 46]. However, some investigators suggest that elevated cytokine levels could be the result rather than the cause of CC. Interleukin-6 (IL-6) may play a role in muscle wasting in certain animal tumors, possibly through both lysosomal (cathepsin) and nonlysosomal (proteasome) pathways [47]. Cytokines that are important in the initiation of the acute phase response (APR) have also been hypothesized in the genesis of CC [14, 46]. The presence of an APR or high circulating levels of proinflammatory cytokines is known to be related to adverse outcome in cancer patients. TNFα has been shown to exert direct catabolic effect on skeletal muscle and adipose tissue and induce muscle atrophy through a depression of protein synthesis and an increase in protein degradation via the ubiquitin-proteasome pathway, and this involves formation of reactive oxygen species leading to activation of NF-κB [31, 48].

More recently, Das et al. [36] demonstrated that genetic ablation of adipose triglyceride lipase and hormone sensitive lipase in tumor-bearing knockout mice prevented fat and muscle loss in CC. However, pharmacological inhibition of metabolic lipases in cancer patients would likely affect other pathways critical to maintaining hepatic lipid homeostasis, insulin secretion, and cardiac function [49–53], making these lipases an impractical therapeutic target. Based on these studies, we hypothesize that interventions targeting *inflammatory pathways in skeletal muscle* are essential to alleviate CC. Targets may include inducers of proteasome expression, enzymes regulating ubiquitination and degradation of myofibrillar proteins, and signaling pathways leading to activation of NF-κB.

More recently, oral administration of $n-3$ fatty acid formulations ($N-3$ FA) has been shown to attenuate tumor growth, weight loss, and/or muscle wasting in animal models of cancer [54, 55]. In a cell culture model of myogenesis, eicosapentaenoic acid (EPA) suppressed increases in the activities of NF-κB, caspase 8, and proteasome in differentiating C2C12 myotubes induced by PIF or TNFα [35, 56]. The deleterious effects of inflammatory cytokine–induced myogenesis have also been shown to be inhibited with EPA [35]. In early clinical trials, we and others have shown improvement in CC with multimodal approaches including adequate nutritional support supplemented with appetite stimulants and supplements with $N-3$ FA [7, 57] and observed stable anthropometrics, nutritional intake, statistically significant increase in serum proteins, functional status, and physical activity with no toxicity related to the study agent. Serum proteasome activity was inhibited in 64% of the subjects receiving treatment discussed in more detail in this chapter [57]. Although these early studies appear promising, interventions to date, including our study, have targeted: (a) heterogeneous cancer patient populations that differed substantially with respect to (b) age range, (c) types/grades/stages of disease, (d) treatment regimens, (e) refractory stages of CC, and failed to use valid, quantifiable biomarkers relevant to the underlying metabolic abnormalities of CC to evaluate effectiveness of interventions [33, 57–59]. Based on these currently available studies, we hypothesize that an integrated, molecular mechanism–based, *multimodal approach* of administration of a standardized dose of $N-3$ FA with an appetite stimulant and a nutritionally adequate diet to lung cancer patients diagnosed with early stage CC will prevent progression of CC, preserve skeletal muscle, and improve function by primarily reducing expression of cytokines and activation of NF-κB and proteasomal pathways and recommended these approaches be validated further in large, prospective clinical trials (Fig. 4.1).

More recently, myostatin, a member of the TGFβ superfamily, which is a key negative regulator of muscle mass in humans and animals, has been evaluated for safety and efficacy for the treatment of CC. Myostatin has been demonstrated to inhibit skeletal protein growth by several mechanisms, primarily through the inhibition of protein synthesis and myoblast differentiation. Myostatin inhibition or genetic ablation increases muscle mass and strength [60]. Deleting myostatin has been reported to attenuate sarcopenia and glucocorticoid-induced muscle atrophy and even improve dystrophic pathology in animals [61–63]. Myostatin acts primarily through the ActRIIB receptor, a transmembrane serine/threonine kinase heterotetramer receptor family member. More recently, novel formulations of an antibody that binds to ActRIIB have been proposed to prevent myostatin engagement, and signal transduction is thus expected to increase muscle mass by preventing the tonic

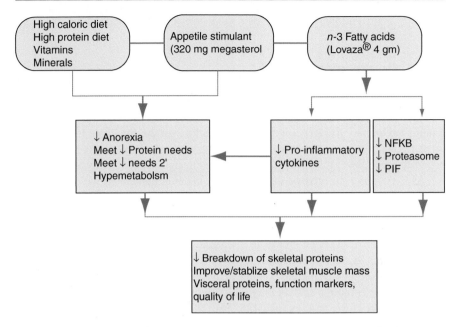

Fig. 4.1 Rationale for a multi-modal approach to reach early stages or cancer cachexla

negative effects of myostatin on muscle growth. These agents are in the early stage of development in clinical trials for the treatment of CC in lung and pancreatic cancer patients.

4.4   Current Therapies for CC

4.4.1   Nutritional Approaches

Initially, the pathophysiology of CC had two principle components – a failure of food intake and a systemic hypermetabolism/hypercatabolism syndrome. Strategies to counteract both hypermetabolism and reduced dietary intake have been demonstrated to be of importance for the survival, function, and quality of life of cancer patients [9]. The superimposed metabolic changes and the rate of depletion of physiological reserves of energy and protein were observed to be significantly increased in CC. These features indicated a need for nutritional support and metabolic management to ensure adequate intake of calories and protein in CC. Additionally, diets adequate in calories from fats and carbohydrates were required in "protein sparing" quantities for muscle anabolism [9, 64]. Protein intake must also be sufficient for wound repair, resistance to infection, and synthesis of enzymes and plasma proteins [5, 16]. Caloric deficits as much as 250–400 cal/day have been observed in CC. Hence, it was logical to infer that traditional approaches such as refeeding and/or supplementing dietary calories and proteins may resolve the issue.

However, interventions providing increased calories and protein have produced retention of fat mass but not muscle mass [65–67].

4.4.1.1 Eicosapentaenoic Acid

Eicosapentaenoic acid (EPA) is an essential $N - 3$ FA that cannot be synthesized completely by mammalian tissue and must be consumed in the diet. These polyunsaturated fats are present in fish oils from cod, sardine, and salmon. There is no established Dietary Reference Intake for $N - 3$ FA, yet the Adequate Intake (AI) is set at 1.6 and 1.1 g/day for men and women, respectively. While intake in the USA occurs at much lower than the proposed AI and no signs of deficiency are observed, the AI is proposed to provide optimal health benefits associated with consuming $N - 3$ FA [35].

Evidence from laboratory and clinical studies has demonstrated that EPA has antitumor and anticachectic effects. Oral administration of fish oil-derived $N - 3$ FA EPA and/or DHA has been shown to attenuate tumor growth, weight loss, and/or muscle wasting in animal models of cancer [54, 55]. In a cell culture model of myogenesis, EPA suppresses increases in the activities of NF-κB, caspase 8, and proteasome in differentiating C2C12 myotubes induced by PIF or TNFα, thereby suppressing apoptosis and necrosis [35, 56]. The deleterious effects of inflammatory cytokines on myogenesis have also been shown to be inhibited by EPA [35, 56]. Several recent laboratory studies indicate that EPA may attenuate protein degradation by preventing NF-κB translocation to the nucleus [10, 34]. Proteolysis-inducing factor (PIF) [25–27] is produced by cachexia-inducing murine and human tumors and stimulates muscle protein degradation directly through activation of the ubiquitin-proteasome pathway. Administration of EPA attenuates PIF-induced protein degradation in cachectic tumor-bearing mice [35]. Thus, EPA is hypothesized to prevent cachexia and preserve muscle by reducing expression of cytokines and activation of NF-κB and proteasomal or other proteolytic pathways.

In early clinical trials, results from $N - 3$ FA administration have been mixed. In a terminal cancer patient population with life expectancy of 2 months, changes in net weight gain, lean body mass, and improved quality of life were noted [57–59, 68, 69]. In a preliminary clinical trial [57], we evaluated the safety, efficacy, and potential mechanism of a multimodal intervention with a nutritionally adequate diet supplemented with an appetite stimulant and a standardized esterified $N - 3$ FA supplement – 4 g Lovaza® administered for 6 weeks to patients with stage II–IV cancer, mostly lung, with early symptoms of CC. Thirty six subjects were recruited and 33 subjects completed the study. We observed stable anthropometrics (Fig. 4.2a), moderate increase in nutritional intake, and significant increase in serum albumin (Fig. 4.2b) from baseline to 6 weeks. A progressive increase from baseline to 6 weeks in both functional status (Karnofsky Scale) and physical activity was also observed with no toxicity related to the study drug. Serum levels of TNFα progressively increased, while IL-6 decreased slightly. We then explored if treatment with 4 g/day Lovaza® results in inhibition of proteasome activity in pre- and posttreatment serum samples from the patients in this trial. Venous blood was collected from

Fig. 4.2 (a) Change in serum albumin levels with Lovaza®. (b) Change in triceps skinfold and mid-arm muscle circumference with Lovaza®

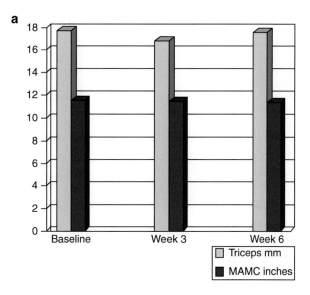

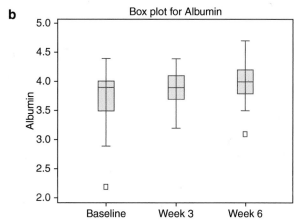

subjects at baseline and 6 weeks postintervention into heparin containing tubes and proteasome assay performed with Proteasome ELISA Kit according to manufacturer's instructions (ENZO Life Sciences). Complete pre- and posttreatment serum samples were available for 14 subjects. Inhibition of proteasome activity in serum samples posttreatment was calculated and plotted based on proteasome activity of pretreatment samples. Figure 4.3 shows that proteasome activity was inhibited by 6–29% in 9 out of 14 patients (64%): Our observations are provocative in that this improvement/stabilization of skeletal and visceral proteins, functional status, and physical activity scores occurred after initial weight loss, diagnosis of cancer, and while on active cytotoxic therapies [57]. In summary, laboratory studies and our

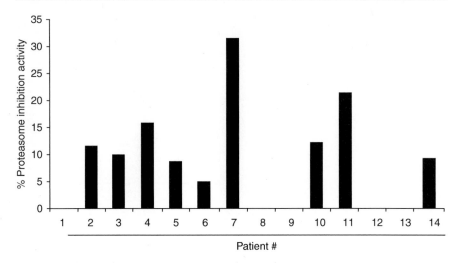

Fig. 4.3 Inhibition of proteasome activity in serum samples in cancer patients post treatment with $n - 3$ fatty acids

preliminary clinical trial [57] collectively indicate that treatment with $n - 3$ FA can attenuate muscle protein degradation and sarcopenia by preventing NF-κB, accumulation in the nucleus, and inhibiting proteasome activity [6, 10, 13, 26–28, 34, 36]. EPA, thus, represents a promising therapeutic agent to prevent degeneration as well as promote regeneration of skeletal muscle mass [56], and further clinical trials are warranted to examine its efficacy for the treatment of CC. It is noteworthy that the molecular mechanism of the effects of $N - 3$ FA has never been validated comprehensively in a well-powered randomized, placebo-controlled clinical trial in a homogeneous cancer patient population with early stages of CC, using objective markers of skeletal protein metabolism, and in a patient population with a relatively better prognosis than those previously targeted.

4.4.2   Appetite Stimulants

To improve food intake, other approaches have included administration of appetite stimulants such as progestogens, cannabinoids, corticosteroids, and antidepressants in addition to nutritional supplementation [47, 70–73]. Appetite stimulants have been shown to ameliorate or slow anorexia and unintentional weight loss in other populations but have not demonstrated improvements in lean body mass or markers of protein metabolism in the cachectic patient. The prevalent treatments to improve patient appetite are orexigenic agents such as megestrol acetate which acts by reducing cytokine production and increasing fat mass [70, 71]. Other common agents include dronabinol, a cannabis derivative demonstrated to enhance appetite and mood in cancer patients [47, 71], though its pharmacokinetics in this population has never been examined. In a preliminary retrospective study of 156 patients diagnosed and treated for CC, we evaluated the prevalence, type, and effectiveness of appetite stimulants and nutritional supplementation used at our Cancer Center. We observed that the most common appetite stimulants used were cannabinoids (50%), steroids (24%), and megestrol acetate (26%). Although an increase in appetite and food intake was observed, we were unable to achieve improvement in skeletal muscle mass with *nutrition support and appetite stimulants alone to treat CC*. Over 33% of these subjects were lung cancer patients, and all were on active treatment [73].

4.4.3   Physical Activity

Other nonpharmacological strategies to preserve muscle and bone mass include increasing physical activity via aerobic or anaerobic exercise [45, 66, 74]. However, the fatigue commonly associated with cancer therapy and cachexia, especially in the elderly [5, 16], prevents many patients from following physical activity regimens. These symptoms are accelerated in the elderly who have relatively lower steroid hormone levels, as a result of "hormonal aging," and lowered physical activity, as a result of treatment-related fatigue that has been demonstrated to contribute to lowered bone mineral density and muscle mass. These age-related conditions may thus be exacerbated, resulting in falls, fractures, and general muscle weakness.

The most prominent feature of wasting from cachexia versus starvation or anorexia is refractoriness to treatment by dietary consumption alone. Although strategies to improve appetite, intake of nutrients, and retain lean body mass (physical activity) have a scientific rationale and merit evaluation, randomized clinical trials with appetite stimulants or supplementation with proteins, calories, and antioxidants have failed to demonstrate reversal of metabolic abnormalities seen in CC [1, 14, 46]. Many studies, including our own, suggest that maintenance of lean body mass and myofibrillar proteins is difficult to achieve in CC, unless the *etiology of the underlying metabolic abnormalities is understood, targeted, and corrected* [1, 14, 46].

4.5   Guidelines for Treatment

Currently, there are no standard agents or therapies established to treat the symptom cluster associated to CC. The following guidelines are considered best practice standards. Improved management of CC may require a *multimodal approach by multidisciplinary teams*. These include specific nutritional guidelines, pharmacotherapy, and physical activity, in addition to monitoring and closely assessing patients for change in status. Figure 4.1 represents a molecular mechanism–based approach that is multimodal targeting the underlying metabolic abnormalities observed in CC.

4.5.1   Nutrition Guidelines

Nutritional assessment must be performed within 24 h of admission of the patient by a registered dietitian/nutritionist.

The goals for nutritional support in a cancer patient on active treatment may be as follows:

- To slow down the wasting process due to hypermetabolism (ensuring adequate nutritional intake and appetite stimulants)
- Attenuating the systemic inflammation
- Attenuating skeletal muscle catabolism or stimulating the muscle protein anabolism ($n - 3$ fatty acid supplementation)
- Prevent or reverse nutrient deficiencies
- Help patients better tolerate treatments
- Minimize nutrition-related side effects and complications
- Maintain strength and energy
- Protect immune function, decreasing the risk of infection
- Aid in recovery and healing
- Maximize quality of life
- Take into consideration patient wishes
- Common symptom clusters in patients with CC:
  - Anorexia
  - Constipation (laxatives, stool softeners, prokinetics based on etiology)
  - Oral pain (lidocaine swishes/Oragel)
  - Nausea and vomiting
  - Early satiety (adopt suggestions provided below)
  - Hypermetabolism
  - Inventory nutritional symptoms and treat consistently integrating both pharmacological and nonpharmacological approaches
1. Screen patient within 24 h of admission. This order for nutritional screening can be a standard order for all cancer patient admissions to avoid delay in timing of screening.
2. In addition to standard nutritional assessment parameters described in Chap. 2, assess all symptoms: gastrointestinal tract: taste alterations, smell alterations, dysphagia, dyspnea, other pain, early satiety, dry mouth, too much saliva production, anorexia, diarrhea, constipation, nausea, vomiting, dehydration, and fatigue; psychosocial: family/caregiver support, depression, and activities of daily living (ADL).
3. Assess current nutritional status and estimate caloric, protein, and multivitamin/mineral needs. There are no specific guidelines that have been evaluated in the cancer patient population. The recommendations provided here are usual standards of care that is provided in this patient population based on best practice standards as follows.
4. Provide adequate nutrition by including "calorie" and "protein" booster education material and nutritional supplements to ensure intake of proteins (recommended 0.8 g–1.0 g/kg/day). Provide dense caloric supplements up to 400 cal/

day containing 1.5 kcal/mL. If intake is insufficient in protein intake, supplement with modular protein supplements, adding this to favorite beverage (http://www.nestle-nutrition.com/Products/Default.aspx; http://abbottnutrition.com/). The choice of nutritional supplements can be based in the personal choice of the patient, patient needs, and tolerance to product as well as other comorbidities.

5. Include a standard multivitamin mineral supplementation to prevent any further deficits and meet increased needs.

6. Assess adequacy of intake and provide an appetite stimulant (megestrol acetate 800 mg/day or alternate) if patient has cancer anorexia to ensure adequate intake and prevent further weight loss.

7. Provide each patient with nutritional guidelines to ensure adequate intake of calories and proteins and a list of suggested high-calorie and high-protein nutritional supplements to choose from, taking into consideration taste alterations, early satiety, nausea, and vomiting that are common symptoms observed in this patient population.

8. Recommend prescription for standardized omega-3 fatty acid supplement if benefits outweigh risks.

9. Alter consistency of foods as needed, based on ability to chew and swallow.

10. Selection of route of feeding may be informed based on general guidelines and criteria provided in Table 2.6.

11. Other tips to enhance nutritional intake:

    - Meal and snack times need to be planned to occur at regular intervals and not in response to the hunger mechanism, which may be absent or altered.
    - Snacks of high calorie and protein density must be planned between meals, such as high-calorie puddings, shakes, high-calorie and protein drink supplements, sandwiches, avocados, and nuts.
    - Plans must be made for special circumstances. If meals need to be missed or delayed due to a test or therapy, snacks or a meal must be planned for consumption after the event/test.
    - High-calorie and protein-dense foods may be essential. Choose high-calorie foods, such as avocados, nuts, pudding, cream soups, cooked cereals, and vegetables with added butter or margarine. Use extra olive oil in salads.
    - Season foods with exotic flavors, fresh herbs, and spices that stimulate appetite. Unless contraindicated, use salt and sweetening as desired.
    - Consider the role of smell, texture, and eye appeal to help stimulate the desire to eat, such as the smell of fresh bread baking or a colorful fruit cup.
    - Use garnishes on foods to increase the visual "eye" appeal.
    - Fresh fruits and vegetables may be more appealing than canned or frozen ones.
    - Experiment with different food textures as crunchy, creamy, and crispy foods.
    - When shopping, recommend choosing foods that are beautiful, colorful, fresh, and full-flavored.
    - If the patient is unable to tolerate red meats, recommend including other protein sources in the diet such as poultry, fish, milk, eggs, bean and legumes, peanut butter, and other nut butters.

4.5.2 Pharmacotherapy

Assessment must be performed within 24 h of admission of the patient by a clinical pharmacist closely working with the registered dietitian.

Appetite Stimulants: Current therapies used to improve appetite and to reduce breakdown of muscle proteins (proteolysis):

1. *Corticosteroids*
   (a) Dexamethasone (Decadron®)
   (b) Methylprednisolone (Solu-Medrol®)
   (c) Prednisone (Deltasone®)
2. *Orexigenic agents*
   (a) Megestrol acetate (Megace®)
3. *Anabolic steroids*
   (a) Medroxyprogesterone acetate (Provera®, Depo-Provera®)
4. *Antiemetic*
   (a) Dronabinol (Marinol®)
5. Antidepressants
6. Experimental therapies
   (a) Proteasome inhibitors: Omega-3 fatty acids Lovaza (GSK)
   (b) Novel formulations of an antibody that binds to ActRIIB (Novartis)

4.5.3 Physical Activity

Since fatigue and poor nutritional status are classic symptoms of CC, patients should proactively receive a comprehensive assessment of physical status by a licensed physical therapist and therapy initated within 24 h of assessment.

1. *Godin Leisure-Time Exercise Questionnaire* weekly to monitor physical activity.
2. *Handgrip Strength Dynamometry Assessment*: A validated tool commonly used to assess handgrip strength is the Jamar dynamometer, which is a fast, reliable, and easy-to-perform device commonly used by our team to measure improvements in functional strength [75]. The Jamar dynamometer has a lower percent coefficient of variation and is thus a more precise device than other handgrip dynamometers.

4.5.4 Markers and Instruments for Patient Monitoring and Assessment of Response to Treatment by the Interdisciplinary Medical Team

1. *Anthropometric measurements* such as participant's height, weight, and body mass index can be performed at admission and at regular intervals established by the medical team.

2. *Body composition by DXA scan*: DXA should be used to assess both total lean body mass (LBM), fat mass (FM), and total bone mineral density (BMD).Total bone mineral density (BMD) is a valid indirect measure of skeletal muscle and patient activity. Total LBM is sometimes called total fat-free mass (FFM) depending upon specific DXA manufacturer. DXA instruments use an X-ray source that generates or is split into two energies to measure bone mineral mass and soft tissue from which fat and fat-free mass are estimated. The exam is quick (1–2 min), precise (0.5–1%), and noninvasive. DXA scanners have the precision required to detect changes in muscle mass as small as 5%. Radiation exposure from DXA scans is minimal. The National Council on Radiation Protection and Measurements (NCRP) has recommended that the annual effective dose limit for infrequent exposure of the general population is 5,000 μSv and that an annual effective dose of 10 μSv be considered a negligible individual dose. The effective dose of a dual-energy X-ray absorptiometry whole body scan on an adult is 2.1 μSv. Studies have shown that quality assurance is an important issue in the use of DXA scans to determine body composition including lean body mass and bone mineral density. DXA instrument manufacturer and model should remain consistent, and their calibration should be monitored throughout treatment. Use of a standardized scan acquisition protocol and appropriate and unchanging scan acquisition and analysis software is essential to achieve consist results.

3. *Dietary intake* must be assessed at baseline and periodical intervals by conducting random weekly, 2-week days +1 weekend day 24-h dietary recalls (gold standard for collecting dietary data) using a 5-step multipass procedure (which has been found to assess mean energy intake within 10% of actual intake) and using the frequently updated University of Minnesota Nutrition Data System-Research version (NDS-R) database for analysis of nutrient composition. Food portion visuals can be provided to patients to estimate portion sizes of foods while monitoring intake.

4. *Symptom log* may be completed daily and collected from patients on a monthly basis. Based on these symptoms, all anticipated and unanticipated, grades of constitutional, dermatological, gastrointestinal (GI), metabolic, and pain symptoms can be continuously monitored including those symptoms affecting nutritional intake and utilization.

5. *Monthly* CMP and CBC should be monitored to assess electrolytes and organ function.

6. *Functional markers (Karnofsky performance score)*: Evaluation of patient functional status and barriers to obtaining adequate nutrients is also necessary. A physical exam combined with personal interview should include the evaluation of functional status such as the ability to chew and swallow, dental or oral problems causing odynophagia or dysphagia, signs of muscle wasting or anasarca, presence of edema, presence of skin or mouth lesion, and ability to perform instrumental activities of daily living (IADLs) such as cooking, shopping, and self-feeding. It is critical to assess activities of daily living, physical activity, exercise, sleep, and ability to work and perform other functional roles.

Limitations in the activities of daily living have been identified secondary to and as a cause of weight loss in cancer patients. Cancer and other chronic diseases pose difficulties specifically for the cancer patient receiving treatment and the elderly in carrying out activities of daily living. A loss of postural and locomotive muscle mass has been observed within 7 days of inactivity. The Karnofsky Performance Scale Index allows patients to be classified as to their functional impairment. This has been used to compare effectiveness of different therapies and to assess the prognosis in individual patients and has been validated in cancer patient populations. Karnofsky Performance Scale Index allows patients to be classified as to their functional impairment. This has been used to compare effectiveness of different therapies and to assess the prognosis in individual patients and has been validated in cancer patient populations.

7. *Biochemical markers of protein status (serum albumin and transferrin)*: Assessment of protein status is critical in the identification and treatment of abnormalities in protein metabolism. There is substantial evidence of the correlation between serum hepatic proteins and inflammation, making these the most relevant biomarkers in CC. Serum transferrin, prealbumin, and albumin have been observed as intermediate endpoint biomarkers and independently associated with worse outcome in cachexia [5, 68]. Measurements of body composition combined with more objective and sensitive measure of protein nutriture are ideal for the biochemical assessment of intravascular and visceral protein stores. We have thus included the three major valid intermediate endpoint biomarkers (IEBs) that represent intravascular and visceral protein pools – transferrin, prealbumin, and albumin – as the biochemical indicators of protein status [76–78]. Although transferrin levels are affected by iron status, serum transferrin, either singly or as part of a multiparameter index, is the strongest predictor of cancer patient morbidity and mortality [76–78].

8. *Immune and inflammatory markers*: Unlike anorexia of aging, in CC, there is a range of metabolic responses triggered by inflammatory and immunological responses. It is believed that the putative mediators of CC are cytokines, and increased expression of tumor necrosis factor and interleukin-6 has been observed in patients with CC. Cytokines will be measured in a panel including IL-1, IL-4, IL-6, IL-8, IL-10, GM-CSF, IFN-κ, TNFα, and CRP (BioRad-Bioplex). All of these biomarkers have been shown to increase with disease, aging, and cytotoxic agents. Though we realize these intermediate endpoint biomarkers of cytokines cannot be reliably interpreted, as over 70% of the subjects as observed in our studies were on active treatment with cytotoxic agents, these variables are important to determine, as they may provide useful information and contribute to the better understanding of the mechanistic process.

9. *Quality of life*: Should be measured at baseline and monthly using the Rand Short Form (SF)-36 (Medical Outcomes Study SF-36) [79]. The SF-36 has been used extensively with both general, high-risk, and cancer populations and has available norms for mail and telephone versions and comparisons between group and individual scores. Scores are calculated and transformed to a 0–100 scale, with higher

scores indicating increased health status. Reliability of the SF-36 scales was measured by Cronbach α coefficient, and the results ranged from 0.78 in general health perceptions to 0.91 in the physical functioning domain.

10. *Erythrocyte n − 3 index*: Red blood cell levels of eicosapentaenoic acid (EPA) and docosahexaenoic acid (DHA) are a reflection of tissue levels and are determined by a complex interplay of metabolism and nutrition. The Omega-3 Index, which is the EPA + DHA content of erythrocytes expressed as a percent of total identified fatty acids, was originally suggested as a marker of increased risk for death from coronary heart disease, but it can also be viewed as an actual risk factor, playing a pathophysiologic role in the disease. Optimal levels appear to be 8% or greater. At this stage of its development, the erythrocyte Omega-3 Index appears to fulfill many of the requirements for both a risk marker and a risk factor. The Omega-3 Index may represent a novel, physiologically relevant, and easily modified variable that could have significant clinical utility. A monthly monitor of these levels will be an excellent indicator of compliance to supplement.

4.5.5   Follow-up

Patients must be seen by a multidisciplinary member of the team on a monthly basis to monitor progress and to review compliance to intervention including diet intake adequacy, symptom logs, change in concomitant medications, and any other issues related to treatment.

4.6   Future Directions

The debilitating symptoms and consequences of cachexia can no longer be accepted as unavoidable sequelae of advanced cancer. Currently, there are no standard treatment guidelines or therapies established to treat the symptom cluster associated with CC. Although early studies appear promising, interventions to date, including our study, have targeted (a) heterogeneous cancer patient populations that differed substantially with respect to (b) age range, (c) types/grades/stages of disease, (d) treatment regimens, (e) refractory stages of CC, and (f) failed to use valid, quantifiable biomarkers relevant to the underlying metabolic abnormalities of CC to evaluate effectiveness of interventions. Improved management of CC may require a multimodal intervention by multidisciplinary teams using a molecular mechanism–based approach. It is beneficial to examine the potential to intervene in molecular pathways to modify metabolic alterations that contribute to wasting, and downregulate transcription factor or cytokine signaling to treat CC. Future studies should focus on evaluating multimodal approaches that are innovative and timely, and provide a robust, well-rationalized, and molecular-based approach for the development of a systematic, safe, and effective treatment of CC.

Summary for the Clinician

Cancer cachexia is a condition, unlike cancer anorexia, nonresponsive to traditional treatment approaches alone, such as increased feeding and appetite stimulants.

Currently, there are no standard agents or therapies established to treat the symptom cluster associated with cancer cachexia – pharmacological or nonpharmacological – and there is no drug registered to address cancer cachexia.

Improved management of CC by clinicians for now may require a multimodal approach by multidisciplinary teams.

These include specific (a) nutritional guidelines, (b) pharmacotherapy with appetite stimulants, and (c) physical activity, in addition to (d) monitoring and closely assessing patients for change in status.

Appetite stimulants and supplementation with proteins, calories, and antioxidants produce some stabilization in functional status and were not contraindicated in most cancer patients on treatment.

Randomized clinical trials, including our trials with appetite stimulants, nutrient supplementation, 5-HT3 antagonists, antioxidants, and Cox-2 inhibitors, alone have failed to reverse the metabolic abnormalities seen in CC.

Several novel drugs are currently being evaluated for treatment of cancer cachexia including $n - 3$ fatty acids, myostatin inhibitors, and combination therapies that attempt to treat the symptom clusters and underlying metabolic abnormalities observed in cancer cachexia.

The guidelines provided are best practice standards based on current evidence in the research literature.

Future studies must focus on understanding the etiology, underlying metabolic abnormalities observed in CC in order to target, treat, and reverse this complex syndrome.

References

1. Ross PJ, Ashley S, Norton A, Priest K, Waters JS, Eisen T et al (2004) Do patients with weight loss have a worse outcome when undergoing chemotherapy for lung cancers? Br J Cancer 90:1905–1911
2. Jatoi A (2008) Weight loss in patient with advanced cancer: effects, causes, and potential management. Curr Opin Support Palliat Care 2(1):45–48
3. Evans WJ, Morley JE, Argilés J, Bales C, Baracos V, Guttridge D, Jatoi A et al (2008) Cachexia: a new definition. Clin Nutr 27(6):793–799, Epud 2008 Aug 21. PMID: 18718696
4. Behl D, Jatoi A (2007) Pharmacological options for advanced cancer patients with loss of appetite and weight. Expert Opin Pharmacother 8(8):1085–1090
5. Morley JE (2002) Pathophysiology of anorexia. Clin Geriatr Med 18(4):661–673, v. Review. PMID: 12608495
6. Melstrom LG, Melstrom KA Jr, Ding XZ, Adrian TE (2007) Mechanisms of skeletal muscle degradation and its therapy in cancer cachexia. Histol Histopathol 22(7):805–814

7. Mantovani G, Macciò A, Madeddu C, Serpe R, Massa E, Dessì M, Panzone F, Contu P (2010) Randomized phase III clinical trial of five different arms of treatment in 332 patients with cancer cachexia. Oncologist 15(2):200–211, Epub 2010 Feb 15

8. Giacosa A, Rondanelli M (2008) Fish oil and treatment of cancer cachexia. Genes Nutr 3(1):25–28

9. Bosaeus I (2008) Nutritional support in multimodal therapy for CC. Support Care Cancer 16(5):447–451, Epub 2008 Jan 15. PMID: 18196284

10. Blum B, Omlin A, Fearon K, Baracos V, Radbruch L, Kaasa S, Strasser F, European Palliative Care Research Collaborative (2010) Evolving classification systems for CC: ready for clinical practice? Support Care Cancer 18(3):273–279, PMID: 20076976

11. Bozzetti F, Mariani L (2009) Defining and classifying CC: a proposal by SCRINIO Working Group. JPEN J Parenter Enteral Nutr 33(4):361–367, Epub 2008 Dec 24. PMID: 19109514

12. Deans DA, Tan BH, Wigmore SJ, Ross JA, de Beaux AC, Paterson-Brown S, Feron KV (2009) The influence of systemic inflammation, dietary intake and stage of disease on rate of weight loss in patients with gastro-esophageal cancer. Br J Cancer 100(1):63–69

13. Hamerman D (2002) Molecular-based therapeutic approaches in treatment of anorexia of aging and CC. J Gerontol A Biol Sci Med Sci 57(8):M511–M518, Review. PMID: 12145364

14. Dewys WD, Begg C, Lavin PT, Band PR, Bennett JM, Bertino JR, Cohen MH, Douglass HO Jr, Engstrom PF, Ezdinli EZ, Horton J, Johnson GJ, Moertel CG, Oken MM, Perlina C, Rosenbaum C, Silverstein MN, Skeel RT, Sponzo RW, Tormey DC (1980) Prognostic effect of weight loss prior to chemotherapy in cancer patients. Eastern Cooperative Oncology Group. Am J Med 69:491–497, PMID: 7424938

15. McMillan DC (2009) Systemic inflammation, nutritional status and survival in patients with cancer. Curr Opin Clin Nutr Metab Care 12(3):223–226

16. Morley JE (2003) Anorexia and weight loss in older persons. J Gerontol A Biol Sci Med Sci 58(2):131–137

17. Kim W, McMurray DN, Chapkin RS (2010) $n - 3$ polyunsaturated fatty acids-physiological relevance of dose. Prostaglandins Leukot Essent Fatty Acids 82(4–6):155–158, Epub 2010 Feb 25. Review

18. Barton BE (2001) IL-6-like cytokines and CC: consequences of chronic inflammation. Immunol Res 23(1):41–58, Review. PMID: 11417859

19. Mantovani G, Madeddu C, Gramignano G, Ferreli L, Massa E, Contu P, Serpe R (2004) Association of serum IL-6 levels with comprehensive geriatric assessment variables in a population of elderly cancer patients. Oncol Rep 11(1):197–206

20. Barber MD, Wigmore SJ, Ross JA, Fearon KC, Tisdale MJ (1998) Proinflammatory cytokines, nutritional support, and the cachexia syndrome: interactions and therapeutic options. Cancer 82(5):1000

21. Evans WJ (2010) Skeletal muscle loss: cachexia, sarcopenia, and inactivity. Am J Clin Nutr 91(4):1123S–1127S, Epub 2010 Feb 17

22. Pickering WP, Price SR, Bircher G, Marinovic AC, Mitch WE, Walls J (2002) Nutrition in CAPD: serum bicarbonate and the ubiquitin-proteasome system in muscle. Kidney Int 61:1286–1292

23. Du J, Wang X, Miereles C et al (2004) Activation of caspase-3 is an initial step triggering accelerated muscle proteolysis in catabolic conditions. J Clin Invest 113:115–123

24. Mantovani G, Maccio A, Mura L, Massa E, Mudu MC, Mulas C et al (2000) Serum levels of leptin and proinflammatory cytokines in patients with advanced-stage cancer at different sites. J Mol Med 78(10):554–561

25. Deans DA, Wigmore SJ, Gilmour H, Tisdale MJ, Fearon KC, Ross JA (2008) Expression of the proteolysis-inducing factor core peptide mRNA is upregulated in both tumour and adjacent normal tissue in gastro-esophageal malignancy. Br J Cancer 98(1):242; author reply 243. PMCID: PMC2361198

26. Wigmore SJ, Todorov PT, Barber MD, Ross JA, Tisdale MJ, Fearon KC (2000) Characteristics of patients with pancreatic cancer expressing a novel cancer cachectic factor. Br J Surg 87(1):53–58

27. Whitehouse AS, Tisdale MJ (2003) Increased expression of the ubiquitin-proteasome pathway in murine myotubes by proteolysis-inducing factor (PIF) is associated with activation of the transcription factor NF-kappaB. Br J Cancer 89(6):1116–1122

28. Mitch WE, Price SR (2001) Transcription factors and muscle cachexia: is there a therapeutic target? Lancet 357(9258):734–735

29. Ciechanover A, Orian A, Schwartz AL (2000) The ubiquitin-mediated proteolytic pathway: mode of action and clinical implications. J Cell Biochem Suppl 34:40–51

30. Voges D, Zwickl P, Baumeister W (1999) The 26S proteasome: a molecular machine designed for controlled proteolysis. Annu Rev Biochem 68:1015–1068

31. Chen S, Fribley A, Wang CY (2002) Potentiation of tumor necrosis factor-mediated apoptosis of oral squamous cell carcinoma cells by adenovirus-mediated gene transfer of NF-kappaB inhibitor. J Dent Res 81:98–102

32. Ghosh S, Karin M (2002) Missing pieces in the NF-kappaB puzzle. Cell 109 Suppl:S81–S96

33. Fearon KC, Van Meyenfeldt MF, Moses AG, Van Geenen R, Roy A, Gouma DJ et al (2003) Effect of a protein and energy dense $N - 3$ fatty acid enriched oral supplement on loss of weight and lean tissue in CC: a randomised double blind trial. Gut 52(10):1479–1486, PMCID: PMC1773823

34. Maltoni M, Fabbri L, Nanni O, Scarpi E, Pezzi L, Flamini E et al (1997) Serum levels of tumor necrosis factor alpha and other cytokines do not correlate with weight loss and anorexia in cancer patients. Support Care Cancer 5(2):130–135; comments in Support Care Cancer. 1997;5(5):422–423. PMID: 9069613

35. Whitehouse AS, Khal J, Tisdale MJ (2003) Induction of protein catabolism in myotubes by 15(S)-hydroxyeicosatetraenoic acid through increased expression of the ubiquitin-proteasome pathway. Br J Cancer 89(4):737–745, PMID: 12915888

36. Das SK, Eder S, Schauer S, Diwoky C, Temmel H, Guertl B, Gorkiewicz G, Tamilarasan KP, Kumari P, Trauner M, Zimmermann R, Vesely P, Haemmerle G, Zechner R, Hoefler G (2011) Adipose triglyceride lipase contributes to cancer-associated cachexia. Science 333(6039):233–238, Epub 2011 Jun 16

37. Fearon KC (2011) Cancer cachexia and fat-muscle physiology. N Engl J Med 365(6):565–567

38. Acharyya S, Ladner KJ, Nelsen LL et al (2004) Cancer cachexia is regulated by selective targeting of skeletal muscle gene products. J Clin Invest 114:370–378

39. Peterson JM, Bakkar N, Guttridge DC (2011) NF-κB signaling in skeletal muscle health and disease. Curr Top Dev Biol 96:85–119

40. Guttridge DC, Mayo MW, Madrid LV, Wang CY, Baldwin AS Jr (2000) NF-kappaB-induced loss of MyoD messenger RNA: possible role in muscle decay and cachexia. Science 289(5488):2363–2366

41. Attaix D, Combaret L, Béchet D, Taillandier D (2008) Role of the ubiquitin-proteasome pathway in muscle atrophy in cachexia. Curr Opin Support Palliat Care 2(4):262–266

42. Fukuda T, Sumi T, Nobeyama H, Yoshida H, Matsumoto Y, Yasui T, Honda K, Ishiko O (2009) Multiple organ failure of tumor-bearing rabbits in cancer cachexia is caused by apoptosis of normal organ cells. Int J Oncol 34(1):61–67

43. Argilés JM, López-Soriano FJ, Busquets S (2007) Mechanisms to explain wasting of muscle and fat in cancer cachexia. Curr Opin Support Palliat Care 1(4):293–298

44. Belizário JE, Lorite MJ, Tisdale MJ (2001) Cleavage of caspases-1, -3, -6, -8 and -9 substrates by proteases in skeletal muscles from mice undergoing cancer cachexia. Br J Cancer 84(8):1135–1140

45. Adamsen L, Quist M, Andersen C, Møller T, Herrstedt J, Kronborg D et al (2009) Effect of a multimodal high intensity exercise intervention in cancer patients undergoing chemotherapy: randomized controlled trial. BMJ 339:b3410

46. Sun LC, Chu KS, Cheng SC, Lu CY, Kuo CH, Hsieh JS et al (2009) Preoperative serum carcinoembryonic antigen, albumin and age are supplementary to UICC staging systems in predicting survival for colorectal cancer patients undergoing surgical treatment. BMC Cancer 9:288

47. Walsh D, Nelson KA, Mahmoud FA (2003) Established and potential therapeutic applications of cannabinoids in oncology. Support Care Cancer 11(3):137–143, Epub 2002 Aug 21. Review. PMID: 12618922

48. Ghosh S, Karin M (2002) Missing pieces in the NF-kappaB puzzle. Cell 109(Suppl): S81–S96

49. Reid BN, Ables GP, Otlivanchik OA, Schoiswohl G, Zechner R, Blaner WS, Goldberg IJ, Schwabe RF, Chua SC Jr, Huang LS (2008) Hepatic overexpression of hormone-sensitive lipase and adipose triglyceride lipase promotes fatty acid oxidation, stimulates direct release of free fatty acids, and ameliorates steatosis. J Biol Chem 283(19):13087–13099, Epub 2008 Mar 12

50. Lass A, Zimmermann R, Oberer M, Zechner R (2011) Lipolysis - a highly regulated multi-enzyme complex mediates the catabolism of cellular fat stores. Prog Lipid Res 50(1):14–27, Epub 2010 Nov 16. Review

51. Wölkart G, Schrammel A, Dörffel K, Haemmerle G, Zechner R, Mayer B (2011) Cardiac dysfunction in adipose triglyceride lipase deficiency: treatment with a PPARα agonist. Br J Pharmacol. doi:10.1111/j.1476–5381.2011.01490.x

52. Wu JW, Wang SP, Alvarez F, Casavant S, Gauthier N, Abed L, Soni KG, Yang G, Mitchell GA (2011) Deficiency of liver adipose triglyceride lipase in mice causes progressive hepatic steatosis. Hepatology 54(1):122–132

53. Schoiswohl G, Schweiger M, Schreiber R, Gorkiewicz G, Preiss-Landl K, Taschler U, Zierler KA, Radner FP, Eichmann TO, Kienesberger PC, Eder S, Lass A, Haemmerle G, Alsted TJ, Kiens B, Hoefler G, Zechner R, Zimmermann R (2010) Adipose triglyceride lipase plays a key role in the supply of the working muscle with fatty acids. J Lipid Res 51(3):490–499, Epub 2009 Nov 25

54. Spencer L, Mann C, Metcalfe M, Webb M, Pollard C, Spencer D, Berry D, Steward W, Dennison A (2009) The effect of omega-3 FAs on tumour angiogenesis and their therapeutic potential. Eur J Cancer 45(12):2077–2086, Epub 2009 Jun 1

55. Smith GI, Atherton P, Reeds DN, Mohammed BS, Rankin D, Rennie MJ, Mittendorfer B (2011) Dietary omega-3 fatty acid supplementation increases the rate of muscle protein synthesis in older adults: a randomized controlled trial. Am J Clin Nutr 93(2):402–412, Epub 2010 Dec 15

56. Magee P, Pearson S, Allen J (2008) The omega-3 fatty acid, eicosapentaenoic acid (EPA), prevents the damaging effects of tumour necrosis factor (TNF)-alpha during murine skeletal muscle cell differentiation. Lipids Health Dis 7:24

57. Kumar NB, Kazi A, Smith T, Crocker T, Yu D, Reich RR, Reddy K, Hastings S, Exterman M, Balducci L, Dalton K, Bepler G (2010) Cancer cachexia: traditional therapies and novel molecular mechanism-based approaches to treatment. Curr Treat Options Oncol 11(3–4):107–117, Review

58. Mantovani G, Macciò A, Madeddu C, Gramignano G, Serpe R, Massa E et al (2008) Randomized phase III clinical trial of five different arms of treatment for patients with CC: interim results. Nutrition 24(4):305–313, Epub 2008 Feb 11

59. Dewey A, Baughan C, Dean T, Higgins B, Johnson I (2007) Eicosapentaenoic acid (EPA, an omega-3 fatty acid from fish oils) for the treatment of CC. Cochrane Database Syst Rev 24(1):CD004597, same as 33

60. Lee SJ, McPherron AC (2001) Regulation of myostatin activity and muscle growth. Proc Natl Acad Sci USA 98(16):9306–9311

61. Siriett V, Salerno MS, Berry C, Nicholas G, Bower R, Kambadur R, Sharma M (2007) Antagonism of myostatin enhances muscle regeneration during sarcopenia. Mol Ther 15(8):1463–1470

62. Bogdanovich S, Perkins KJ, Krag TO, Whittemore LA, Khurana TS (2005) Myostatin propeptide-mediated amelioration of dystrophic pathophysiology. FASEB J 19(6):543–549

63. Bogdanovich S, Krag TO, Barton ER, Morris LD, Whittemore LA, Ahima RS, Khurana TS (2002) Functional improvement of dystrophic muscle by myostatin blockade. Nature 420(6914):418–421

64. Blackburn GL, Moldawer LL, Usui S, Bothe A Jr, O'Keefe SJ, Bistrian BR (1979) Branched chain amino acid administration and metabolism during starvation, injury, and infection. Surgery 86(2):307–315

65. Hart DW, Wolf SE, Herndon DN et al (2002) Energy expenditure and caloric balance after burn: increased feeding leads to fat rather than lean mass accretion. Ann Surg 235:152–161

66. Couch M, Lai V, Cannon T, Guttridge D, Zanation A, George J, Hayes DN, Zeisel S, Shores C (2007) Cancer cachexia syndrome in head and neck cancer patients: part I. Diagnosis, impact on quality of life and survival, and treatment. Head Neck 29(4):401–411, PMID: 17285641

67. Fearon KC, von Meyenfeldt M, Moses AG, Van Geenen R, Roy A, Gouma DJ, Giacosa A, Van Gossum A, Bauer J, Barber MD, Aaronson NK, Voss AC, Tisdale MJ (2003) Effect of a protein and energy dense $n - 3$ fatty acid enriched oral supplement on weight and lean tissue in CC: a randomized double blind trial. Gut 52(10):1479–1486, PMCID: PMC1773823

68. Barber MD, Fearon KC, Tisdale MJ, McMillan DC, Ross JA (2001) Effect of a fish oil-enriched nutritional supplement on metabolic mediators in patients with pancreatic CC. Nutr Cancer 40(2):118–124

69. Fearon KC, Barber MD, Moses AG, Ahmedzai SH, Taylor GS, Tisdale MJ, Murray GD (2006) Double-blind, placebo-controlled, randomized study of eicosapentaenoic acid diester in patients with CC. J Clin Oncol 24(21):3401–3407

70. Karcic E, Philpot C, Morley JE (2002) Treating malnutrition with megestrol acetate: literature review and review of our experience. J Nutr Health Aging 6(3):191–200, Review. PMID: 12152625

71. Morley JE (2002) Orexigenic and anabolic agents. Clin Geriatr Med 18(4):853–866, Review. PMID: 12608509

72. Desport JC, Gory-Dalabaere G, Blanc-Vincent MP, Bachmann P, Béal J, Benamouzig R, Colomb V, Kere D, Melchior JC, Nitenberg G, Raynard B, Schneider S, Senesse P, FNCLCC (2003) Standards, options and recommendations for the use of appetite stimulants in oncology (2000). Br J Cancer 89 Suppl 1:S98–S100, PMID: 12915909

73. Kumar NB, Hopkins K (2007) A retrospective study of nutritional supplementation and appetite stimulants in the treatment of Cancer Cachexia. Abstract. Proceedings of Research Day, Moffitt Cancer Center

74. Al-Majid S, Waters H (2008) The biological mechanisms of cancer-related skeletal muscle wasting: the role of progressive resistance exercise. Biol Res Nurs 10(1):7–20

75. Trutschnigg B, Kilgour RD, Reinglas J et al (2008) Precision and reliability of strength. (Jamar vs. Biodex handgrip) and body composition (dual-energy X-ray absorptiometry vs bioimpedance analysis) measurements in advanced cancer patients. Appl Physiol Nutr Metab 33:1232–1239

76. Guerra LT, Rosa AR, Romani RF, Gurski RR, Schirmer CC, Kruel CD (2009) Serum transferrin and serum prealbumin as markers of response to nutritional support in patients with esophageal cancer. Nutr Hosp 24(2):241–242, PMID: 19593499

77. Neyra NR, Hakim RM, Shyr Y, Ikizler TA (2000) Serum transferrin and serum prealbumin are early predictors of serum albumin in chronic hemodialysis patients. J Ren Nutr 10(4):184–190

78. Beguin Y (2003) Soluble transferrin receptor for the evaluation of erythropoiesis and iron status. Clin Chim Acta 329:9–22

79. Garratt AM, Ruta DA, Abdalla MI, Buckingham JK, Russell IT (1993) The SF36 health survey questionnaire: an outcome measure suitable for routine use within the NHS? BMJ 306(6890):1440–1444

Oral Mucositis

5

Core Messages

Oral mucositis refers to erythematous and ulcerative lesions of the oral mucosa observed in patients with cancer being treated with chemotherapy and/or with radiation therapy to fields involving the oral cavity. Oral mucositis, the breakdown of the mucosal lining of the oropharynx, occurs as a result of a toxic insult to the normal epithelium of the oral mucosa. Mucositis is also defined as inflammatory lesions of the oral and/or gastrointestinal tract caused by high-dose cancer therapies. The gastrointestinal tract mucositis refers to the expression of mucosal injury across the continuum of oral and gastrointestinal mucosa, from the mouth to the anus.

Oral mucositis is a common treatment-limiting side effect of cancer therapy that may have a significant impact on quality of life, patient distress, delays in treatment administration, dose-limiting toxicity, reductions in dose intensity, interruption, or discontinuance of cancer therapy, contributing to poor treatment outcomes and significantly increasing cost to the health-care system.

Nearly all (100%) patients undergoing myeloablative therapy for stem cell or bone marrow transplantation experience oral mucositis. Traditionally, mucositis has been associated more with hematologic malignancies than with solid tumors, because the incidence of severe mucositis has been much higher with the high-dose chemotherapy regimens used in hematologic malignancies. However, mucositis also occurs in populations receiving standard-dose chemotherapy and in the treatment of other solid tumors, although these symptoms vary in intensity from those observed in hematological malignancies. It is reported that oral mucositis affects up to 80% of patients receiving radiation for head and neck malignancies.

Recent research on the etiology of mucositis indicates a multifactorial basis with a combination of treatment- and patient-related factors contributing to mucosal injury.

N.B. Kumar, *Nutritional Management of Cancer Treatment Effects*,
DOI 10.1007/978-3-642-27233-2_5, © Springer-Verlag Berlin Heidelberg 2012

Cancer treatment–related factors contributing to mucositis can include chemotherapy, radiation therapy, biologic therapy, myeloablative therapy, duration of therapy, combination therapies, fractionation radiation schedules, previous history of radiation treatment, salivary gland dysfunction, graft-versus-host disease, bone marrow status, and oral microflora.

Patient-related factors can include age, nutritional status, oral health, oral microflora, inflammation, and salivary function.

Genetic, molecular factors include cellular- and tissue-based changes, activation of NF-κB, upregulation of genes that control synthesis of inflammatory cytokines, interleukin-1, activation of enzymes that increase the rate of apoptosis, chemical insult to the mucosa, ulceration penetrating to the submucosa, loss of function and pain, cell-wall products from colonizing bacteria stimulate macrophages to release additional cytokines, and presentation of oral symptoms and functional disturbances (erythema, ulceration) and pain.

Oral mucositis is the most distressing complication of cancer therapy affecting several cancer patient populations, which is also contributing to other symptom clusters such as life-threatening systemic sepsis and other infections during periods of profound immunosuppression, dysphagia, anorexia, weight loss, depression, and pain.

5.1   Definition

With the emergence of new paradigms for cancer treatment and advances in diagnostic technology, the effectiveness of cancer treatments has increased significantly. However, these advances have also been associated to an increase in the incidence of several associated short- and long-term side effects. Oral mucositis refers to erythematous and ulcerative lesions of the oral mucosa observed in patients with cancer being treated with chemotherapy and/or with radiation therapy to fields involving the oral cavity [1]. Oral mucositis, the breakdown of the mucosal lining of the oropharynx, occurs as a result of a toxic insult to the normal epithelium of the oral mucosa [2–4]. The terms oral mucositis and stomatitis are often used interchangeably at the clinical level, but they do not reflect identical processes. Oral mucositis describes inflammation of oral mucosa resulting from chemotherapeutic agents or ionizing radiation typically manifested as erythema or ulcerations and may be exacerbated by local factors [1, 5, 6]. Stomatitis, on the other hand, refers to any inflammatory condition of oral tissue, including mucosa, dentition/periapices, and periodontium, and includes infections of oral tissues as well as mucositis. Most cancer treatment–induced mucositis are not limited only to the oral cavity and may affect several regions of the gastrointestinal tract. Mucositis is also defined as inflammatory lesions of the oral and/or gastrointestinal tract caused by high-dose cancer therapies. The gastrointestinal tract mucositis refers to the expression of mucosal injury across the continuum of oral and gastrointestinal mucosa, from the mouth to the anus [7]. Oral mucositis is a common treatment-limiting side effect of cancer therapy that may have a significant impact on quality of life, patient distress, delays in treatment administration, dose-limiting toxicity, reductions in dose intensity, interruption or discontinuance of cancer therapy contributing to poor treatment outcomes and significantly increasing cost to the health-care system [3, 4, 8]. In one study, approximately 16% of patients receiving radiation therapy for head and neck cancer were hospitalized due to mucositis. Further, 11% of the patients receiving radiation therapy for head and neck cancer had unplanned breaks in radiation therapy due to severe mucositis [9]. Oral mucositis is the most distressing complication of cancer therapy affecting several cancer patient populations, also contributing to other symptom clusters such as life-threatening systemic sepsis and other infections during periods of profound immunosuppression, dysphagia, anorexia, weight loss, depression, and pain [1, 8]. Several similarities and differences exist between radiation therapy– and chemotherapy- or combination therapy–induced mucositis, with each having specific time to occurrence and location, thus requiring targeting strategies for risk prediction, prevention, and treatment [3, 4]. Mucositis is also defined as inflammatory lesions of the oral and/or gastrointestinal tract caused by high-dose cancer therapies. The gastrointestinal tract mucositis refers to the expression of mucosal injury across the continuum of oral and gastrointestinal mucosa, from the mouth to the anus [7]. However, since the etiology and hence the treatment strategies may vary significantly, the focus of this chapter will be limited to oral mucositis. The chapter on radiation enteritis will include the management of mucositis of the other segments of the GI tract.

5.2 Prevalence

Nearly all (100%) patients undergoing myeloablative therapy for stem cell or bone marrow transplantation experience oral mucositis [10]. Others have reported that approximately 75–80% of patients who receive high-dose chemotherapy prior to hematopoietic cell transplantation develop clinically significant oral mucositis [11]. Ninety-nine percent of patients receiving hematopoietic stem cell transplant (SCT) experienced oral mucositis and 67.4% of them had a WHO oral mucositis grade of 3 or 4 [12]. Traditionally, mucositis has been associated more with hematologic malignancies than with solid tumors, because the incidence of severe mucositis has been much higher with the high-dose chemotherapy regimens used in hematologic malignancies. However, mucositis also occurs in populations receiving standard-dose chemotherapy and in the treatment of other solid tumors, although these symptoms vary in intensity from those observed in hematological malignancies [1, 8, 10]. In population studies of prevalence, 51% receiving chemotherapy for solid tumors or lymphoma developed oral and/or GI mucositis [13]. For all tumor sites, chemotherapy with 5-fluorouracil (5-FU), capecitabine, or tegafur leads to a high rate (e.g., 20–50%) of alimentary tract mucositis. Recently, chemotherapy with methotrexate and other antimetabolites leads to a 20–60% rate of alimentary tract mucositis according to the drug's given dose per cycle [7]. Irinotecan is associated with severe

GI mucositis in over 20% of patients. On the other hand, in patients receiving radiation therapy for head and neck cancer will develop some degree of oral mucositis. It is reported that oral mucositis affects up to 80% of patients receiving radiation for head and neck malignancies [14] and approximately 40% of patients undergoing chemotherapy [15]. Severe oral mucositis occurred in 29–66% of all patients receiving radiation therapy for head and neck cancer [13, 16]. The common symptoms are erythema, burning sensation, increased sensitivity to hot and spicy foods, and white patches on mucus membranes of the cheeks, lips, tongue, and palette followed by ulcers leading to poor or inability to consume foods orally [17]. Mucositis is self-limited when uncomplicated by infection and typically heals within 2–4 weeks after cessation of cytotoxic chemotherapy.

5.3   Etiology

5.3.1   Patient- and Treatment-Related Etiology of Mucositis

Recent research on the etiology of mucositis indicates a multifactorial basis with a combination of treatment- and patient-related factors contributing to mucosal injury. Cytotoxic treatments, radiation therapy, biological therapies, and combination therapies have been implicated in the etiology of mucositis and severity of this symptom. The cytotoxic drugs most frequently associated with stomatotoxic toxicity include bleomycin, cytarabine, doxorubicin, etoposide, 5-fluorouracil, ifosfamide, mercaptopurine, methotrexate, paclitaxel, vinblastine, vincristine, and vinorelbine [18–20]. Additionally, high-dose methotrexate, etoposide, and melphalan are implicated in the most severe forms of mucositis [21, 22]. Additionally, several biologic products impact the severity and extent of mucositis, including epidermal growth factor, tumor necrosis factor-α, and cytokines such as granulocyte macrophage colony-stimulating factor and interleukin-1 [23]. Hyperfractionated radiation therapy has been demonstrated to produce the most severe forms of mucositis [22, 24]. Erythematous mucositis typically appears 7–10 days after initiation of high-dose cancer therapy and has the potential for increased toxicity with escalating dose or treatment duration. The incidence of oral mucositis was especially high in patients with primary tumors in the oral cavity, oropharynx or nasopharynx, those who also received concomitant chemotherapy, those who received a total dose over 5,000 cGy, and those who were treated with altered fractionation radiation schedules (e.g., more than one radiation treatment per day) [1]. Other factors include previous history of radiation treatment, salivary gland dysfunction, microbial flora, and graft-versus-host disease [5]. The combination of treatment-related effects and cytokines leads to mucosal atrophy, collagen breakdown, and eventual ulceration of the mucosa. Radiation and chemotherapy also alter normal oral microbial flora and salivary quantity and composition [25]. Although several treatment regimens have been shown to cause mucositis, there is still a great deal of patient variation in the severity of mucositis, even among patients

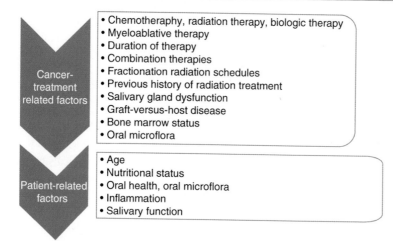

Fig. 5.1 Etiology of mucositis

receiving identical treatment regimens. Although it is not clear to what extent patient factors correlate with mucositis prevalence, several patient-related factors are identified in the literature. More recently, drugs such as bevacizumab have been implicated to decrease the VEGF levels in saliva and delay wound healing in oral mucositis [26]. Patient's age, nutritional status, oral health, oral microflora, inflammation, and salivary function [27] are other factors contributing to the severity of symptoms (Fig. 5.1).

5.3.2   Biologic Development of Mucositis

More recently, a molecular-based etiology of mucositis has evolved in which mucositis involves a complex series of molecular, cellular, and tissue-based changes with a certain degree of genetic involvement [28–31]. The development and progression of the various phases of mucositis are interdependent and mediated by the action of cytokines, chemotherapy, oral bacterial flora, and bone marrow status [6]. The biological development of mucositis is characterized in part by upregulation of NF-κB, inflammatory cytokines (e.g., tumor necrosis factor-α), and interleukin-1 in addition to epithelial basal cell injury. During the initial phase, free radicals break DNA strands and cause a small proportion of cells to die quickly. Tissue injury from activation of numerous biologic control mechanisms characterizes the second and third phases. Transcription factors such as NF-κB are activated and upregulate the genes that control synthesis of cytokines. Both chemotherapy and radiation treatment activate enzymes that increase the rate of apoptosis, which further adds to the chemical insults to the mucosa. Ulceration penetrating through the epithelium into the submucosa occurs in the fourth phase and creates the loss of function and pain that are cardinal symptoms of mucositis. Also in this phase, cell-wall products from colonizing bacteria stimulate macrophages to release additional cytokines [6]. With the varying baseline genetic and physical condition, cancer and stage of diagnosis, treatments, and other comorbidities, the complexity and severity of the process varies significantly, thus establishing the need for the development and implementation of personalized therapies for the treatment of this complex symptom.

5.4   Current Therapies for Mucositis

5.4.1   Assessment and Early Identification of Oral Mucositis

Assessment and treatment of mucositis should be performed and implemented using a multiprofessional approach to clinical care, research, and education associated with mucosal injury in cancer patients. Oral management has been observed to be critical in this patient population [32]. In a study comparing planned oral management on the severity of oral mucositis during hematopoietic SCT, Yamagata et al. [33] reported a significant oral mucositis score in those subjects receiving oral management and care from a dentist compared to the control group. Their study showed that oral management may decrease the occurrence or oral mucositis in this population and that it was important to include an oral management provider such as a dentist, dental hygienist in this setting, in addition to oncology teams. A long experience of observation of the trajectory of cancer treatment–induced mucositis and a comprehensive knowledge of the molecular-based causation of the lesion have contributed to the development of early screening, identification, and treatment to ameliorate the symptoms of mucositis. For example, erythematous mucositis typically appears 7–10 days after initiation of high-dose cancer therapy. It is also anticipated that there is a significant potential for mucosal toxicity with escalating dose or treatment duration in clinical trials that demonstrate gastrointestinal mucosal toxicity. Similarly, high-dose chemotherapy, such as that used in the treatment of leukemia and hematopoietic stem cell transplant regimens, may produce severe mucositis. Thus, proactive, systematic assessment and early identification of lesions [34–36] for specific treatments should be part of standard of care. Since there is no single intervention that completely prevents or treats all symptoms associated with mucositis, combined strategies seem to be required to ensure more successful outcomes. Additionally, screening and education for fastidious oral hygiene, pain management, nutritional care, and other supportive care measures are important to minimize the severity of the lesion.

The basic goals of this screening are to obtain a collective measurement of oral symptoms, signs, and functional disturbances. Accurate pretreatment assessment, fastidious oral cavity hygiene, and frequent review of symptoms during treatment [37] have been observed to be critical. A variety of assessment scales exist in an effort to standardize measurements of mucosal integrity and for the measurement of oral mucositis, allowing for grading of the level of stomatitis by characterizing alterations in lips, tongue, mucous membranes, gingiva, teeth, pharynx, quality of saliva, and voice [7, 34–36]. On the other hand, there are only a limited number of instruments for indirect measurements of gastrointestinal mucositis. Excellent examples of these instruments are the measures of indirect outcomes of mucosal injury, including diarrhea due to radiation enteritis. Oral diagnosis of mucositis is based on the symptoms the patient is experiencing and the appearance of the tissues of the mouth following treatment. Red burn-like sores or ulcers throughout the mouth accompanied by pain are enough to diagnose mucositis. Several instruments are available to gauge severity of oral mucositis. The most commonly used are the World Health Organization (WHO) Oral Toxicity score [30] and the National Cancer Institute Common Toxicity Criteria (NCI-CTC) for Oral Mucositis [31]. While the NCI system has separate scores for appearance (erythema and ulceration) and function (pain and ability to eat solids, liquids, or nothing by mouth), the WHO score combines both elements into a single score that grades the severity of the condition from 0 (no oral mucositis) to 4 (swallowing not possible such that patient needs supplementary nutrition). One of the earliest instruments developed was the Oral Mucositis Assessment Scale (OMAS) which provides an objective assessment of oral mucositis based on assessment of the appearance and extent of redness and ulceration in various areas of the mouth [38]. This scale has demonstrated high reproducibility between observers, responsive over time, and accurate in recording symptoms associated with mucositis and continues to be used in clinical settings.

5.4.2   Treatment Approaches with Immunomodulators, Amino Acids, and Vitamins

Several amino acid, vitamins, and immunomodulating formulations that have been demonstrated to protect normal tissue from an array of oxidative insults have been examined for the treatment of oral mucositis. In a previous report of a summary of evidence on effectiveness of treatment strategies for oral mucositis, the Mucositis Study Group of the Multinational Association of Supportive Care in Cancer/International Society for Oral Oncology recommended the use of recombinant human keratinocyte growth factor-1 (palifermin) to prevent oral mucositis in patients receiving high-dose CT and total body irradiation followed by stem cell transplantation for hematological malignancies. This group also suggests that granulocyte macrophage colony-stimulating factor mouthwash not be used for the prevention of oral mucositis in the transplant setting with high-dose CT and autologous or allogeneic stem cell transplantation [39]. Use of traditional mouthwashes to obtain mechanical cleaning of the oral cavity and administration of some agents like benzydamine, imidazole antibiotics, tryazolic antimycotics, povidone iodine, keratinocyte growth factor, and vitamin E seem to reduce the intensity of mucositis [37]. The evidence of efficacy of oral supplemental glutamine outside of research protocols has not been established [40]. In early studies evaluating the dextro-isomer of the common amino acid L-methionine, D-methionine (D-met)'s capacity to selectively prevent radiation-induced oral mucositis using in vitro cell culture models, as well as an in vivo model of radiation injury to the oral mucosa in C3H mice, [41] demonstrated that D-met protected normal tissues, but not tumor cells, in culture from radiation-induced cell death; it also protected normal cells from radiation-induced mucosal injury in a murine model but did not alter tumor response to therapy. More recently, antrum mucosal protein (AMP)-18 and a synthetic peptide surrogate, which exhibit cell protective and mitogenic properties in vitro and in vivo models of gastrointestinal epithelial cell injury has been examined for the management of oral mucositis. It has been hypothesized that the mucosal barrier–protective effects may be mediated by AMP-18's capacity to increase accumulation of specific tight junction (TJ) and adherens junction proteins, and also protect against their loss after injury [42, 43]. Results demonstrated that AMP peptide prevented radiation-induced oral mucositis in a murine model, and thus the importance of epithelial junctional integrity in the pathogenesis of OM demonstrates that AMP-18, by targeting TJ proteins through the activation of cholecystokinin-B/gastrin receptor (CCKBR), could provide a novel strategy for the prevention and treatment of oral mucositis. More recently, platelet-derived growth factors (PDGFs) have been shown to have a high capability for tissue healing and may play a role in repairing the mucosal barrier. In an attempt to develop a mucoadhesive formulation to administer platelet lysate to oral cavity prolonging contact time of platelet lysate with oral mucosa, Del Fante et al. demonstrated that in both in vitro and early preliminary clinical trials, GVPL has optimal mucoadhesive and healing enhancer properties maintained over time (up to 14 days); preliminary clinical results also suggest that oral application of platelet lysate–loaded mucoadhesive formulation is feasible, safe, well tolerated, and effective, although larger controlled randomized study is needed [44]. A novel immunomodulating peptide (SCV-07) in attenuating the course of radiation-induced mucositis in an established animal model of oral mucositis showed [45] that SCV-07 reduced the severity and duration of both acute and fractionated radiation–induced OM. Similarly, when radiation and chemotherapy were used to induce oral mucositis, treatment with SCV-07 significantly reduced the duration of ulcerative oral mucositis. Other interventions with sucralfate were effective in reducing the severity of mucositis [40]. In an effort to reduce toxicities [46] with pralatrexate, vitamin supplementation with folic acid and vitamin B12 supplementation have been administered to patients with previously treated NSCLC. However, mucositis continued to be a dose-limiting toxicity of pralatrexate, and this study failed to demonstrate that vitamin supplementation prevents mucositis. Interventions with aloe vera, amifostine, intravenous glutamine, granulocyte macrophage-colony stimulating factor, honey, laser, and antibiotic lozenges containing polymyxin/tobramycin/amphotericin (PTA) showed weaker evidence of benefit [40].

5.4.3 Physical Approaches for the Prevention and Treatment of Oral Mucositis

Additionally, physical approaches like cryotherapy and low-energy helium-neon laser or the use of modern radiotherapy techniques with the exclusion of the oral cavity from radiation fields have been shown to be efficacious in preventing mucositis onset [37]. Cryotherapy (ice chips) [47, 48] has consistently shown some benefit in preventing mucositis in early phase I–II clinical trials [2, 49]. However, cryotherapy during MTX administration does not reduce severe oral mucositis in patients undergoing myeloablative allogeneic HSCT [50]. Simões et al. [51] examined varying doses of LPT protocols for management of oral mucositis and observed that all protocols of LPT led to the maintenance of oral mucositis scores in the same levels until the last RT session. Moreover, LPT three times a week also maintained the pain levels. However, the patients submitted to once-a-week LPT had significant pain increase, and the association of low/high LPT led to increased healing time. In a more recent study, Simões et al. [51, 52] demonstrated that laser phototherapy (LPT) used for oral mucositis could influence xerostomia symptoms and hyposalivation of patients undergoing RT and can be beneficial as an auxiliary therapy for hypofunction of salivary glands. Mouthwashes with allopurinol and phototherapy with low-energy laser can be used as treatment. Ruiz-Esquide [53] summarized that local cryotherapy with ice chips and phototherapy with low-energy laser may be useful as preventive measures. However, in addition to these physical approaches, radiotherapy and special radiation administration techniques should contribute to minimizing mucosal injury.

5.4.4 Treatment Approaches of Related Symptom Clusters to Oral Mucositis

Worthington also reviewed treatments for candidiasis in patients with cancer receiving radiation or chemotherapy and observed some benefit of antifungal drugs, especially when absorbed in the gastrointestinal tract. However, these reviews concluded that larger, well-designed clinical trials were needed to claim or refute this efficacy [40]. Similarly, patient-controlled analgesia failed to demonstrate any difference in pain control compared to continuous infusion method [54]. However, fewer opiates were used by patients during self-administration. Pain control should always be optimized with the use of patient-controlled analgesia and topical use of morphine Ruiz-Esquide [53]. Others have explored the use of mouthwash to reduce severity and further infections with oral mucositis, combining several combinations, such as salt and soda, chlorhexidine, and "magic" mouthwash (lidocaine, Benadryl, and Maalox) and others, [18] and observed cessation of the signs and symptoms of mucositis within 12 days. No significant differences in time for the cessation of the signs and symptoms were observed among the three groups. Similar mixtures of mouthwashes including specific combinations, primarily to control pain transiently while feeding orally, have been tested by nutritionists and nursing personnel caring for this patient population, showing some benefit with symptom management. Yen et al. observed that phenylbutyrate mouthwash significantly mitigates oral mucositis during chemoradiotherapy or radiotherapy in patients with head and neck cancers [55]. There is also weak evidence that allopurinol mouthwash compared to placebo can reduce severity of oral mucositis [54]. In a systematic review of [56] chlorhexidine mouthwash for preventing chemotherapy-induced oral mucositis, results failed to detect any beneficial effects of chlorhexidine as compared with sterile water or NaCl 0.9%. Additionally, patients complained about negative side effects of chlorhexidine, including teeth discoloration and alteration of taste, in two of the five studies on chlorhexidine. However, in a more recent review, it was observed that chlorhexidine may play a part in reducing oral mucosal damage during chemotherapy for children with cancer, possibly due to a reduction in oral microflora and plaque [57]. In conclusion, the results of the present study suggest that the prophylactic use of 0.12% chlorhexidine gluconate also reduced the frequency of oral mucositis and oral pathogens in children with ALL [58].

5.5 Guidelines for Assessment and Treatment of Oral Mucositis

Aggressive cancer therapy places patients at greater risk for oral mucositis and resulting treatment-related complications. Prevention and/or treatment of such oral sequelae has often been overlooked as a priority of the treatment team. There are no single standard therapies that have been proven to be effective in the prevention and management of oral mucositis, and they vary considerably among institutions. Since it is clear that several similarities and differences exist between radiation therapy– and chemotherapy- or combination therapy–induced mucositis, with each having specific time to occurrence and location, there is a need for targeting management strategies for risk prediction, prevention, and treatment. From the vast body of literature, it is clear that the basic principles of treatments that have been evaluated for the prevention and management of oral mucositis have been to screen proactively and predict/detect lesions early and reduce tumor-related factors, taking into consideration common patient-related factors while targeting the biological basis of the manifestation of the symptoms. Change in treatment technologies such as radiotherapy techniques with the exclusion of the oral cavity from radiation fields has been evaluated in addition to targeting other symptom clusters that occur along with oral mucositis such as pain and infections. Treatment regimens have thus included early identification and prediction, several chemical as well as physical strategies, and combination approaches for the prevention and treatment of oral mucositis. The following guidelines are thus best practice standards based on the current research literature.

5.5.1   Assessment of Mucositis

It is predictable that certain patient populations are more vulnerable than others for the development of oral mucositis. The timeline from start of treatment to appearance of early oral lesions are also predictable with certain cancer treatment, Erythematous mucositis typically appears 7–10 days after initiation of high-dose cancer therapy. It is also anticipated that there is a significant potential for mucosal toxicity with escalating dose or treatment duration in clinical trials that demonstrate gastrointestinal mucosal toxicity. Similarly, high-dose chemotherapy, such as that used in the treatment of leukemia and hematopoietic stem cell transplant regimens, may produce severe mucositis. These patients must be considered high risk, and thus a proactive mucositis assessment must be incorporated as standard of care. Cancer patients who are to receive chemotherapy, radiation, immunotherapy, combination radiochemotherapies, or bone marrow transplantation must be screened thoroughly for all oral symptoms and nutritional status by a multidisciplinary team including a dentist. The basic goals of this screening are to obtain a collective measurement of oral symptoms, signs, and functional disturbances.

Several mucositis evaluation scales are available. These include the National Cancer Institute Common Toxicity Criteria (NCI-CTC) for Oral Mucositis, WHO scale, and the Oral Mucositis Assessment Scale (OMAS). While the NCI system has separate scores for appearance (erythema and ulceration) and function (pain and ability to eat solids, liquids, or nothing by mouth), the WHO score combines both elements into a single score that grades the severity of the condition from 0 (no oral mucositis) to 4 (swallowing not possible such that patient needs supplementary nutrition). One of the earliest instruments developed was the Oral Mucositis Assessment Scale (OMAS) which provides an objective assessment of oral mucositis based on assessment of the appearance and extent of redness and ulceration in various areas of the mouth. This scale has demonstrated high reproducibility between observers, responsive over time, and accurate in recording symptoms associated with mucositis and continues to be used in clinical settings.

Based on initial screening and course of treatment, frequent review of symptoms during treatment should be planned. Patients at high risk must receive education for fastidious oral hygiene, pain management, and nutritional alterations to minimize the severity of the lesion.

5.5.2 Dental Care Guidelines

A referral to the dentist prior to start of care may help manage oral mucositis in most patients. Since oral management is critical for this patient, any oral infections and oral hygiene issues must be resolved prior to start of treatment by an oral management provider such as a dentist or dental hygienist in this setting. Referral to a dentist must include details regarding current diagnosis, plan of treatment, start date of treatment, limitations of use of medications including antibiotics, and other specific information that will assist the dentist to if teeth are ill fitting; patients should be referred to the dentist to ensure proper fitting. Additionally, assure that if dentures or other prosthesis for teeth are used, such as partials; patients have these always available and use them.

- Fastidious mouth care must be followed to prevent any infections or decay.
- Any scaling, cleaning, tooth extraction, or repair of cavities should be done before cancer therapy begins.
- Extractions should be completed at least 2 weeks before therapy to give the area of trauma a chance to heal; ill-fitting dentures should be adjusted or replaced; any periodontal or dental work needs to be coordinated with the oncologist.
- Benadryl elixir, lozenges, and analgesics may help reduce mouth pain.
- Swishing with one teaspoon of viscous Xylocaine (hold in the mouth for 1 min and then spit out) before meals. Patients should be cautioned about accidentally biting inside of cheeks due to oral numbness.
- Frequent use of gentle mouthwash may help reduce the discomfort or pain. A solution of one teaspoon baking soda and salt dissolved in warm water should be used instead of commercial mouthwashes, which may be irritating to the oral mucosa.
- Patients should be instructed to avoid hydrogen peroxide.
- Patients need to use a soft bristle toothbrush and soften it by soaking first in warm water prior to brushing.
- Damage to the mucosa can facilitate some infections, such as candida or herpes simplex. Patients should be instructed to examine their mouth daily for irritation or white spots.
- If brushing the teeth is painful, cotton swabs or Toothettes, a sponge-tipped stick impregnated with dentifrice, may be used. Lemon glycerine swabs may make the mouth feel clean, but the glycerine can dehydrate and dry the mouth.
- Using a gentle Waterpik to cleanse the mouth may be helpful but must be used with caution since the pressure of the waterjet may irritate oral tissues.
- Brushing the teeth with a paste of baking soda and water may be less irritating than using a commercial toothpaste.
- Biotene toothpaste® has been found to be less irritating to the oral mucosa.

5.5.3 Pharmacotherapy

- Although several amino acids and immunomodulators have shown promise in vitro and in animal models, there is only weak evidence of benefit at this time. Well-powered clinical trials are needed to confirm safety and efficacy for the management of cancer treatment–related oral mucositis [40].

- Cryotherapy (ice chips) [47, 48] has consistently shown some benefit in preventing mucositis in early phase I–II clinical trials. However, cryotherapy during MTX administration does not reduce severe oral mucositis in patients undergoing myeloablative allogeneic HSCT.
- Laser phototherapy (LPT) used for oral mucositis could influence xerostomia symptoms and hyposalivation of patients undergoing radiation therapy and can be beneficial as an auxiliary therapy for hypofunction of salivary glands. Laser phototherapy led to the maintenance of oral mucositis scores in the same levels until the last RT session. Moreover, LPT three times a week also maintained the pain levels. However, the patients submitted to once-a-week LPT had significant pain increase, and the association of low/high LPT led to increased healing time.
- Since oral mucositis can be complicated with fungal infections, specifically candidiasis in patients with cancer receiving radiation or chemotherapy, use of antifungal drugs that can be absorbed in the gastrointestinal tract has been found to beneficial in reduce complications.
- Since pain is a common symptom cluster occurring with oral mucositis, patient-controlled analgesia or continuous infusion method with opiates has demonstrated relief and must be evaluated and considered for pain management.
- Recombinant human keratinocyte growth factor-1 (palifermin) to prevent oral mucositis in patients receiving high-dose CT and total body irradiation followed by stem cell transplantation for hematological malignancies is now recommended.
- Use of traditional mouthwashes to obtain mechanical cleaning of the oral cavity and administration of some agents like benzydamine, imidazole antibiotics, tryazolic antimycotics, povidone iodine, keratinocyte growth factor, and vitamin E seem to reduce the intensity of mucositis. Other interventions with sucralfate were effective in reducing the severity of mucositis. Use of mouthwash has been shown to reduce severity and further infections with oral mucositis. Several combinations such as salt and soda, chlorhexidine, and "magic" mouthwash (lidocaine, Benadryl, and Maalox) and others have produced cessation of the signs and symptoms of mucositis within 12 days. Phenylbutyrate and allopurinol mouthwash significantly mitigates oral mucositis during chemoradiotherapy or radiotherapy in patients with head and neck cancers.

5.5.4 Nutrition Guidelines

Nutritional assessment must be performed within 24 h of admission of the patient by a registered dietitian/nutritionist.

1. Screen patient within 24 h of admission. This order for screening has been a standard order for all cancer patient admissions to avoid delay in timing of screening.
2. Assess all symptoms: Gastrointestinal tract: taste alterations, smell alterations, dysphagia, dyspnea, other pain, early satiety, dry mouth, too much

saliva production, anorexia, diarrhea, constipation, nausea, vomiting, dehydration, and fatigue; anthropometrics: height, weight, recent weight loss, grip strength, and others (mid arm muscle circumference, body composition [DEXA]); psychosocial: family/caregiver support, depression, and ADL.

3. Assess current nutritional status and estimate caloric, protein, and multivitamin/mineral needs.

4. Provide adequate nutrition by including "calorie" and "protein" booster education material and nutritional supplements to ensure intake of proteins (recommended 0.8–1.0 g/kg/day). Provide dense caloric supplements up to 400 cal/day containing 1.5 kcal/mL; if intake is insufficient in proteins, supplement with modular protein supplements, adding this to favorite beverage (http://www.nestle-nutrition.com/Products/Default.aspx; http://abbottnutrition.com/). The choice of nutritional supplements can be based in the personal choice of the patient, patient needs, tolerance to product as well as other comorbidities.

5. Include a standard multivitamin mineral supplementation to prevent any further deficits and meet increased needs.

6. Assess adequacy of intake and provide an appetite stimulant (megestrol acetate 320–800 mg/day or alternate) if patient has cancer anorexia to ensure adequate intake and prevent further weight loss.

7. Provide each patient with nutritional guidelines to ensure adequate intake of calories and proteins and a list of suggested high-caloric and high-protein nutritional supplements to choose from, taking into consideration taste alterations, early satiety, nausea, and vomiting that are common symptoms observed in this patient population.

8. Proactive measures to provide alternate mode of nutritional support must be planned during acute phase of treatment when it would be a greater risk to feed patient via the oral route.

9. Selection of route of feeding may be informed based on general guidelines and criteria provided in Table 2.6.

10. Other specific guidelines for patients with mucositis:
    • Provide soft bland foods, such as creamed soups, cooked cereals, macaroni and cheese, yogurt, pudding, mashed potatoes, eggs, custard, casseroles, cheesecake, and milk shakes.
    • Add high-calorie, high-protein supplements if intake in inadequate. High-protein diet, such as pudding pops or frozen modular protein-calorie supplements, may be well tolerated.
    • Patients may tolerate cold foods better as they may act as a local oral anesthetic.
    • Few studies have demonstrated that around-the-clock or periodic administration of oral glutamine may decrease both the severity and duration of mucositis. The patient can be advised to swish and swallow this mixture. If renal or hepatic function is impaired, this amino acid supplement may be contraindicated.
    • Blend and moisten foods with gravy, butter, cream, or sauces.
    • Soften foods, such as bread, by soaking in milk.

- To bypass mouth sores, a straw can be used.
- The following foods may be avoided:
  - Tart, acidic foods and juices such as tomatoes, grapefruit, lemons, and oranges, and pickles, which can burn the mouth.
  - Salty foods, which can burn sensation.
  - Hot, spicy, coarse, or rough foods, including toast, dry crackers, and potato chips.
  - Alcoholic beverages and tobacco, which irritate the lining of the mouth.
  - Any medication that contains alcohol, such as mouthwashes or cough syrups.
  - Patients using anesthetic jelly must be cautioned to be especially careful consuming the above foods, as they may not feel any irritation and could injure the mucosa.

5.5.5 Physical Activity

Since fatigue and poor nutritional status are classic symptoms of CC, patients should proactively receive a comprehensive assessment of physical status by a licensed physical therapist and therapy initiated within 24 h of assessment.
1. *Godin Leisure-Time Exercise Questionnaire* weekly to monitor physical activity.
2. *Handgrip strength dynamometry assessment*: A validated tool commonly used to assess handgrip strength is the Jamar dynamometer, which is a fast, reliable, and easy-to-perform device commonly used by our team to measure improvements in functional strength. The Jamar dynamometer has a lower percentage coefficient of variation and is thus a more precise device than other handgrip dynamometers.

5.5.6 Markers and Instruments for Patient Monitoring and Assessment of Response to Treatment by the Interdisciplinary Medical Team

1. *Anthropometric measurements* such as participant's height, weight, and body mass index can be performed at admission and at regular intervals established by the medical team. Skeletal muscle function is a central determinant of functional capacity in humans. Loss of muscle as seen in CC results in poor function and decreased survival rate following critical illness. Muscle size is therefore considered an important marker of functional status in studies of sarcopenia/cachexia.
2. *Body composition by DXA scan*: DXA should be used to assess both total lean body mass (LBM), fat mass (FM), and total bone mineral density (BMD).Total bone mineral density (BMD) is a valid indirect measure of skeletal muscle and patient activity. Total LBM is sometimes called total fat-free mass (FFM), depending upon specific DXA manufacturer. DXA instruments use an x-ray source that generates or is split into two energies to measure bone mineral mass and soft tissue from which fat and fat-free mass are estimated. The exam is quick

(1–2 min), precise (0.5–1%), and noninvasive. DXA scanners have the precision required to detect changes in muscle mass as small as 5%. Radiation exposure from DXA scans is minimal. The National Council of Radiation Protection and Measurements (NCRP) has recommended that the annual effective dose limit for infrequent exposure of the general population is 5,000 µSv and that an annual effective dose of 10 µSv be considered a negligible individual dose. The effective dose of a dual-energy x-ray absorptiometry whole body scan on an adult is 2.1 µSv. Studies have shown that quality assurance is an important issue in the use of DXA scans to determine body composition including lean body mass and bone mineral density. DXA instrument manufacturer and model should remain consistent and their calibration should be monitored throughout treatment. Use of a standardized scan acquisition protocol and appropriate and unchanging scan acquisition and analysis software is essential to achieve consist results.

3. *Dietary intake* must be assessed at baseline and at regularly scheduled intervals by conducting random weekly, 2 weekdays + 1 weekend day, 24-h dietary recalls (gold standard for collecting dietary data) using a 5-step multipass procedure [33, 34] (which has been found to assess mean energy intake within 10% of actual intake) and using the frequently updated University of Minnesota Nutrition Data System for Research (NDSR) version database for analysis of nutrient composition. Food portion visuals can be provided to patients to estimate portion sizes of foods while monitoring intake.

4. *Symptom log* may be completed daily and collected from patients on a monthly basis. Based on these symptoms, all anticipated and unanticipated grades of constitutional, dermatological, gastrointestinal (GI), metabolic, and pain symptoms can be continuously monitored including those symptoms affecting nutritional intake and utilization.

5. *Monthly* CMP and CBC should be monitored to assess electrolytes and organ function.

6. *Functional markers (Karnofsky performance score)*: Evaluation of patients' functional status and barriers to obtaining adequate nutrients is also necessary. A physical exam combined with personal interview should include the evaluation of functional status such as the ability to chew and swallow, dental or oral problems causing odynophagia or dysphagia, signs of muscle wasting or anasarca, presence of edema, presence of skin or mouth lesion, and ability to perform instrumental activities of daily living (IADLs) such as cooking, shopping, and self-feeding. It is critical to assess activities of daily living, physical activity, exercise, sleep, and ability to work and perform other functional roles. Limitations in the activities of daily living have been identified secondary to and as a cause of weight loss in cancer patients. Cancer and other chronic diseases pose difficulties specifically for the cancer patient receiving treatment and the elderly in carrying out activities of daily living. A loss of postural and locomotive muscle mass has been observed within 7 days of inactivity. The Karnofsky Performance Scale Index allows patients to be classified as to their functional impairment. This has been used to compare effectiveness of different therapies and to assess the prognosis in individual patients and has been validated in cancer patient

populations. Karnofsky Performance Scale Index allows patients to be classified as to their functional impairment. This has been used to compare effectiveness of different therapies and to assess the prognosis in individual patients and has been validated in cancer patient populations.

7. *Biochemical markers of protein status (serum albumin and transferrin)*: Assessment of protein status is critical in the identification and treatment of abnormalities in protein metabolism. There is substantial evidence of the correlation between serum hepatic proteins and inflammation, making these the most relevant biomarkers in cancer patient populations. Serum transferrin, prealbumin, and albumin have been observed as intermediate endpoint biomarkers and independently associated with clinical outcomes. Measurements of body composition combined with more objective and sensitive measure of protein nutriture are ideal for the biochemical assessment of intravascular and visceral protein stores. We have thus included the three major valid intermediate endpoint biomarkers (IEBs) that represent intravascular and visceral protein pools–transferrin, prealbumin, and albumin–as the biochemical indicators of protein status. Although transferrin levels are affected by iron status, serum transferrin, either singly or as part of a multiparameter index, is the strongest predictor of cancer patient morbidity and mortality.

8. *Immune and inflammatory markers*: A range of metabolic responses triggered by inflammatory and immunological responses in cancer patients. Cytokines can be measured in a panel including IL-1, IL-4, IL-6, IL-8, IL-10, GM-CSF, IFN-κ, TNF-α, and CRP (Bio-Rad–Bio-Plex). All of these biomarkers have been shown to increase with disease, aging, and cytotoxic agents. Though we realize these intermediate endpoint biomarkers of cytokines cannot be reliably interpreted, as over 70% of the subjects as observed in our studies were on active treatment with cytotoxic agents, these variables are important to determine, as they may provide useful information and contribute to the better understanding of the mechanistic process.

9. *Quality of life* should be measured at baseline and monthly using the Rand Short Form (SF)-36 (Medical Outcomes Study SF36). The SF-36 has been used extensively with general, high-risk, and cancer populations and has available norms for mail and telephone versions and comparisons between group and individual scores. Scores are calculated and transformed to a 0–100 scale, with higher scores indicating increased health status. Reliability of the SF-36 scales was measured by Cronbach α coefficient, and the results ranged from 0.78 in general health perceptions to 0.91 in the physical functioning domain.

5.5.7   Follow-up

Patients must be seen by the multidisciplinary team on a monthly basis to monitor progress and to review compliance to intervention including diet intake adequacy, symptom logs, change in concomitant medications, and any other issues related to treatment. Improved management of malnutrition with nutritional therapy may require a multimodal intervention by multidisciplinary teams using a comprehensive and integrated approach. Initial screening and knowledge of treatment trajectory of the cancer patient should guide a plan for reassessment at regularly planned intervals. Subjective and objective data on progress and response to nutritional therapy may be assessed using the indicators used in the comprehensive nutritional assessment. Newly developed symptoms resulting from treatment or progression of disease may require additional monitoring or revision of nutritional therapy. Reassessment/reevaluation for monitoring and evaluation of nutritional therapy must include monitoring of clinical, functional, dietary, and behavioral outcomes that were identified by the comprehensive nutritional assessment.

5.6   Future Directions

As novel cytotoxic, radiation, immunotherapy, and combination therapies evolve, there is a continued need for research evaluating strategies for preventing or mitigating the symptoms related to oral mucositis. The evidence of efficacy of current treatment regimens needs further validation in well-powered clinical trials, targeted to and specific to cancers and treatment regimens. In spite of focused interventions, responders and nonresponders to treatment present a greater challenge. Future studies using personalized medicine approaches for the treatment of mucositis with the identification of specific gene clusters to discriminate these groups will be valuable [59].

> **Summary for the Clinician**
> Aggressive cancer therapy places patients at greater risk for oral mucositis and resulting sequelae of complications and treatment-related consequences. There are no single standard therapies that have been proven to be effective in the prevention and management of oral mucositis, and they vary considerably among institutions.
>
> Assessment and treatment of mucositis should be performed and implemented using a multiprofessional approach to clinical care, research, and education associated with mucosal injury in cancer patients, including oral management with dental professionals.
>
> Proactive and systematic screening, assessment, and early identification of oral lesions for specific treatments should be part of standard of care. The basic goal of this screening is to obtain a collective measurement of oral symptoms, signs, and functional disturbances.
>
> It is predictable that certain patient populations are more vulnerable than others for the development of oral mucositis. These patients must be considered high risk, and thus, a proactive mucositis assessment must be incorporated as standard of care.
>
> Patients at high risk must receive education for fastidious oral hygiene, pain management, and nutrition to minimize the severity of the lesion.

Several mucositis evaluation scales are available. These include the National Cancer Institute Common Toxicity Criteria (NCI-CTC) for Oral Mucositis, WHO scale, and the Oral Mucositis Assessment Scale (OMAS).

Current treatment strategies can include the use of recombinant human keratinocyte growth factor-1 (palifermin), mouthwashes to include phenylbutyrate, allopurinol and other antibacterial and antifungal medications, as well as lidocaine, to prevent and manage oral mucositis.

Cryotherapy (ice chips) has consistently shown some benefit in preventing mucositis in early phase I–II clinical trials. However, cryotherapy during MTX administration does not reduce severe oral mucositis in patients undergoing myeloablative allogeneic HSCT.

Laser phototherapy (LPT) used for oral mucositis could influence xerostomia symptoms and hyposalivation of patients undergoing radiation therapy and can be beneficial as an auxiliary therapy for hypofunction of salivary glands.

Most institutions use a combination of these therapies to prevent and manage cancer patients with oral mucositis.

As novel cytotoxic, radiation, immunotherapy, and combination therapies evolve, there is a continued need for research evaluating strategies for preventing or mitigating the symptoms related to oral mucositis.

The evidence of efficacy of current treatment regimens need further validation in well-powered clinical trials, targeted to and specific to cancers and treatment regimens. In spite of focused interventions, responders and nonresponders to treatment present a greater challenge. Future studies using personalized medicine approaches for the treatment of mucositis with the identification of specific gene clusters to discriminate these groups will be valuable.

References

1. Lalla RV, Brennan MT, Schubert MM (2011) Oral complications of cancer therapy. In: Yagiela JA, Dowd FJ, Johnson BS et al (eds) Pharmacology and therapeutics for dentistry, 6th edn. St. Louis, Mosby Elsevier, pp 782–798
2. Beaven AW, Shea TC (2007) Recombinant human keratinocyte growth factor palifermin reduces oral mucositis and improves patient outcomes after stem cell transplant. Drugs Today (Barc) 43(7):461–473
3. Keefe DM, Peterson DE, Schubert MM (2006) Developing evidence-based guidelines for management of alimentary mucositis: process and pitfalls. Support Care Cancer 14(6):492–498, Epub 2006 Apr 7
4. Keefe DM (2006) Mucositis management in patients with cancer. Support Cancer Ther 3(3):154–157
5. Sonis ST (1998) Mucositis as a biological process: a new hypothesis for the development of chemotherapy-induced stomatotoxicity. Oral Oncol 34(1):39–43 [PUBMED Abstract]
6. Sonis ST, Elting LS, Keefe D et al (2004) Perspectives on cancer therapy-induced mucosal injury: pathogenesis, measurement, epidemiology, and consequences for patients. Cancer 100(9 Suppl):1995–2025 [PUBMED Abstract]

7. Peterson DE, Bensadoun RJ, Lalla RV, McGuire DB (2011) Supportive care treatment guidelines: value, limitations, and opportunities. Semin Oncol 38(3):367–373
8. Epstein JB, Klasser GD (2006) Emerging approaches for prophylaxis and management of oropharyngeal mucositis in cancer therapy. Expert Opin Emerg Drugs 11(2):353–373
9. Trotti A, Bellm LA, Epstein JB et al (2003) Mucositis incidence, severity and associated outcomes in patients with head and neck cancer receiving radiotherapy with or without chemotherapy: a systematic literature review. Radiother Oncol 66(3):253–262
10. Silverman S Jr (2007) Diagnosis and management of oral mucositis. J Support Oncol 5(2 Suppl 1):13–21
11. Vera-Llonch M, Oster G, Ford CM, Lu J, Sonis S (2007) Oral mucositis and outcomes of allogeneic hematopoietic stem-cell transplantation in patients with hematologic malignancies. Support Care Cancer 15(5):491–496
12. Wardley AM, Jayson GC, Swindell R, Morgenstern GR, Chang J, Bloor R, Fraser CJ, Scarffe JH (2000) Prospective evaluation of oral mucositis in patients receiving myeloablative conditioning regimens and haemopoietic progenitor rescue. Br J Haematol 110(2):292–299
13. Elting LS, Cooksley CD, Chambers MS, Garden AS (2007) Risk, outcomes, and costs of radiation-induced oral mucositis among patients with head-and-neck malignancies. Int J Radiat Oncol Biol Phys 15:68(4):1110–1120. Epub 2007 Mar 29
14. Rubenstein EB, Peterson DE, Schubert M, Keefe D, McGuire D, Epstein J, Elting LS, Fox PC, Cooksley C, Sonis ST, Mucositis Study Section of the Multinational Association for Supportive Care in Cancer; International Society for Oral Oncology (2004) Clinical practice guidelines for the prevention and treatment of cancer therapy-induced oral and gastrointestinal mucositis. Cancer 100(9 Suppl):2026–2046
15. Wojtaszek C (2000) Management of chemotherapy-induced stomatitis. Clin J Oncol Nurs 4(6):263–270
16. Vera-Llonch M, Oster G, Hagiwara M, Sonis S (2006) Oral mucositis in patients undergoing radiation treatment for head and neck carcinoma. Cancer 106(2):329–336
17. Sonis ST (2009) Mucositis: the impact, biology and therapeutic opportunities of oral mucositis. Oral Oncol 45(12):1015–1020, Epub 2009 Oct 13. Review
18. Dodd MJ, Dibble SL, Miaskowski C, MacPhail L, Greenspan D, Paul SM, Shiba G, Larson P (2000) Randomized clinical trial of the effectiveness of 3 commonly used mouthwashes to treat chemotherapy-induced mucositis. Oral Surg Oral Med Oral Pathol Oral Radiol Endod 90(1):39–47
19. Raber-Durlacher JE, Weijl NI, Abu Saris M, de Koning B, Zwinderman AH, Osanto S (2000) Oral mucositis in patients treated with chemotherapy for solid tumors: a retrospective analysis of 150 cases. Support Care Cancer 8(5):366–371
20. Brown CG, Wingard J (2004) Clinical consequences of oral mucositis. Semin Oncol Nurs 20(1):16–21, Review
21. Kwong KK (2004) Prevention and treatment of oropharyngeal mucositis following cancer therapy: are there new approaches? Cancer Nurs 27(3):183–205, Review
22. Harris DJ (2006) Cancer treatment-induced mucositis pain: strategies for assessment and management. Ther Clin Risk Manag 2(3):251–258
23. Epstein JB, Schubert MM (2003) Oropharyngeal mucositis in cancer therapy. Review of pathogenesis, diagnosis, and management. Oncology (Williston Park) 17(12):1767–1779; discussion 1779–1782, 1791–1792. Review
24. Palazzi M, Tomatis S, Orlandi E, Guzzo M, Sangalli C, Potepan P, Fantini S, Bergamini C, Gavazzi C, Licitra L, Scaramellini G, Cantu' G, Olmi P (2008) Effects of treatment intensification on acute local toxicity during radiotherapy for head and neck cancer: prospective observational study validating CTCAE, version 3.0, scoring system. Int J Radiat Oncol Biol Phys 70(2):330–337, Epub 2007 Sep 19
25. Turhal NS, Erdal S, Karacay S (2000) Efficacy of treatment to relieve mucositis-induced discomfort. Support Care Cancer 8(1):55–58
26. Takahashi H, Sato M, Tsukada K, Tsuchiya S, Tanda S (2011) A retrospective study of oral adverse events with colorectal cancer chemotherapy using bevacizumab. Gan To Kagaku Ryoho 38(6):959–962

27. Barasch A, Gordon S, Geist RY, Geist JR (2003) Necrotizing stomatitis: report of 3 Pseudomonas aeruginosa-positive patients. Oral Surg Oral Med Oral Pathol Oral Radiol Endod 96(2):136–140

28. Ezzeldin HH, Diasio RB (2008) Predicting fluorouracil toxicity: can we finally do it? J Clin Oncol 26(13):2080–2082 [PUBMED Abstract]

29. Schwab M, Zanger UM, Marx C et al (2008) Role of genetic and nongenetic factors for fluorouracil treatment-related severe toxicity: a prospective clinical trial by the German 5-FU Toxicity Study Group. J Clin Oncol 26(13):2131–2138 [PUBMED Abstract]

30. Werbrouck J, De Ruyck K, Duprez F et al (2009) Acute normal tissue reactions in head-and-neck cancer patients treated with IMRT: influence of dose and association with genetic polymorphisms in DNA DSB repair genes. Int J Radiat Oncol Biol Phys 73(4):1187–1195 [PUBMED Abstract]

31. Hahn T, Zhelnova E, Sucheston L et al (2010) A deletion polymorphism in glutathione-S-transferase mu (GSTM1) and/or theta (GSTT1) is associated with an increased risk of toxicity after autologous blood and marrow transplantation. Biol Blood Marrow Transplant 16(6):801–808 [PUBMED Abstract]

32. Keefe DM, Schubert MM, Elting LS, Sonis ST, Epstein JB, Raber-Durlacher JE, Migliorati CA, McGuire DB, Hutchins RD, Peterson DE (2007) Mucositis Study Section of the Multinational Association of Supportive Care in Cancer and the International Society for Oral Oncology. Updated clinical practice guidelines for the prevention and treatment of mucositis. Cancer 109(5):820–831

33. Yamagata K, Arai C, Sasaki H, Takeuchi Y, Onizawa K, Yanagawa T, Ishibashi N, Karube R, Shinozuka K, Hasegawa Y, Chiba S, Bukawa H (2011) The effect of oral management on the severity of oral mucositis during hematopoietic SCT. Bone Marrow Transplant. doi:10.1038/bmt.2011.171 [Epub ahead of print]

34. Schubert MM, Williams BE, Lloid ME et al (1992) Clinical assessment scale for the rating of oral mucosal changes associated with bone marrow transplantation. Development of an oral mucositis index. Cancer 69(10):2469–2477 [PUBMED Abstract]

35. McGuire DB, Peterson DE, Muller S et al (2002) The 20 item oral mucositis index: reliability and validity in bone marrow and stem cell transplant patients. Cancer Invest 20(7–8):893–903 [PUBMED Abstract]

36. Schubert MM (2000) Oro-pharyngeal mucositis. In: Atkinson K (ed) Clinical bone marrow and blood stem cell transplantation, 2nd edn. Cambridge University Press, Cambridge, pp 812–820

37. Alterio D, Jereczek-Fossa BA, Fiore MR, Piperno G, Ansarin M, Orecchia R (2007) Cancer treatment-induced oral mucositis. Anticancer Res 27(2):1105–1125

38. Sonis ST, Eilers JP, Epstein JB et al (1999) Validation of a new scoring system for the assessment of clinical trial research of oral mucositis induced by radiation or chemotherapy. Mucositis Study Group. Cancer 85:2103–2113

39. von Bültzingslöwen I, Brennan MT, Spijkervet FK, Logan R, Stringer A, Raber-Durlacher JE, Keefe D (2006) Growth factors and cytokines in the prevention and treatment of oral and gastrointestinal mucositis. Support Care Cancer 14(6):519–527, Epub 2006 Apr 21

40. Worthington HV, Clarkson JE, Eden OB (2011) Interventions for preventing oral mucositis for patients with cancer receiving treatment. Cochrane Database Syst Rev 19(2):CD000978, Cochrane Database Syst Rev 2007;(4):CD000978

41. Vuyyuri SB, Hamstra DA, Khanna D, Hamilton CA, Markwart SM, Campbell KC, Sunkara P, Ross BD, Rehemtulla A (2008) Evaluation of D-methionine as a novel oral radiation protector for prevention of mucositis. Clin Cancer Res 14(7):2161–2170

42. Toback FG, Walsh-Reitz MM, Musch MW, Chang EB, Del Valle J, Ren H, Huang E, Martin TE (2003) Peptide fragments of AMP-18, a novel secreted gastric antrum mucosal protein, are mitogenic and motogenic. Am J Physiol Gastrointest Liver Physiol 285(2):G344–G353

43. Chen P, Lingen M, Sonis ST, Walsh-Reitz MM, Toback FG (2011) Role of AMP-18 in oral mucositis. Oral Oncol 47(9):831–839, Epub 2011 Jul 6

44. Del Fante C, Perotti C, Bonferoni MC, Rossi S, Sandri G, Ferrari F, Scudeller L, Caramella CM (2011) Platelet lysate mucoadhesive formulation to treat oral mucositis in graft versus host

disease patients: a new therapeutic approach. AAPS PharmSciTech 12(3):893–899, Epub 2011 Jul 6

45. Watkins B, Pouliot K, Fey E, Tuthill C, Sonis S (2010) Attenuation of radiation- and chemo-radiation-induced mucositis using gamma-D-glutamyl-L-tryptophan (SCV-07). Oral Dis 16(7):655–660

46. Azzoli CG, Patel JD, Krug LM, Miller V, James L, Kris MG, Ginsberg M, Subzwari S, Tyson L, Dunne M, May J, Huntington M, Saunders M, Sirotnak FM (2011) Pralatrexate with vitamin supplementation in patients with previously treated, advanced Non-small cell lung cancer: safety and efficacy in a phase 1 trial. J Thorac Oncol 6(11):1915–1922

47. No authors listed (2008) Oral mucositis due to cancer treatments. Orodental hygiene and ice cubes. Prescrire Int 17(93):33–35

48. Karagözo lu S, Filiz Ulusoy M (2005) Chemotherapy: the effect of oral cryotherapy on the development of mucositis. J Clin Nurs 14(6):754–765

49. McDonnell AM, Lenz KL (2007) Palifermin: role in the prevention of chemotherapy- and radiation-induced mucositis. Ann Pharmacother 41(1):86–94, Epub 2006 Dec 26

50. Gori E, Arpinati M, Bonifazi F, Errico A, Mega A, Alberani F, Sabbi V, Costazza G, Leanza S, Borrelli C, Berni M, Feraut C, Polato E, Altieri MC, Pirola E, Loddo MC, Banfi M, Barzetti L, Calza S, Brignoli C, Bandini G, De Vivo A, Bosi A, Baccarani M (2007) Cryotherapy in the prevention of oral mucositis in patients receiving low-dose methotrexate following myeloablative allogeneic stem cell transplantation: a prospective randomized study of the Gruppo Italiano Trapianto di Midollo Osseo nurses group. Bone Marrow Transplant 39(6):347–352, Epub 2007 Feb 5

51. Simões A, Eduardo FP, Luiz AC, Campos L, Sá PH, Cristófaro M, Marques MM, Eduardo CP (2009) Laser phototherapy as topical prophylaxis against head and neck cancer radiotherapy-induced oral mucositis: comparison between low and high/low power lasers. Lasers Surg Med 41(4):264–270

52. Simões A, de Campos L, de Souza DN, de Matos JA, Freitas PM, Nicolau J (2010) Laser phototherapy as topical prophylaxis against radiation-induced xerostomia. Photomed Laser Surg 28(3):357–363

53. Ruiz-Esquide G, Nervi B, Vargas A, Maíz A (2011) Treatment and prevention of cancer treatment related oral mucositis. Rev Med Chil 139(3):373–381, Epub 2011 Aug 25

54. Dodd MJ, Dibble SL, Miaskowski C, MacPhail L, Greenspan D, Paul SM, Shiba G, Larson P (2000) Randomized clinical trial of the effectiveness of 3 commonly used mouthwashes to treat chemotherapy-induced mucositis. Oral Surg Oral Med Oral Pathol Oral Radiol Endod 90(1):39–47

55. Yen SH, Wang LW, Lin YH, Jen YM, Chung YL (2011) Phenylbutyrate mouthwash mitigates oral mucositis during radiotherapy or chemoradiotherapy in patients with head and neck cancer. Int J Radiat Oncol Biol Phys

56. Potting CM, Uitterhoeve R, Op Reimer WS, Van Achterberg T (2006) The effectiveness of commonly used mouthwashes for the prevention of chemotherapy-induced oral mucositis: a systematic review. Eur J Cancer Care (Engl) 15(5):431–439

57. Nashwan AJ (2011) Use of chlorhexidine mouthwash in children receiving chemotherapy: a review of literature. J Pediatr Oncol Nurs 28(5):295–299

58. Soares AF, Aquino AR, Carvalho CH, Nonaka CF, Almeida D, Pinto LP (2011) Frequency of oral mucositis and microbiological analysis in children with acute lymphoblastic leukemia treated with 0.12% chlorhexidine gluconate. Braz Dent J 22(4):312–316

59. Alterovitz G, Tuthill C, Rios I, Modelska K, Sonis S (2011) Personalized medicine for mucositis: Bayesian networks identify unique gene clusters which predict the response to gamma-d-glutamyl-l-tryptophan (SCV-07) for the attenuation of chemoradiation-induced oral mucositis. Oral Oncol 47(10):951–955

Nausea and Vomiting in Cancer

6

Core Messages

Nausea is a subjective phenomenon of an unpleasant, wavelike sensation experienced in the back of the throat and/or the epigastrium often culminating in vomiting (emesis). Vomiting is the forceful expulsion of the contents of the stomach, duodenum, or jejunum through the oral cavity. Vomiting can serve the function of emptying a noxious chemical from the gut, and nausea appears to play a role in a conditioned response to avoid ingestion of offending substances.

Nausea and vomiting (N&V) are common in advanced cancer patients and are dreaded more than the symptom of pain. Nausea and vomiting are ranked as the most severe side effects to chemotherapy by cancer patients [7]. Chemotherapy- and radiotherapy-induced nausea and vomiting are the most common, intractable, and unpleasant side effects in patients undergoing treatment for cancer.

Symptoms of nausea and vomiting have been shown to result in severe malnutrition, anorexia, interruption of serial treatments, poor treatment outcomes, psychological distress, esophageal tears, fractures, wound dehiscence, withdrawal from potentially useful and curative antineoplastic treatment, and degeneration of self-care and functional ability.

Nausea and vomiting have been documented to affect some 60% of cancer patients at some stage in their illness. Risk factors for CINV include patient gender and age, past history of CINV, plus the emetogenicity and administration schedule of chemotherapy. Research has documented that the incidence of acute and delayed postchemotherapy nausea and vomiting is greater than 50%, even after antiemetic prophylaxis.

The potential factors contributing to N&V in cancer patients include tumor-induced (cranial, gastrointestinal, metabolic), drug-induced, cytotoxic chemotherapy, and radiation-induced and psychological mechanisms [24]. Chronic nausea in the advanced cancer setting is often multifactorial in origin.

N.B. Kumar, *Nutritional Management of Cancer Treatment Effects*,
DOI 10.1007/978-3-642-27233-2_6, © Springer-Verlag Berlin Heidelberg 2012

The relative contribution from these multiple pathways culminating in N&V symptoms is complex and is postulated to account for the variable emetogenicity (intrinsic emetogenicity and mitigating factors [i.e., dosage, administration route, and exposure duration]) and emetogenic profile (i.e., time to onset, symptom severity, and duration) of agents.

Although the sensory pathways for nausea and vomiting are generally well understood (e.g., vagal and vestibular inputs), the pivotal problem of defining the convergent neural circuitry that generates nausea and vomiting is still largely unsolved. Future research focused on solving this puzzle would likely provide a significant resource of information for designing effective treatments to control nausea and vomiting and yield significant insight into understanding gut-brain communication.

6.1   Definition/Description

Although nausea and vomiting are important as biological systems for drug side effects, disease comorbidities, and defenses against food poisoning [1], these are distressing side effects of chemotherapy most feared by cancer patients. Nausea and vomiting are common in advanced cancer patients and dreaded more than the symptom of pain [2, 3]. Nausea is a subjective phenomenon of an unpleasant, wavelike sensation experienced in the back of the throat and/or the epigastrium often culminating in vomiting (emesis). Vomiting is the forceful expulsion of the contents of the stomach, duodenum, or jejunum through the oral cavity. Vomiting can serve the function of emptying a noxious chemical from the gut, and nausea appears to play a role in a conditioned response to avoid ingestion of offending substances. Retching is the gastric and esophageal movements of vomiting without expulsion of vomitus and is also referred to as dry heaves. A vomit (expulsion of gastric contents) is usually preceded by several retching responses, but retching and vomiting can occur separately [4] and involve different sets of muscles. During a retch, thoracic pressure is decreased and abdominal pressure is increased, which may serve to position gastric contents and overcome esophageal resistance [4]. Conversely, a vomit occurs with increased thoracic and abdominal pressure. Unlike a simple reflex, the occurrence of which can be predicted from the intensity of stimulation, the threshold for the emetic response is more variable. The response is modifiable by experience and can be conditioned [5, 6]. Symptoms of nausea and vomiting (N&V) have been shown to result in severe malnutrition, anorexia, interruption of serial treatments, poor treatment outcomes, psychological distress, esophageal tears, fractures, wound dehiscence, withdrawal from potentially useful and curative antineoplastic treatment, and degeneration of self-care and functional ability. Nausea and vomiting are ranked as the most severe side effects to chemotherapy by cancer patients [7].

Chemotherapy- and radiotherapy-induced nausea and vomiting are the most common, intractable, and unpleasant side effects in patients undergoing treatment for cancer [8].

6.2   Prevalence

Despite advances in pharmacologic and nonpharmacologic management, N&V remain two of the more distressing and feared side effects to cancer patients and their families, and incidence may be underestimated by health professionals. Nausea and vomiting have been recognized as a consistent cancer treatment symptom cluster across multiple studies examining the concept of co-occurring symptoms of cancer [9–14]. N&V has been documented to affect some 60% of cancer patients at some stage in their illness [9–15]. In spite of the development of several mechanism-based targeted therapies to treat N&V in cancer patient populations, N&V continue to be among the most distressing side effects of chemotherapy(chemotherapy-induced nausea and vomiting [CINV]) [8, 16] and radiation therapy(radiation-induced nausea and vomiting [RINV]) [17, 18]. Risk factors for CINV include patient gender and age, past history of CINV, plus the emetogenicity and administration schedule of chemotherapy [19]. Research has documented that the incidence of acute and delayed postchemotherapy nausea and vomiting is greater than 50% [20, 21], even after antiemetic prophylaxis. DE most commonly occurs within the first 24–48 h of chemotherapy administration and can persist for 2–5 days. Olanzapine, which has been used anecdotally for chronic nausea in advanced cancer patients, might be a useful treatment for the prevention of delayed emesis in chemotherapy patients [22]. Gastrointestinal side effects can also complicate radiation therapy in cancer patients. RINV is also observed to be common among patients receiving palliative radiotherapy for bone metastases, especially during delayed phase [23]. Even with the best antiemetic pharmacological agents, 60–70% of cancer patients continue to experience nausea and vomiting when undergoing cancer treatments [17, 18], establishing the need for continuous assessment of these symptoms in this patient population and using additional, prophylactic, integrative, nonpharmacological approaches for supportive care and improvement of quality of life.

6.3   Etiology/Common Causes

Significant progress has been made in our understanding the neurophysiologic mechanisms that control nausea and vomiting in cancer. However, the relative contribution of the multiple pathways culminating in N&V symptoms is complex and continues to be an unsolved puzzle and is postulated to account for the variable emetogenicity (intrinsic emetogenicity and mitigating factors [i.e., dosage, administration route, and exposure duration]) and emetogenic profile (i.e., time to onset, symptom severity, and duration) of agents. Overall, the potential factors contributing to N&V in cancer patients include tumor-induced (cranial, gastrointestinal, metabolic), drug-induced, cytotoxic chemotherapy, radiation-induced, and psychological mechanisms [24]. Chronic nausea in the advanced cancer setting is often multifactorial in origin [25–27]. The relative contribution from these multiple pathways culminating in N&V symptoms is complex and is postulated to account for the variable emetogenicity (intrinsic emetogenicity and mitigating factors [i.e., dosage, administration route, and exposure duration]) and emetogenic profile (i.e., time to onset, symptom severity, and duration) of agents.

6.3.1   Neurophysiology of Nausea and Vomiting

Significant progress has been made in our understanding the neurophysiologic mechanisms that control nausea and vomiting. Although both are controlled or mediated by the central nervous system, nausea is mediated through the autonomic nervous system and vomiting results from the stimulation of a complex reflex that is coordinated by a putative true vomiting center, potentially located in the dorsolateral reticular formation near the medullary respiratory centers. Although the sensory pathways for nausea and vomiting are generally well understood (e.g., vagal and vestibular inputs), the pivotal problem of defining the convergent neural circuitry that generates nausea and vomiting is still largely unsolved [1]. It is believed that the vomiting center receives multiple and convergent afferent stimulation from several central neurologic pathways, including the following [25, 27]: (a) a chemoreceptor trigger zone (CTZ); (b) the cerebral cortex and the limbic system in response to sensory stimulation (particularly smell and taste), psychological distress, and pain; (c) the vestibular-labyrinthine apparatus of the inner ear in response to body motion; and (d) peripheral stimuli from visceral organs and vasculature (via vagal and spinal sympathetic nerves) as a result of exogenous chemicals and endogenous substances that accumulate during inflammation, ischemia, and irritation. The CTZ is located in the area postrema, one of the circumventricular regions of the brain on the dorsal surface of the medulla oblongata at the caudal end of the fourth ventricle. Unlike vasculature within the blood–brain diffusion barrier, the area postrema is highly vascularized with fenestrated blood vessels, which lack tight junctions (zonae occludentes) between capillary endothelial cells. The CTZ is anatomically specialized to readily sample elements present in the circulating blood and cerebrospinal fluid (CSF) [26, 28]. Currently, evidence indicates that acute emesis following chemotherapy is initiated by the release of neurotransmitters from cells that are susceptible to the presence of toxic substances in the blood or CSF. Area postrema cells in the CTZ and enterochromaffin cells within the intestinal mucosa are implicated in initiating and propagating afferent stimuli that ultimately converge on central structures corresponding to a vomiting center. The relative contribution from these multiple pathways culminating in N&V symptoms is complex and is postulated to account for the variable emetogenicity (intrinsic emetogenicity and mitigating factors [i.e., dosage, administration route, and exposure duration]) and emetogenic profile (i.e., time to onset, symptom severity, and duration) of agents. Although the sensory pathways for nausea and vomiting are generally well understood (e.g., vagal and vestibular inputs), the pivotal problem of defining the convergent neural circuitry that generates nausea and vomiting is still largely unsolved [1]. Future research focused on solving this puzzle would likely provide a significant resource of information for designing effective treatments to control nausea and vomiting and yield significant insight into understanding gut-brain communication [1].

6.3.2   Cytotoxic Chemotherapy and Radiation-Induced Mechanisms

Nausea and vomiting is a frequent side effect of cancer therapy such as chemotherapy and radiation. CINV involves coordination of several organs of the gastrointestinal tract and the peripheral and central nervous systems. Many neurotransmitters are involved in this process, and the predominant receptors are serotonin, neurokinin-1, and dopamine receptors [19]. In general, nausea and vomiting are symptoms classified under four major types, based on the etiology and timing of occurrence: (a) Acute N&V: N&V experienced during the first 24-h period after chemotherapy administration is considered acute N&V [27]. (b) Delayed (or late) N&V: N&V that occurs more than 24 h after chemotherapy administration is considered delayed, or late, N&V. Delayed N&V is associated with cisplatin, cyclophosphamide, and other drugs (e.g., doxorubicin and ifosfamide) given at high doses or on 2 or more consecutive days. (c) Anticipatory nausea and vomiting (ANV): ANV is nausea and/or vomiting that occurs prior to the beginning of a new cycle of chemotherapy in response to conditioned stimuli such as the smells, sights, and sounds of the treatment room. ANV is a classically conditioned response that typically occurs after three or four prior chemotherapy treatments, following which the person experienced acute or delayed N&V. (d) Chronic N&V is seen in advanced cancer patients associated with a variety of potential etiologies.

Because cells of the GI tract are dividing quickly, they are quite sensitive to radiation therapy. Radiation to the brain is believed to stimulate the brain's vomiting center or chemoreceptor trigger zone. Similar to chemotherapy, radiation dose factors also play a role in determining the possible occurrence of N&V. In general, the higher the daily fractional dose and the greater the amount of tissue that is irradiated, the higher the potential for N&V. In addition, the larger the amount of GI tract irradiated (particularly for fields that include the small intestine and stomach), the higher the potential for N&V. Total body irradiation before bone marrow transplant, for example, has a high probability of inducing N&V as acute side effects. Prevalence of N&V from radiation may be acute and self-limiting, usually occurring 30 min to several hours after treatment. Patients report that symptoms improve on days that they are not being treated. There are also cumulative effects that may occur in patients receiving radiation therapy to the GI tract [27]. Research in this patient population is limited with few prospective, randomized clinical trials limiting development of guidelines for this population.

6.3.3 Tumor-Induced Nausea and Vomiting

Nausea and vomiting can also be induced by raised intracranial pressure (from metastatic brain disease or primary brain tumors, malignant bowel obstruction, and gastroduodenal ulcers) [29]. Nausea relieved by vomiting or induced by nutritional intake is usually due to gastroparesis, gastric outlet obstruction, or SB obstruction [2]. Emesis is an instinctive defense reaction caused by the somatoautonomic nerve reflex, which is integrated in the medulla oblongata. Continuous severe nausea unrelieved by vomiting is usually caused by medications or metabolic abnormalities related to tumors. Patients receiving radiation to the gastrointestinal (GI) tract or brain have the greatest potential for nausea and vomiting (emesis) (N&V) as side effects. In addition, metabolic abnormalities such as hypercalcemia, hyponatremia, uremia, dehydration [29], and infections of the mouth, pharynx, or esophagus can contribute to these symptoms.

6.3.4 Drugs Contributing to Nausea and Vomiting

Medications cause nausea and vomiting via the chemoreceptor trigger zone, such as opiates, digoxin, L-dopa, nonsteroidal anti-inflammatory drugs, by damaging the gastric mucosa; antibiotics such as tetracycline, metronidazole, erythromycin, sulfonamides, and selective serotonin reuptake inhibitor (SSRI) antidepressants may contribute to N&V in cancer patients. In addition, alcohol acts directly on the chemoreceptor trigger zone and via gastric mucosal damage to cause nausea [30]. In the case of opioids, nausea frequently resolves spontaneously a few days after initiation of treatment, although in some cases it may persist. Nausea has also been reported resulting from the accumulation of active opioid metabolites (morphine-6-glucuronide) [28], and patients with impaired renal function may be at increased risk. Since opioids are a common contributor of constipation in this population, most patients are routinely placed on prophylactic laxative regimens. Failure to do so may contribute to increase in symptoms of nausea and vomiting due to constipation, especially in those with cancer cachexia-anorexia in advanced cancer [31–34]. The autonomic dysfunction that often accompanies this syndrome results in decreased GI motility, early satiety, and chronic nausea [24].

6.3.5 Psychological Etiology

Fear of death, pain, treatment-related effects or the recurrence of the illness of tumor in cancer patients has consistently demonstrated increased distress in the patient population. Nausea, like many other symptoms, may have psychological undercurrents that either exacerbate or induce chronic nausea [29]. The role of classical conditioning in patients' anticipatory nausea and vomiting is well known. Nausea and vomiting manifest unconditionally after a nauseogenic experience [35]. Although initially, nausea and vomiting occur during and after the administration of cytotoxic

Fig. 6.1 Etiology of nausea and vomiting in cancer

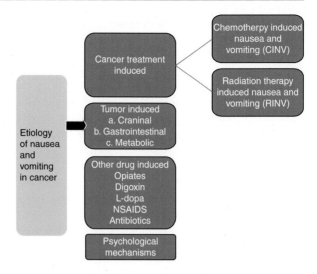

drugs (posttreatment nausea and vomiting) as unconditioned responses (UR). However, when reexposed to the stimuli that usually signal the chemotherapy session and its drug infusion, anywhere from 10% to 30% of patients report symptoms called anticipatory nausea (AN) and/or anticipatory vomiting (ANV). Anticipatory nausea/vomiting is hypothesized to be acquired by Pavlovian conditioning and, consequently, may be alleviated by conditioning techniques [6, 35, 36]. More recently, efforts have been made to determine the possible conditioning effects on posttreatment nausea [37]. In studies examining the contribution of anticipatory (conditioned) nausea to patients' subsequent posttreatment nausea, results revealed a significant correlation between the intensity of anticipatory nausea in the clinic prior to their treatment infusion and subsequent posttreatment nausea [37–39]. Thus, once established, conditioned nausea and vomiting may contribute to the severity of subsequent posttreatment nausea and vomiting in patients receiving repeated cycles of chemotherapy for cancer. In a study to investigate the prevalence of anticipatory nausea (AN), its associated factors, and its impact on quality of life (QOL) among ambulatory cancer patients receiving chemotherapy, Akechi et al. [40] demonstrated that the presence of AN was also significantly associated with most domains of patient outcomes, including psychological distress, perceived needs, and QOL even after adjustments for age, gender, performance status, and psychological distress. Vomiting may follow nausea and be brought on by treatment or food and other odors (Fig. 6.1).

6.4   Current Treatment of Nausea and Vomiting

Due to the complex and multietiological basis contributing to the symptoms of nausea and vomiting during treatment, it may be important to utilize a systematic, stepwise approach, combining both pharmacological and nonpharmacological management of these symptoms [41–43]. In a systematic review of the treatment of nausea and vomiting in cancer, Davis [43] found 93 articles with only 14 that were randomized clinical trials, of which most were of low-quality, unblinded, small sample sizes and lack randomization. Current treatment strategies include clinical assessment of the pathophysiological component of the emetogenic pathway that is being triggered and selecting an antiemetic drug that blocks the key receptors involved. A comprehensive assessment obtaining a thorough history and physical examination are essential first steps to define the severity of the symptoms and determine the underlying etiology. Current treatment of nausea and vomiting are mostly based on etiology. Currently, the primary method of treatment is pharmacological, with current recommendations based on the etiology, knowledge of the emetogenic pathways, and matching of the emetogenic stimulus with the drug most likely to act on the relevant receptors [41]. Once the most likely etiology is determined, the medical team can identify the mechanism contributing to these symptoms, the specific transmitters, and receptors by which this etiology is triggering nausea and vomiting. Based on this assessment, the pharmacological management may focus on intervention with appropriate antagonist to the implicated receptors. This is often complicated by the difficulty in identifying the cause(s) and specific transmitters and the fact that many antiemetics work on multiple receptors. If symptoms are refractory despite adequate dosage and around-the-clock prophylactic administration, an empirical trial combining several therapies to block multiple emetic pathways should be attempted. Therapy is then changed to rotation to medications which bind to multiple receptors (broad spectrum antiemetics), the addition of another antiemetic to a narrow-spectrum antiemetic (a serotonin receptor antagonist such as tropisetron to a phenothiazine), rotation to a different class of antiemetic (tropisetron for a phenothiazine), or in-class drug rotation [2, 42]. Additionally, since oral administration of medication is not always feasible, alternate routes such as rectal suppositories, subcutaneous infusions, and orally dissolvable tablets should be considered [42]. Although these are current clinical practice guidelines, based on the most current reviews, there was no evidence that multiple emetics based on etiology of emesis were any better than a single emetic. There is also poor evidence for dose response, intraclass or interclass drug switch, or antiemetic combinations in those individuals failing to respond to the initial antiemetic [43, 44]. Based on this review, antiemetic studies and published guidelines are largely based on expert opinion and have moderate to weak evidence at best establishing the need for prospective randomized clinical trials of single emetics as well as old and more recently developed agents [44] to establish evidence-based guidelines. Additionally, to date, both empirical and etiology-based therapies have similar overall efficacy.

6.4.1   Pharmacological Approaches

Over the past two decades, more effective and better-tolerated pharmacologic agents have been developed to prevent chemotherapy-induced nausea and vomiting. Selective 5-HT3 antagonists, neurokinin-1 antagonists, and corticosteroids are at present the most effective therapeutic agents. Recommended antiemetic regimens for highly emetogenic chemotherapy and moderately emetogenic chemotherapy with a high risk of delayed CINV include a serotonin antagonist, dexamethasone, and aprepitant. Metoclopramide had modest evidence of effectiveness based on these studies [43], followed by phenothiazines and tropisetron [2]. Aprepitant has been shown to have a significant role in the management of CINV, as it allows the majority of patients to complete their chemotherapies without significant morbidity [45]. The recommended antiemetic regimen of aprepitant, a 5-HT(3) RA, and a corticosteroid is safe. The combination of aprepitant, a 5-HT(3) RA, and dexamethasone is now the gold standard of antiemetic treatment in prevention of CINV induced by HEC or by the combination of an anthracycline and cyclophosphamide. The intravenous formulation of aprepitant used as a single dose is expected to be of benefit to cancer patients [46]. Other moderately emetogenic chemotherapy requires a serotonin antagonist and dexamethasone. Medications for breakthrough symptoms include dopamine antagonists, lorazepam, metoclopramide, haloperidol, droperidol, and other agents. Options for treatment of refractory CINV include olanzapine, dronabinol, nabilone, and gabapentin. New evidence from noncontrolled studies supports the use of olanzapine, casopitant, and gabapentin in controlling the symptoms of CINV [19, 47]. Billo et al. [48] completed a review to compare efficacy of different serotonin receptor antagonists (5-HT(3) RAs) in the control of acute and delayed emesis induced by highly emetogenic chemotherapy. Ondansetron and granisetron appear to be equivalent drugs for the prevention of acute and delayed emesis following the use of highly emetogenic chemotherapy. According to one single trial, the combination of palonosetron and dexamethasone was superior to granisetron and dexamethasone in controlling delayed emesis. However, more evidence is needed before palonosetron could become the candidate 5-HT(3) RA for the control of delayed emesis induced by highly emetogenic chemotherapy [48]. Palonosetron, a unique second-generation 5-HT3 receptor antagonist, has been demonstrated to control emesis related to chemotherapy-induced nausea and vomiting (CINV). In a study to evaluate the efficacy and tolerability of single administration of palonosetron followed by a single dose of dexamethasone on day 1 in patients with breast cancer (BC) or colorectal cancer (CRC) receiving moderate emetogenic chemotherapy (MEC), adequately controlled CINV during the entire period of emetic risk [49]. To reduce side effects of corticosteroid-containing antiemetic regimens, tailoring antiemetic schedules to specific requirements of different patients could be of benefit. In a study to evaluate the possibility to reduce the total dose of corticosteroids administered with palonosetron, Aapro et al. [50] observed no significant reduction in antiemetic control during the 5-day period or an impact on patient functioning. Granisetron is a highly selective serotonin 5-HT(3) receptor antagonist for the prevention of chemotherapy-induced nausea and vomiting. The transdermal granisetron system delivers continuous granisetron (3.1 mg/day) into the systemic circulation (via passive diffusion) for up to 7 days, with maximum absorption reached within 48 h. Transdermal granisetron was generally well tolerated in clinical trials, with few adverse events being treatment related [51]. Randomized clinical trials have demonstrated anywhere from 49% to 60% control of acute CINV using transdermal granisetron, thus its effectiveness and safety in controlling acute emesis induced by chemotherapy with both moderate and high emetogenic potential [52]. A more recent meta-analysis by Salvo et al. [53] summarized data from 46 studies, with 9 included in the review of moderate quality, continuing to demonstrate lack of prospective randomized clinical trials using this agent. Findings showed that 5-hydoxytryptamine-3 RAs were superior to placebo and other emetics for prevention of emesis but not for nausea prevention and delayed N&V [53]. Retrospective studies evaluating antiemetic therapies in radiation therapy patients have shown that patients receiving prophylactic antiemetics with tropisetron + dexamethasone completed RT with lower intensity of N&V and lower ECOG PS scores compared to groups that received other antiemetic treatments [54]. Hydroxytryptamine-3 (5-HT3) receptor antagonists plus dexamethasone have significantly improved the control of acute nausea and vomiting, but delayed nausea and vomiting remains a significant clinical problem. Combined neurokinin-1 receptor antagonists with 5-HT3 antagonists and steroids are observed to be better in the control of both acute and delayed emesis. However, the use of these antiemetics is observed to possess inherent side effects. Corticosteroids have not been demonstrated to be effective, except in bowel obstruction. Other treatments that improve symptoms of N&V with malignant bowel obstruction that have been found to be effective are venting gastrostomy and octreotide [2].

In a recent update, the American Society of Clinical Oncology (ASCO) guideline for antiemetics in oncology [38], a systematic review of the medical literature including MEDLINE; the Cochrane Collaboration Library; and meeting materials from ASCO and the Multinational Association for Supportive Care in Cancer were all searched. Primary outcomes of interest were complete response and rates of any vomiting or nausea. Thirty-seven trials met prespecified inclusion and exclusion criteria for this systematic review. Two systematic reviews from the Cochrane Collaboration were identified; one surveyed the pediatric literature. The other compared the relative efficacy of the 5-hydroxytryptamine-3 (5-HT3) antagonists. Based on this review, it is recommended that combined anthracycline and cyclophosphamide regimens are reclassified as highly emetic. Patients who receive this combination or any highly emetic agents should receive a 5-HT3 antagonist, dexamethasone, and a neurokinin-1 (NK1) receptor antagonist. A large trial validated the equivalency of fosaprepitant, a single-day formulation, with aprepitant; either therapy is appropriate. Preferential use of palonosetron is recommended for moderate emetic risk regimens, combined with dexamethasone. For low-risk agents, patients can be offered dexamethasone before the first dose of chemotherapy. Patients undergoing high-emetic-risk radiation therapy should receive a 5-HT3 antagonist before each fraction and for 24 h after treatment and may receive a 5-day course of dexamethasone before fractions 1–5.

6.4.2 Nonpharmacological Approaches

Even with the best antiemetic pharmacological agents, 60% of cancer patients continue to experience nausea and vomiting when undergoing chemotherapy treatments. Several plant-based medications, as well as therapies such as acupressure, acupuncture, and hypnosis, have been integrated along with traditional interventions with antiemetics to manage nausea and vomiting. Although no single nonpharmacological approach has been deemed effective to manage cancer-related nausea and vomiting, several of these have a rationale for integration with traditional pharmacological interventions with antiemetics.

6.4.2.1 Botanicals for Management of Nausea and Vomiting

Botanicals such as *Scutellaria baicalensis*, Korean red ginseng, American ginseng berry, *Ganoderma lucidum*, *Zingiber officinale*, grape-seed extract, and the oil of *Mentha spicata* are reported to be effective in the treatment of nausea and vomiting mostly in preclinical studies. Of these, ginger has also been evaluated for its efficacy in humans with mixed results, continuing to emphasize aspects that need further investigations for these plants to be of use in clinics in the future [8].

Ginger has been used in the treatment of nausea related to multiple causes, including chemotherapy-induced nausea and vomiting [55]. Although use of ginger has been shown to have no additional toxicities, studies are mixed with regard to effectiveness in reducing cancer treatment–induced nausea and vomiting. In preclinical studies, Sharma et al. [56] demonstrated varying formulations of ginger's antiemetic effect. Using acetone and ethanolic extract of ginger (*Zingiber officinale*, Roscoe, Zingiberaceae) against cisplatin-induced emesis in dogs, doses of 100, 200, and 500 mg/kg (p.o.), and ginger juice, in the doses of 2 and 4 mL/kg, was investigated against cisplatin effect on gastric emptying in rats. All three ginger preparations significantly reversed cisplatin-induced delay in gastric emptying. The ginger juice and acetone extract were more effective than the 50% ethanolic extract. The reversal produced by the ginger acetone extract was similar to that caused by the 5-HT3 receptor antagonist ondansetron; however, ginger juice produced better reversal than ondansetron. The authors concluded that ginger, an antiemetic for cancer chemotherapy, may also be useful in improving the gastrointestinal side effects of cancer chemotherapy [56]. In a review of trials with ginger, daily doses of up to 6 g, ginger seems to be a drug with few side effects [57]. In small prospective trials, high-protein meals with ginger reduced the delayed nausea of chemotherapy and reduced use of antiemetic medications. Protein with ginger holds the potential of representing a novel, nutritionally based treatment for the delayed nausea of chemotherapy [58]. More recently, in well-designed randomized clinical trials, ginger supplementation at a daily dose of 0.5–1.0 g significantly aids in reduction of the severity of acute chemotherapy-induced nausea in adult cancer patients [18]. Ginger root powder was effective in reducing severity of acute and delayed CINV as additional therapy to ondansetron and dexamethasone in patients receiving high-emetogenic chemotherapy [59]. However, ginger was observed to provide no additional benefit for reduction in the prevalence or severity of acute or delayed CINV when given with 5-HT3 receptor agonist and/or aprepitant in a randomized double-blind, placebo-controlled trial [55].

6.4.2.2 Acupressure for Management of Nausea and Vomiting

Several randomized, placebo-controlled clinical trials have assessed the effect of acupressure applied to the pericardium 6 (P6 or Neiguan) acupuncture point with a

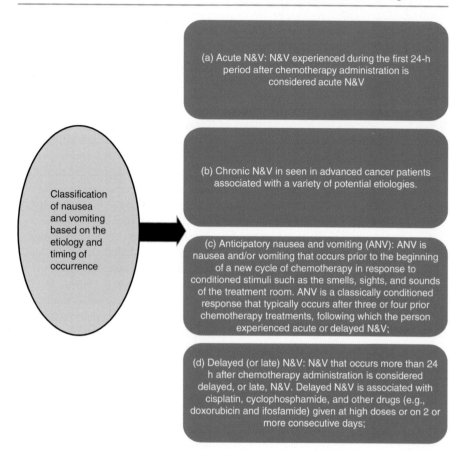

Fig. 6.2 Classification of nausea and vomiting based on the etiology and timing of occurrence

wristband on nausea-vomiting in addition to the standard antiemetic medications used to prevent nausea-vomiting due to chemotherapy in gynecologic and breast cancer patients. The findings from these studies have consistently demonstrated that acupressure applied to P6 acupuncture point with wristbands may be effective in reducing chemotherapy-related nausea and may decrease the antiemetic use after chemotherapy [60]. It was found that nausea and retching experience, and nausea, vomiting, and retching occurrence and distress were all significantly lower in the experimental group compared to the control group ($p < 0.05$). The only exception was with the vomiting experience, which was close to significance ($p = 0.06$) [61]. Acupressure at the P6 point is a value-added technique in addition to pharmaceutical management for women undergoing treatment for breast and gynecological cancers to reduce the amount and intensity of delayed CINV [62]. Research thus supports the safety and effectiveness of self-administered acupressure for the treatment of chemotherapy-induced nausea and vomiting when used in conjunction with current antiemetic drugs for relief of the nausea and vomiting resulting from chemotherapy [17] (Fig. 6.2).

6.5   Guidelines for the Management of Nausea and Vomiting

Due to complex and multifactorial nature, preventing and treating N&V continues to present a challenge. Despite the progress, uncontrolled vomiting and inadequately controlled nausea remain as major problems in several cancer patients. Nonetheless, complete prevention of treatment-induced nausea and vomiting should be a realistic goal for most patients. Clinicians underestimate the incidence of nausea, which is not as well controlled as emesis. The following guidelines are considered best practice standards based on available review of the current research literature. Due to the multifactorial etiology of nausea and vomiting, there is no single standard of therapy established to treat the symptoms in cancer patients. Diagnosis and management of nausea and vomiting requires timely and careful screening using detailed history and clinical examination by integrated, multidisciplinary teams consisting of treating oncologists (surgeons, radiation oncologists, medical oncologists), dentists, speech pathologist, clinical pharmacist, psychosocial worker, physical therapist, radiologist, and dietitian for comprehensive symptom assessment, established nutritional guidelines, pharmacotherapy, psychosocial intervention, in addition to monitoring and closely assessing patients for change in status. In addition, the intervention must be proactive and based on ongoing evaluations to monitor patient's change in status based on disease stage, response to treatment, and treatment outcomes, as well as use of concomitant medications.

6.5.1   Assessment

Proactive and systematic screening, assessment, and early identification of high-risk populations for specific treatments should be part of standard of care. The basic goal of this screening is to obtain a collective measurement of gastrointestinal symptoms, signs, and functional disturbances, including pain. A comprehensive history that includes determining the frequency and effectiveness of bowel movements and laxative therapy is essential. Concurrent medications should be reviewed, and the frequency and nature of N&V should be documented. Several assessment tools are available to assess nature and extent of nausea and vomiting in cancer patients. Screening and follow-up evaluation can be made utilizing the National Cancer Institute Common Toxicity Criteria (NCI-CTC). Continued symptom monitoring throughout therapy is recommended [38]. A thorough *physical examination* should attempt to exclude bowel obstruction, fecal impaction, dehydration, and raised intracranial pressure. History and physical examination are poor at determining the extent of constipation. A plain flat-plate X-ray of the abdomen can be very useful to this end. Surgical X-ray views of the abdomen may be helpful if a bowel obstruction is suspected.

6.5.2   Pharmacologic Interventions

Interventions with antiemetics are the mainstay of treatment of nausea and vomiting in clinical oncology. Based on the etiology, pharmacological interventions can include benzodiazepines, 5-HT3 receptor antagonists, corticosteroids, and NK1 receptor antagonists. Selection of antiemetics should be based on emetic potential of the chemotherapy agent(s) as well as patient factors, taking into consideration the potential causes of nausea and emesis in patients with cancer that may be contributing factors. Oral and IV antiemetics are equally effective. The period of expected nausea and vomiting should be covered with appropriate antiemetics (anticipatory, acute, and delayed period for at least 4 days). It is recommended that the lowest efficacious dose of the antiemetics should be used. If nausea is due to poor motility, prevent/treat as indicated with promotility drugs along with antiemetics.

6.5.3   Nutrition Guidelines

Although evidence is limited, experts recommend the following additional guidelines for dietary interventions in patients receiving chemotherapy to minimize nausea and vomiting based on best practice standards.

Nutritional screening must be performed within 24 h of admission of the patient by a registered dietitian/nutritionist.

1. Screen patient within 24 h of admission. This order for screening has been a standard order for all cancer patient admissions to avoid delay in timing of screening;
2. Assess all symptoms: Gastrointestinal tract–taste alterations, smell alterations, dysphagia, dyspnea, other pain, early satiety, dry mouth, too much saliva production, anorexia, diarrhea, constipation, nausea, vomiting, dehydration, fatigue, height, weight, recent weight loss, anthropometrics, grip strength, psychosocial/family/caregiver support, depression, ADL, and others (midarm muscle circumference, body composition [DEXA]).
3. Screen and assess current nutritional status and estimate caloric, protein, and multivitamin/mineral needs (Refer to Chap. 2).
4. Provide adequate nutrition by including "calorie" and "protein" boosters education material and nutritional supplements to ensure intake of proteins (recommended 0.8–1.0g/kg/day). Provide dense caloric supplements up to 400 cal/day containing 1.5 kcal/mL; if intake is insufficient in proteins, supplement with modular protein supplements, adding this to favorite beverage. (http://www.nestle-nutrition.com/Products/Default.aspx;   http://abbottnutrition.com/) The choice of nutritional supplements can be based in the personal choice of the patient, patient needs, tolerance to product, as well as other comorbidities.
5. Include a standard multivitamin mineral supplementation to prevent any further deficits and meet increased needs.
6. Assess adequacy of intake and provide an appetite stimulant (megestrol acetate 20 mL or 800 mgs/day or alternate) if patient has cancer anorexia to ensure adequate intake and prevent further weight loss.
7. Provide each patient with nutritional guidelines to ensure adequate intake of calories and proteins and a list of suggested high-caloric and high-protein

nutritional supplements to choose from, taking into consideration taste alterations, early satiety, nausea, and vomiting that are common symptoms observed in
this patient population.

8. Proactive measures to provide alternate mode of nutritional support must be
planned during acute phase of treatment when it would be a greater risk to feed
patient via the oral route. Selection of route of feeding may be informed based on
general guidelines and criteria provided in Table 2.6.

9. Other strategies to improve nutritional intake:

- Time dose of antiemetics prior to meals so that the effect is present during and
  after meals.
- Recommend smaller, more frequent meals and snacks such as toast, crackers,
  and chips as nausea is lessened when the stomach is not empty.
- Recommend that patients avoid going for long periods of time without food.
- Recommend reduction of strong, aromatic stimuli and flavors in foods.
  Recommend avoiding food preparation or food preparation areas.
- Recommend that patients avoid foods that are spicy, fatty, or highly salty.
- Several foods are considered "comfort foods" specific to each patient (e.g.,
  oatmeal, macaroni, and cheese). Include these as needed.
- Crackers can be kept at bedside if nausea is a problem in the morning or fol-
  lowing a nap.
- Recommend that the patient eat in a well-ventilated room, with no food odors.
  Advise patients to eat in the dining room or other room rather than in the
  kitchen.
- Best-tolerated foods include:
- Bland foods such as cream of wheat or rice, or oatmeal
- Boiled potatoes or noodles
- Low-fat protein sources such as skinned chicken, turkey, eggs, or tofu that are
  baked or broiled, not fried
- Canned peaches, pears, apple sauce, or other soft, bland fruits and
  vegetables
- Clear liquids such as apple and cranberry juice, low-salt broth, teas, and caf-
  feine-free carbonated drinks.
- Teas such as ginger and peppermint (avoid peppermint if reflux is a problem),
  served lukewarm or cold, have been well tolerated by patients with nausea.
- Drinking with a straw may help to manage odors.
- Suggest that patients maintain a diary and track nausea and what triggers it,
  such as specific foods, events, surroundings, etc. See if there is a pattern, and
  if so, try to change that pattern.
- Suggest patient rest sitting up after a meal for about an hour–watching TV,
  reading a magazine, talking with loved ones, or enjoying a pet may distract
  from thinking about nausea.
- Avoid fried, greasy, and rich foods.
- Avoid forcing patients to eat their favorite foods as they may develop an aversion to these favorite foods, particularly if eaten within the time pre- and
  postreceiving chemotherapy.

- Patient should not eat or drink anything until the vomiting is under control (risk of aspiration).
- Recommend trying small amounts of clear liquids such as water or bouillon, apple or cranberry juice, fruit ices without fruit pieces, ginger ale or 7-Up, gelatin desserts, popsicles, sports drinks such as Gatorade, vegetable broth, and teas.
- Begin with one teaspoon of food every 10 min, gradually increasing the amount to one tablespoon every 20 min, and then try two tablespoons every 30 min or as tolerated.
- Once these liquids are tolerated, try a softer diet with bland foods such as mashed potatoes, pureed fruits, smoothies, fruit nectars, yogurts, and cereals with milk or soy.
- Practice behavioral modification techniques such as meditation, imagery, and other relaxation techniques. Several studies have demonstrated that behavioral techniques such as relaxation, meditation, imagery, and listening to favorite music may reduce symptoms.
- Avoid hot, spicy foods or other dishes that might upset your stomach or gastrointestinal tract.
- Assure that fluids and electrolytes are replaced (8–10 cups of fluids recommended per day).
- Avoid foods for at least 2 h before treatment.
- Acupressure (i.e., seasickness wristbands) has been demonstrated to reduce symptoms of nausea.

6.5.4 Markers and Instruments for Patient Monitoring and Assessment of Response to Treatment by the Interdisciplinary Medical Team

1. *Anthropometric measurements* such as participant's height, weight, and body mass index can be performed at admission and at regular intervals established by the medical team.
2. *Body composition by DXA scan*: DXA should be used to assess both total lean body mass (LBM), fat mass (FM), and total bone mineral density (BMD).Total bone mineral density (BMD) is a valid indirect measure of skeletal muscle and patient activity. Total LBM is sometimes called total fat-free mass (FFM), depending upon specific DXA manufacturer. DXA instruments use an X-ray source that generates or is split into two energies to measure bone mineral mass and soft tissue from which fat and fat-free mass are estimated. The exam is quick (1–2 min), precise (0.5–1%), and noninvasive. DXA scanners have the precision required to detect changes in muscle mass as small as 5%. Radiation exposure from DXA scans is minimal. The National Council of Radiation Protection and Measurements (NCRP) has recommended the annual effective

dose limit for infrequent exposure of the general population is 5,000 μSv and that an annual effective dose of 10 μSv be considered a negligible individual dose. The effective dose of a dual-energy X-ray absorptiometry whole body scan on an adult is 2.1 μSv. Studies have shown that quality assurance is an important issue in the use of DXA scans to determine body composition including lean body mass and bone mineral density. DXA instrument manufacturer and model should remain consistent, and their calibration should be monitored throughout treatment. Use of a standardized scan acquisition protocol and appropriate and unchanging scan acquisition and analysis software is essential to achieve consist results.

3. *Dietary intake* must be assessed at baseline and periodical intervals by conducting random weekly, 2 weekdays + 1 weekend day, 24-h dietary recalls (gold standard for collecting dietary data) using a 5-step multipass procedure (which has been found to assess mean energy intake within 10% of actual intake) and using the frequently updated University of Minnesota Nutrition Data System for Research (NDSR) version database for analysis of nutrient composition. Food portion visuals can be provided to patients to estimate portion sizes of foods while monitoring intake.

4. *Symptom log* may be completed daily and collected from patients on a monthly basis. Based on these symptoms, all anticipated and unanticipated grades of constitutional, dermatological, gastrointestinal (GI), metabolic, and pain symptoms can be continuously monitored including those symptoms affecting nutritional intake and utilization.

5. *CMP and CBC*: Monthly CMP and CBC should be monitored to assess electrolytes and organ function.

6. *Functional markers* (*Karnofsky performance score*): Evaluation of patients' functional status and barriers to obtaining adequate nutrients is also necessary. A physical exam combined with personal interview should include the evaluation of functional status such as the ability to chew and swallow, dental or oral problems causing odynophagia or dysphagia, signs of muscle wasting or anasarca, presence of edema, presence of skin or mouth lesion, and ability to perform instrumental activities of daily living (IADLs) such as cooking, shopping, and self-feeding. It is critical to assess activities of daily living, physical activity, exercise, sleep, and ability to work and perform other functional roles. Limitations in the activities of daily living have been identified secondary to and as a cause of weight loss in cancer patients. Cancer and other chronic diseases pose difficulties specifically for the cancer patient receiving treatment and the elderly in carrying out activities of daily living. A loss of postural and locomotive muscle mass has been observed within 7 days of inactivity. The Karnofsky Performance Scale Index allows patients to be classified as to their functional impairment. This has been used to compare effectiveness of different therapies and to assess the prognosis in individual patients and has been validated in cancer patient populations.

7. *Godin Leisure-Time Exercise Questionnaire* weekly to monitor physical activity.

8. *Handgrip strength dynamometry assessment*: A validated tool commonly used to assess handgrip strength is the Jamar dynamometer, which is a fast, reliable, and easy-to-perform device commonly used by our team to measure improvements in functional strength. The Jamar dynamometer has a lower percentage coefficient of variation and is thus a more precise device than other handgrip dynamometers.

9. *Biochemical markers of protein status (serum albumin and transferrin)*: Assessment of protein status is critical in the identification and treatment of abnormalities in protein metabolism. There is substantial evidence of the correlation between serum hepatic proteins and inflammation, making these the most relevant biomarkers in cancer patient populations. Serum transferrin, prealbumin, and albumin have been observed as intermediate endpoint biomarkers and independently associated with clinical outcomes. Measurements of body composition combined with more objective and sensitive measure of protein nutriture are ideal for the biochemical assessment of intravascular and visceral protein stores. We have thus included the three major valid intermediate endpoint biomarkers (IEBs) that represent intravascular and visceral protein pools–transferrin, prealbumin and albumin–as the biochemical indicators of protein status. Although transferrin levels are affected by iron status, serum transferrin, either singly or as part of a multiparameter index, is the strongest predictor of cancer patient morbidity and mortality.

10. *Immune and inflammatory markers*: A range of metabolic responses triggered by inflammatory and immunological responses in cancer patients. Cytokines can be measured in a panel including IL-1, IL-4, IL-6, IL-8, IL-10, GM-CSF, IFNκ, TNF-α, and CRP (Bio-Rad–Bio-Plex). All of these biomarkers have been shown to increase with disease, aging, and cytotoxic agents. Though we realize these intermediate endpoint biomarkers of cytokines cannot be reliably interpreted, as over 70% of the subjects as observed in our studies were on active treatment with cytotoxic agents, these variables are important to determine, as they may provide useful information and contribute to the better understanding of the mechanistic process.

11. *Quality of life* should be measured at baseline and monthly using the Rand Short Form (SF)-36 (Medical Outcomes Study SF36) [63]. The SF-36 has been used extensively with general, high-risk, and cancer populations and has available norms for mail and telephone versions and comparisons between group and individual scores. Scores are calculated and transformed to a 0–100 scale, with higher scores indicating increased health status. Reliability of the SF-36 scales was measured by Cronbach α coefficient, and the results ranged from 0.78 in general health perceptions to 0.91 in the physical functioning domain.

6.5.5 Dentist

Referral to a dentist must include details regarding current diagnosis, plan of treatment, start date of treatment, limitations of use of medications including antibiotics, and other specific information that will assist the dentist to treat patient periodically to prevent tooth decay during this period. Fastidious mouth care must be followed to prevent any infections or decays.

6.5.6 Follow-up

Patients must be seen by the multidisciplinary team on a regularly scheduled basis to monitor progress and to review compliance to intervention including diet intake adequacy, symptom logs, change in concomitant medications, and any other issues related to treatment. Improved management of malnutrition with nutritional therapy may require a multimodal intervention by multidisciplinary teams using a comprehensive and integrated approach. Initial screening and knowledge of treatment trajectory of the cancer patient should guide a plan for reassessment at regularly planned intervals. Subjective and objective data on progress and response to nutritional therapy may be assessed using the indicators used in the comprehensive nutritional assessment. Newly developed symptoms resulting from treatment or progression of disease may require additional monitoring or revision of nutritional therapy. Reassessment/reevaluation for monitoring and evaluation of nutritional therapy must include monitoring of clinical, functional, dietary, and behavioral outcomes that were identified by the comprehensive nutritional assessment

6.6 Future Directions

In spite of most patients receiving antiemetics to prevent emesis and lessen nausea while undergoing cancer therapy, patients continue to report nausea. It may be critical to continue to fully understand the mechanistic pathway, using a multidisciplinary approach, that contribute to both nausea and vomiting more clearly and identify multimodal approaches based on these mechanisms. In addition, prospective randomized clinical trials to examine the role of antiemetics in patients undergoing chemotherapy and radiation therapy and combination therapies are still lacking to support current recommendations. Future trials should take into consideration symptom clusters observed in cancer treatment and use comprehensive assessment of co-occurring symptoms along with nausea and vomiting. Multimodal treatment regimens, combining pharmacological and nonpharmacological approaches in the management of these symptoms by multidisciplinary teams, may hold promise and has the maximum potential to make important strides in managing these symptom clusters in this cancer patient population.

Summary for the Clinician

There are no single standard pharmacological therapies that have been proven to be effective in the prevention and management of nausea and vomiting in cancer patients. Due to its complex and multifactorial nature, preventing and treating N&V continues to present a challenge. Nonetheless, complete prevention of treatment-induced nausea and vomiting should be a realistic goal for most patients.

Clinicians underestimate the incidence of nausea, which is not as well controlled as emesis.

Proactive and systematic screening, assessment, and early identification of high-risk populations for specific treatments should be part of standard of care. The basic goal of this screening is to obtain a collective measurement of gastrointestinal symptoms, signs, and functional disturbances, including pain. A comprehensive history that includes determining the frequency and effectiveness of bowel movements and laxative therapy is essential. Concurrent medications should be reviewed, and the frequency and nature of N&V should be documented. Several assessment tools are available to assess nature and extent of nausea and vomiting in cancer patients. Screening and follow-up evaluation can be made utilizing the National Cancer Institute Common Toxicity Criteria (NCI-CTC).

Continued symptom monitoring throughout therapy is recommended, using a multiprofessional approach to clinical care, research, and education.

Physical examination should attempt to exclude bowel obstruction, fecal impaction, dehydration, and raised intracranial pressure. History and physical examination are poor at determining the extent of constipation. A plain flatplate X-ray of the abdomen can be very useful to this end. Surgical X-ray views of the abdomen may be helpful if a bowel obstruction is suspected.

Currently, the primary method of treatment is pharmacological, with current recommendations based on the etiology, knowledge of the emetogenic pathways, and matching of the emetogenic stimulus with the drug most likely to act on the relevant receptors. Additionally, since oral administration of medication is not always feasible, alternate routes such as rectal suppositories, subcutaneous infusions, and orally dissolvable tablets should be considered.

If symptoms are refractory despite adequate dosage and around-the-clock prophylactic administration, an empirical trial combining several therapies to block multiple emetic pathways should be attempted. Therapy is then changed to rotation to medications which bind to multiple receptors (broad-spectrum antiemetics), the addition of another antiemetic to a narrow-spectrum antiemetic (a serotonin receptor antagonist such as tropisetron to a phenothiazine), rotation to a different class of antiemetic (tropisetron for a phenothiazine), or in-class drug rotation.

Based on the etiology, pharmacological interventions can include benzodiazepines, 5-HT3 receptor antagonists, corticosteroids, and NK1 receptor antagonists. Selection of antiemetics should be based on emetic potential of the chemotherapy agent(s) as well as patient factors, taking into consideration the potential causes of nausea and emesis in patients with cancer that may be contributing factors. Oral and IV antiemetics are equally effective. The period of expected nausea and vomiting should be covered with appropriate antiemetics (anticipatory, acute, and delayed period for at least 4 days). It is recommended that the lowest efficacious dose of the antiemetics should be used. If nausea is due to poor motility, prevent/treat as indicated with promotility drugs along with antiemetics.

Even with the best antiemetic pharmacological agents, 60% of cancer patients continue to experience nausea and vomiting when undergoing chemotherapy treatments. Several nonpharmacological approaches using plant-based medications, as well as therapies such as acupressure, acupuncture, and hypnosis, have been integrated along with traditional interventions with antiemetics to manage nausea and vomiting. Although no single nonpharmacological approach has been deemed effective to manage cancer-related nausea and vomiting, acupressure has shown to be effective in controlling N&V when integrated with pharmacological interventions with antiemetics.

References

1. Horn CC (2008) Why is the neurobiology of nausea and vomiting so important? Appetite 50(2–3):430–434, Epub 2007 Oct 11
2. Ang SK, Shoemaker LK, Davis MP (2010) Nausea and vomiting in advanced cancer. Am J Hosp Palliat Care 27(3):219–225
3. Jiménez A, Madero R, Alonso A, Martínez-Marín V, Vilches Y, Martínez B, Feliu M, Díaz L, Espinosa E, Feliu J (2011) Symptom clusters in advanced cancer. J Pain Symptom Manage 42(1):24–31
4. Andrews PL, Hawthorn J (1988) The neurophysiology of vomiting. Baillieres Clin Gastroenterol 2(1):141–168
5. Grélot L, Milano S, Portillo F, Miller AD (1993) Respiratory interneurons of the lower cervical (C4-C5) cord: membrane potential changes during fictive coughing, vomiting, and swallowing in the decerebrate cat. Pflugers Arch 425(3–4):313–320
6. Stockhorst U, Steingrueber HJ, Enck P, Klosterhalfen S (2006) Pavlovian conditioning of nausea and vomiting. Auton Neurosci 129(1–2):50–57
7. Herrstedt J, Dombernowsky P (2007) Anti-emetic therapy in cancer chemotherapy: current status. Basic Clin Pharmacol Toxicol 101(3):143–150
8. Haniadka R, Popouri S, Palatty PL, Arora R, Baliga MS (2011) Medicinal plants as antiemetics in the treatment of cancer: a review. Integr Cancer Ther
9. Wickham R (1999) Nausea and vomiting. In: Yarbo CH, Frogge MH, Goodman M (eds) Cancer symptom management, 2nd edn. Jones and Bartlett Publishers, Sudbury, pp 228–263
10. Coates A, Abraham S, Kaye SB et al (1983) On the receiving end – patient perception of the side-effects of cancer chemotherapy. Eur J Cancer Clin Oncol 19(2):203–208, PUBMED Abstract
11. Craig JB, Powell BL (1987) The management of nausea and vomiting in clinical oncology. Am J Med Sci 293(1):34–44, PUBMED Abstract

12. Passik SD, Kirsh KL, Rosenfeld B et al (2001) The changeable nature of patients' fears regarding chemotherapy: implications for palliative care. J Pain Symptom Manage 21(2):113–120, PUBMED Abstract
13. Grunberg SM, Deuson RR, Mavros P et al (2004) Incidence of chemotherapy-induced nausea and emesis after modern antiemetics. Cancer 100(10):2261–2268, PUBMED Abstract
14. Kirkova J, Aktas A, Walsh D, Rybicki L, Davis MP (2010) Consistency of symptom clusters in advanced cancer. Am J Hosp Palliat Care 27(5):342–346
15. Glare PA, Dunwoodie D, Clark K, Ward A, Yates P, Ryan S, Hardy JR (2008) Treatment of nausea and vomiting in terminally ill cancer patients. Drugs 68(18):2575–2590
16. Rhodes VA, McDaniel RW (2001) Nausea, vomiting, and retching: complex problems in palliative care. CA Cancer J Clin 51(4):232–248
17. Collins KB, Thomas DJ (2004) Acupuncture and acupressure for the management of chemotherapy-induced nausea and vomiting. J Am Acad Nurse Pract 16(2):76–80
18. Ryan JL, Heckler CE, Roscoe JA, Dakhil SR, Kirshner J, Flynn PJ, Hickok JT, Morrow GR (2011) Ginger (*Zingiber officinale*) reduces acute chemotherapy-induced nausea: a URCC CCOP study of 576 patients. Support Care Cancer
19. Lohr L (2008) Chemotherapy-induced nausea and vomiting. Practice of oncology: recent advances. Cancer 14(2):85–93
20. Liau CT, Chu NM, Liu HE, Deuson R, Lien J, Chen JS (2005) Incidence of chemotherapy-induced nausea and vomiting in Taiwan: physicians' and nurses' estimation vs. patients' reported outcomes. Support Care Cancer 13(5):277–286, Epub 2005 Mar 16
21. Neymark N, Crott R (2005) Impact of emesis on clinical and economic outcomes of cancer therapy with highly emetogenic chemotherapy regimens: a retrospective analysis of three clinical trials. Support Care Cancer 13(10):812–818, Epub 2005 Apr 15
22. Passik SD, Kirsh KL, Theobald DE, Dickerson P, Trowbridge R, Gray D, Beaver M, Comparet J, Brown J (2003) A retrospective chart review of the use of olanzapine for the prevention of delayed emesis in cancer patients. J Pain Symptom Manage 25(5):485–488
23. Dennis K, Nguyen J, Presutti R, Deangelis C, Tsao M, Danjoux C, Barnes E, Sahgal A, Holden L, Jon F, Wong S, Chow E (2011) Prophylaxis of radiotherapy-induced nausea and vomiting in the palliative treatment of bone metastases. Support Care Cancer
24. Bruera E, Catz Z, Hooper R et al (1987) Chronic nausea and anorexia in advanced cancer patients: a possible role for autonomic dysfunction. J Pain Symptom Manage 2(1):19–21, Winter
25. Baines MJ (1998) Nausea, vomiting, and intestinal obstruction. In: Fallon M, O'Neill B (eds) ABC of palliative care. BMJ Books, London, pp 16–18
26. Stephenson J, Davies A (2006) An assessment of aetiology-based guidelines for the management of nausea and vomiting in patients with advanced cancer. Support Care Cancer 14(4):348–353
27. Pereira J, Bruera E (1996) Chronic nausea. In: Bruera E, Higginson I (eds) Cachexia-anorexia in cancer patients. Oxford University Press, New York, pp 23–37
28. Hagen NA, Foley KM, Cerbone DJ et al (1991) Chronic nausea and morphine-6-glucuronide. J Pain Symptom Manage 6(3):125–128
29. Ripamonti C, Bruera E (2002) Chronic nausea and vomiting. In: Ripamonti C, Bruera E (eds) Gastrointestinal symptoms in advanced cancer patients. Oxford University Press, New York, pp 169–174
30. Cheifetz AS, Brown A, Currey A, Moss AC (2011) Nausea and vomiting definitions and neurophysiology. American handbook of gastroenterology and hepatology. Oxford University Press, Inc., New York, pp 52–54
31. Bruera E, Suarez-Almazor M, Velasco A et al (1994) The assessment of constipation in terminal cancer patients admitted to a palliative care unit: a retrospective review. J Pain Symptom Manage 9(8):515–519
32. Derby S, Portenoy RK (1997) Assessment and management of opioid-induced constipation. In: Portenoy RK, Bruera E (eds) Topics in palliative care, vol 1. Oxford University Press, New York, pp 95–112

33. Culpepper-Morgan JA, Inturrisi CE, Portenoy RK et al (1992) Treatment of opioid-induced constipation with oral naloxone: a pilot study. Clin Pharmacol Ther 52(1):90–95
34. Sykes NP (1991) Oral naloxone in opioid-associated constipation. Lancet 337(8755):1475
35. Stockhorst U, Enck P, Klosterhalfen S (2007) Role of classical conditioning in learning gastro-intestinal symptoms. World J Gastroenterol 13(25):3430–3437, Review
36. Stockhorst U, Spennes-Saleh S, Körholz D, Göbel U, Schneider ME, Steingrüber HJ, Klosterhalfen S (2000) Anticipatory symptoms and anticipatory immune responses in pediat-ric cancer patients receiving chemotherapy: features of a classically conditioned response? Brain Behav Immun 14(3):198–218
37. Bovbjerg DH (2006) The continuing problem of post chemotherapy nausea and vomiting: contributions of classical conditioning. Auton Neurosci 129(1–2):92–98, Epub 2006 Aug 14
38. Basch E, Prestrud AA, Hesketh PJ, Kris MG, Feyer PC, Somerfield MR, Chesney M, Clark-Snow RA, Flaherty AM, Freundlich B, Morrow G, Rao KV, Schwartz RN, Lyman GH (2011) Antiemetics: American society of clinical oncology clinical practice guideline update. J Oncol Pract 7(6):395–398, Posted ahead of on www.jco.org on Sept 26
39. Watson M, Meyer L, Thomson A, Osofsky S (1998) Psychological factors predicting nausea and vomiting in breast cancer patients on chemotherapy. Eur J Cancer 34(6):831–837
40. Akechi T, Okuyama T, Endo C, Sagawa R, Uchida M, Nakaguchi T, Sakamoto M, Komatsu H, Ueda R, Wada M, Furukawa TA (2010) Anticipatory nausea among ambulatory cancer patients undergoing chemotherapy: prevalence, associated factors, and impact on quality of life. Cancer Sci 101(12):2596–2600. doi:10.1111/j.1349-7006.2010.01718.x., Epub 2010 Sep 6
41. Hamling K (2011) The management of nausea and vomiting in advanced cancer. Int J Palliat Nurs 17(7):321–327
42. Wood GJ, Shega JW, Lynch B, Von Roenn JH (2007) Management of intractable nausea and vomiting in patients at the end of life: "I was feeling nauseous all of the time… nothing was working". JAMA 298(10):1196–1207
43. Davis MP, Hallerberg G, Palliative Medicine Study Group of the Multinational Association of Supportive Care in Cancer (2010) A systematic review of the treatment of nausea and/or vom-iting in cancer unrelated to chemotherapy or radiation. J Pain Symptom Manage 39(4):756–767, Review
44. Harris DG (2010) Nausea and vomiting in advanced cancer. Br Med Bull 96:175–185, Epub 2010 Sep 30
45. Sankhala KK, Pandya DM, Sarantopoulos J, Soefje SA, Giles FJ, Chawla SP (2009) Prevention of chemotherapy induced nausea and vomiting: a focus on aprepitant. Expert Opin Drug Metab Toxicol 5(12):1607–1614
46. Ruhlmann CH, Herrstedt J (2011) Safety evaluation of aprepitant for the prevention of chemotherapy-induced nausea and vomiting. Expert Opin Drug Saf 10(3):449–462, Epub 2011 Mar 21
47. Navari RM (2009) Pharmacological management of chemotherapy-induced nausea and vomit-ing: focus on recent developments. Drugs 69(5):515–533. doi:10.2165/00003495-200969050-00002, Review
48. Billio A, Morello E, Clarke MJ (2010) Serotonin receptor antagonists for highly emetogenic chemotherapy in adults. Cochrane Database Syst Rev 20(1):CD006272
49. Brugnatelli S, Gattoni E, Grasso D, Rossetti F, Perrone T, Danova M (2011) Single-dose palonosetron and dexamethasone in preventing nausea and vomiting induced by moderately emetogenic chemotherapy in breast and colorectal cancer patients. Tumori 97(3):362–366. doi:10.1700/912.10035
50. Aapro M, Fabi A, Nolè F, Medici M, Steger G, Bachmann C, Roncoroni S, Roila F (2010) Double-blind, randomised, controlled study of the efficacy and tolerability of palonosetron plus dexamethasone for 1 day with or without dexamethasone on days 2 and 3 in the preven-tion of nausea and vomiting induced by moderately emetogenic chemotherapy. Ann Oncol 21(5):1083–1088, Epub 2010 Jan 15
51. Duggan ST, Curran MP (2009) Transdermal granisetron. Drugs 69(18):2597–2605

52. Tuca A (2009) Use of granisetron transdermal system in the prevention of chemotherapy-induced nausea and vomiting: a review. Cancer Manag Res 2:1–12
53. Salvo N, Doble B, Khan L, Amirthevasar G, Dennis K, Pasetka M, Deangelis C, Tsao M, Chow E (2012) Prophylaxis of radiation-induced nausea and vomiting using 5-hydroxytryptamine-3 serotonin receptor antagonists: a systematic review of randomized trials. Int J Radiat Oncol Biol Phys 1:82(1):408–417, Epub 2010 Nov 13
54. Mystakidou K, Kouloulias V, Nikolaou V, Tsilika E, Lymperopoulou G, Balafouta M, Kouvaris I, Kelekis A, Gouliamos A (2010) A comparative study of prophylactic antiemetic treatment in cancer patients receiving radiotherapy. J BUON 15(1):29–35
55. Zick SM, Ruffin MT, Lee J, Normolle DP, Siden R, Alrawi S, Brenner DE (2009) Phase II trial of encapsulated ginger as a treatment for chemotherapy-induced nausea and vomiting. Support Care Cancer 17(5):563–572, Epub 2008 Nov 13
56. Sharma SS, Gupta YK (1998) Reversal of cisplatin-induced delay in gastric emptying in rats by ginger (zingiber officinale). J Ethnopharmacol 62(1):49–55
57. Betz O, Kranke P, Geldner G, Wulf H, Eberhart LH (2005) Is ginger a clinically relevant antiemetic? A systematic review of randomized controlled trials. Forsch Komplementarmed Klass Naturheilkd 12(1):14–23
58. Levine ME, Gillis MG, Koch SY, Voss AC, Stern RM, Koch KL (2008) Protein and ginger for the treatment of chemotherapy-induced delayed nausea. J Altern Complement Med 14(5):545–551
59. Pillai AK, Sharma KK, Gupta YK, Bakhshi S (2011) Anti-emetic effect of ginger powder versus placebo as an add-on therapy in children and young adults receiving high emetogenic chemotherapy. Pediatr Blood Cancer 56(2):234–238. doi:10.1002/pbc.22778, Epub 2010 Sep 14
60. Taspinar A, Sirin A (2010) Effect of acupressure on chemotherapy-induced nausea and vomiting in gynecologic cancer patients in Turkey. Eur J Oncol Nurs 14(1):49–54, Epub 2009 Sep 11
61. Molassiotis A, Helin AM, Dabbour R, Hummerston S (2007) The effects of P6 acupressure in the prophylaxis of chemotherapy-related nausea and vomiting in breast cancer patients. Complement Ther Med 15(1):3–12, Epub 2006 Sep 27
62. Dibble SL, Luce J, Cooper BA, Israel J, Cohen M, Nussey B, Rugo H (2007) Acupressure for chemotherapy-induced nausea and vomiting: a randomized clinical trial. Oncol Nurs Forum 34(4):813–820
63. Garratt AM, Ruta DA, Abdalla MI, Buckingham JK, Russell IT (1993) The SF36 health survey questionnaire: an outcome measure suitable for routine use within the NHS? BMJ 306(6890):1440–1444

Cancer-Related Fatigue (CRF)

Core Messages

Cancer-related fatigue (CRF) is a disabling and distressing symptom defined as a subjective report of tiredness that is associated with cancer or its treatment, is persistent, extends in duration or severity beyond that which might be expected based on a subject's recent physical activity, and is severe enough to cause distress and interfere with usual functioning.

Patients with cancer often describe fatigue based on four physical changes: decreased physical performance, unusual or extreme tiredness, feelings of weakness, and unusual need for rest.

Fatigue in cancer patients has been reported to be accompanied by loss of drive, lack of energy, depressive mood, and loss of vigor and vitality; it is unresponsive to rest and sleep.

CRF and related symptoms can thus affect the quality of life during cancer treatment as well as survival, with effects on productivity, family functioning, as well as both physiological and psychological comorbidity. Fatigue has been reported to predict survival time of terminal cancer patients.

Fatigue is reported by as many as 40% of cancer patients at the time of diagnosis, up to 90% of those treated with radiation, and up to 80% of those treated with chemotherapy.

CRF has been observed to have a multifactorial etiology with significant individual variability in its clinical expression, determinants, and sequelae.

Although the pathogenesis of fatigue is not well understood, several physiological and psychological factors have been shown to contribute to CRF.

Physiological factors include tumor-induced and treatment-induced fatigue; other comorbidities such as anemia, heart failure, muscle-energy metabolism, and hypothyroidism; medications like opioids; and declining nutritional status.

Physiological factors include tumor-induced and treatment-induced fatigue; other comorbidities such as anemia, heart failure, muscle-energy metabolism, and hypothyroidism; medications like opioids; and declining nutritional status.

N.B. Kumar, *Nutritional Management of Cancer Treatment Effects*,
DOI 10.1007/978-3-642-27233-2_7, © Springer-Verlag Berlin Heidelberg 2012

These physiological symptoms have a significant impact on physical inactivity, cancer pain, neuroimmunologic changes, abrupt loss of steroid hormones, and insomnia including disruption of circadian rhythm sleep.

Psychological factors include depression and distress.

Environmental factors such as hospitalization and change in environment can be attributed to related psychological distress, also contributing to fatigue.

7.1   Definition

Cancer-related fatigue (CRF) is a disabling and distressing symptom defined as a subjective report of tiredness that is associated with cancer or its treatment, is persistent, extends in duration or severity beyond that which might be expected based on a subject's recent physical activity, and is severe enough to cause distress and interfere with usual functioning [1]. Fatigue has been characterized both from a psychological as well as from a physiological perspective. Patients with cancer often describe fatigue based on four physical changes: decreased physical performance, unusual or extreme tiredness, feelings of weakness, and unusual need for rest [2–4]. Fatigue in cancer patients has been reported to be accompanied by loss of drive, lack of energy, depressive mood, and loss of vigor and vitality; it is unresponsive to rest and sleep [5, 6]. The National Comprehensive Cancer Network [1] defines cancer-related fatigue (CRF) as "a persistent, subjective sense of tiredness related to cancer or cancer treatment that interferes with usual functioning." These symptoms are persistent, disproportionate to the level of exertion, and typically not relieved by rest. CRF has a multifactorial etiology, significant individual variability in its clinical expression, determinants, and sequelae [7], thus complicating standard treatment strategies and requiring individual treatment approaches for this symptom in this population. With significant impact on physical function and ability to perform activities of daily living as well as psychological distress, the impact of CRF on a cancer patient's quality of life (QOL) is profound [8–10]. Fatigue has also been reported to have an impact on the patient's ability to work and consequently may add to the financial burden of the cancer patient. These effects can extend to caregivers and family members, who may also have to reduce their working capacity in order to provide additional care for a patient with CRF [11]. CRF and related symptoms can thus affect the quality of life during cancer treatment as well as survival with effects on productivity, family functioning, as well as both physiological and psychological comorbidity. Fatigue has been reported to predict survival time of terminal cancer patients [12, 13].

7.2   Prevalence

Cancer-related fatigue (CRF) is highly prevalent across the cancer continuum from a cancer patient's diagnosis and treatment through survivorship and end of life [7]. Cancer-related fatigue (CRF) is a significant clinical problem for more than ten million adults diagnosed with cancer each year worldwide [6]. CRF is the most common symptom reported by cancer patients and survivors of cancer [13–16]. With significant differences in individual physiology, heterogeneity in terms of definition of fatigue, stage of tumor, and treatment variations, the prevalence of self-reported fatigue varies widely in this patient population. Overall, 50–90% of cancer patients experience fatigue [17–21]. A significantly greater proportion of patients are receiving chemotherapy, radiotherapy, biologic response modifiers, or antilogous transplantation [22]. Fatigue is reported by as many as 40% of cancer patients at the time of diagnosis, up to 90% of those treated with radiation, and up to 80% of those treated with chemotherapy. However, few other studies have observed no difference in level of fatigue as a function of type of treatment [13, 23]. Fatigue is common in many several types of malignancies, including breast, prostate, leukemia, and lung carcinoma, and is reported to occur in patients who do not receive treatments [21] before, during, and after therapy [15, 24, 25]. Cancer-related fatigue can also persist long after remission in about a third of survivors of cancer [11, 26, 27]. Some patients reported continued clinical levels of fatigue (40%) even 12 months postdiagnosis [28]. Objective symptoms of fatigue is reported in a large population of adult survivors of various childhood cancers, including acute lymphocytic leukemia, central nervous system tumors, Hodgkin lymphoma, soft-tissue sarcomas, and bone tumors, as compared with their siblings [29]. Patients with advanced-stage tumor report significant fatigue. Fatigue is reported in about 90% of breast cancer patients receiving radiation and chemotherapy, a common problem for breast cancer patients [30–37], regardless of whether the cancer is invasive [33], with residual fatigue often persisting for as long as 10 years after treatments [13, 26, 27]. Similarly, fatigue was present in 60% of Hodgkin's disease patients who had been free of cancer for 5 years [38]. Two fifths of men with biochemically controlled prostate cancer on long-term ADT and almost one third of recurrence-free prostate cancer survivors report CRF that interferes with function [39]. CRF is also common in cancer outpatients and is associated with type of disease and treatment, as well as with emotional distress, although not equivalent conditions [39]. In addition to neurologic symptoms, fatigue is commonly reported in patients with primary brain tumors during radiation therapy and in long-term survivors of low-grade brain tumors which may reduce daily functioning and quality of life, with sleep disturbance being a significant predictor of fatigue [40–42]. Fatigue is common among all patients receiving biological modifiers interferon or interleukin-2 [43]. Fatigue is thus a prevalent and significant problem in clinical oncology.

7.3   Etiology of Fatigue in Cancer

CRF has been observed to have a multifactorial etiology with significant individual variability in its clinical expression, determinants, and sequelae. Although the pathogenesis of fatigue is not well understood, several physiological and psychological factors have been shown to contribute to CRF. Physiological factors include tumor-induced and treatment-induced fatigue; other comorbidities such as anemia,

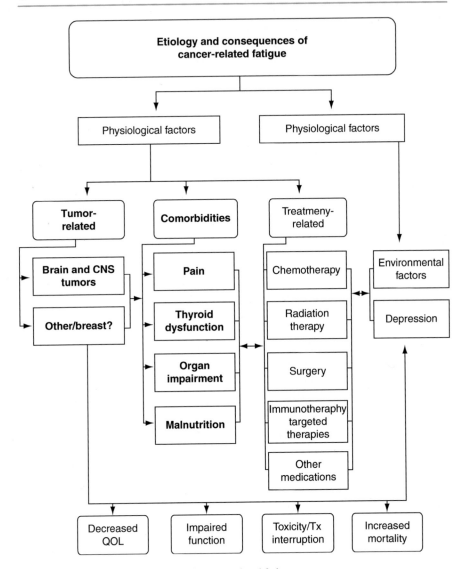

Fig. 7.1 Etiology and consequences of cancer-related fatigue

heart failure, muscle-energy metabolism, and hypothyroidism; medications like opioids; and declining nutritional status. These physiological symptoms have a significant impact on physical inactivity, cancer pain, neuroimmunologic changes, abrupt loss of steroid hormones, and insomnia including disruption of circadian rhythm sleep. Psychological factors include depression and distress. Environmental factors such as hospitalization and change in environment can be attributed to related psychological distress, also contributing to fatigue (Fig. 7.1).

7.3.1   Physiological Factors

7.3.1.1 Tumor-Related Fatigue

Fatigue is commonly reported in patients with primary brain tumors and other central nervous system tumors producing long-term disabling effects [44]. In examining the pathogenesis of fatigue, several studies have examined the mechanism of increased immune inflammatory activity specifically interleukin-6, interleukin-1 receptor antagonist, C-reactive protein, neopterin, and soluble tumor necrosis factor receptor-II [45–47] in breast and prostate cancer patients. Increased cytokines likely contribute to the symptoms of asthenia, fatigue, and lethargy, as supported in animal models of cytokine-induced sickness behavior [48, 49] and in humans [50]. Other studies demonstrate a change in the regulation of cortisol by the hypothalamic pituitary adrenal axis. One key study put fatigued and nonfatigued breast cancer survivors through a stress battery in a laboratory setting. Nonfatigued survivors mounted a significant cortisol increase in response to acute stress, while fatigued survivors had a much blunted response [51]. Others have shown that fatigued breast cancer survivors have flattened cortisol slopes, having higher levels of cortisol at the end of the day than do nonfatigued survivors [52]. It is the dysregulation of the hypothalamic-pituitary-adrenal (HPA) axis that may account for the prolonged inflammatory cytokine milieu; understanding the body's response to numerous chronic stressors in cancer may help in managing fatigue [53, 54]. To date, these concepts have not been examined in large, well-powered randomized clinical trials.

Fatigue is commonly reported in patients with primary brain tumors during radiation therapy and in long-term survivors of low-grade brain tumors which may reduce daily functioning and quality of life, with sleep disturbance being a significant predictor of fatigue [40–42, 55]. Fatigue, nausea, drowsiness, and poor appetite showed an overall increase in symptom severity over time; whereas fatigue, drowsiness, and poor appetite were experienced to some extent by a greater proportion of patients at week 12 compared with baseline in brain tumor patients demonstrating a variable incidence of these symptom clusters [55]. It has also been shown that functional impairments of organ systems and tissues affected by cancer such as brain, muscle, gut, liver, bone marrow, vasculature, lung kidneys, pancreas, thyroid, associated neurotransmitter, and hormone dysregulation contribute to CRF [12, 26, 56–58]. The association between thyroid disorders and risk of breast cancer has long been a subject of debate. Although several studies have shown the association between thyroid disease and predisposition to breast cancer [59–61], others have not shown this association [62–64]. However, most of these studies identified thyroid disease from clinical histories and medical records and therefore did not consider specific, reliable indices of thyroid function. Epidemiological studies have shown geographical variations in the prevalence of breast cancer and attribute this variation at least in part to thyroid function [65]. Japanese women suffering from Hashimoto's thyroiditis (chronic lymphocytic thyroiditis) have reportedly a fivefold increase in breast cancer risk compared to those without evidence of autoimmune thyroid disease [66]. In contrast, when the association of Hashimoto's thyroiditis and breast cancer was studied in the USA [67], this risk was not evident. Recent studies have reported an increased prevalence of antithyroid antibodies in patients with breast cancer [59]. Research has, in addition, demonstrated that clinically evident nontoxic goiter is significantly more common in breast cancer patients than in age-matched controls [61]. Thyroid dysfunction is also an important problem in patients receiving high-dose chemotherapy and bone marrow transplantation (BMT) [68]. Hypothyroidism is one of the most common forms of thyroid disorders after BMT, which is considered immune-mediated thyroid injury contributing to the development of posttransplant hypothyroidism. These thyroid hormone changes may be mediated in part by cytokines and inflammatory mediators, interfering with the peripheral conversion of T4 to T3, the active and potent thyroid hormone. Although the classic clinical spectrum of hypothyroidism with symptoms of lethargy and myxedema is well known to the practitioner, it is rarely seen in today's clinical practice [69]. In contrast, practitioners frequently see patients with very mild thyroid dysfunction. Unlike patients with overt hypothyroidism, these patients have normal levels of thyroxine and triiodothyronine and only mild elevation in thyrotropin levels. This condition is commonly termed "subclinical hypothyroidism" or "mild hypothyroidism" [69, 70]. Several pathogenic factors may explain this association. Firstly, since both breast cancer and hypothyroidism may have a genetic predisposition, the genetic association cannot be discounted. The presence of an iodine pump in both the thyroid and the breast [71] makes the association of the effect of thyroid on breast biologically plausible [72]. Clinical trials have shown a resolution of fibrocystic breast disease and breast pain in women treated with elemental iodine [73]. In a retrospective follow-up study of cancer mortality of 7,338 women, Goldman et al. [74] observed an increased cancer mortality in a subgroup of breast cancer patients with thyroid disease. Additionally, the degree of thyroid function disturbance correlates with low levels of thyroid hormones and poor prognosis in severe illnesses. Thus, the potential for the existence of mild or subclinical hypothyroidism in breast cancer patients and the progression of this mild hypothyroidism to potentially overt hypothyroidism during chemotherapy are biologically plausible and cannot be discounted. In a study to characterize symptom clusters related to chemotherapy in breast cancer patients, we observed significant increase in symptoms of fatigue, weight gain, amenorrhea, lowered physical activity, or lethargy, all of which are also clinical symptoms observed in hypothyroidism. The symptoms were progressive from baseline to end of chemotherapy and at 6 months postchemotherapy from baseline. In addition, 20–25% of the patients screened were already diagnosed with clinical hypothyroidism at diagnosis and were not included in this observational study. The high incidence of hypothyroidism observed in this patient population is significant, compared to the 4–10% observed in American women of the same age group [75]. Based on the results of our study, we hypothesize that breast cancer patients may be a subgroup of women who are at increased risk of subclinical and clinical hypothyroidism at diagnosis and prior to treatment. We are currently examining the prevalence of hypothyroidism in breast cancer patients compared to controls in a longitudinal study to characterize these phenomena further.

7.3.1.2 Treatment-Related Fatigue (Surgery, Chemotherapy, Radiation Therapy, Immunotherapy)

Tumor therapy including chemotherapy, immunotherapy, and radiotherapy have been associated with inflammation and the production of an associated array of proinflammatory and sleep-modulatory cytokines, including TNF-α, IL-1β, and IL-6 [76–79]. Chemotherapeutic drugs paclitaxel, tamoxifen, and cisplatin increase serum levels of sleep-modulatory cytokines in cancer patients [34, 80]. The effects of treatment, including surgical complications, neurotoxic effects of radiation and debility caused by chemotherapy in brain tumors and other neurological tumors have been observed to be profound with increasing severity with increasing age [44]. Surgical patients such as breast cancer patients report a high incidence of postoperative fatigue observed in clinical practice, improve with time with the exception of additional cancer treatments [81]. Chemotherapeutic agents such as taxanes cause neurotoxicity, which contribute to increased fatigue, although the interactions of neurotoxicity and fatigue can be complex and not well understood [82, 83]. Chemotherapeutic drugs paclitaxel, tamoxifen, and cisplatin increase serum levels of sleep-modulatory cytokines in cancer patients [34, 80, 83], which with other cytokines have been also associated with insomnia leading to chronic fatigue [50, 80, 84, 85]. Persistent and increased fatigue has been observed in breast cancer patients with circulating levels of inflammatory cytokines that were up to five times higher compared with those patients who did not report fatigue [86]. Altered glucocorticoid response to stress [85] has also been reported in cancer survivors with fatigue, contributing to both to altered immune activation and problems with sleep [86]. In addition to treatment with chemotherapy being a predictor of fatigue, this can be exacerbated by the symptom cluster of pain, depression, and/or anxiety [87, 88]. Additionally, since biotherapy exposes patients with cancer to exogenous and endogenous cytokines [89–91], fatigue is a dose-limiting toxicity of treatment with a variety of biotherapeutic agents.

Fatigue has also been consistently reported with radiation exposure and is reported as being one of the most common and activity-limiting side effects of radiation therapy for cancer [92–94]. Studies to date have focused on breast and prostate cancer patients receiving radiation therapy and have demonstrated, in sum, significant variability in timing of fatigue and potential contributors [94]. From these studies, it is clear that most patients report increase in fatigue increases throughout radiation therapy, peaking around midcourse; it remains at this level until radiation therapy is completed, improving somewhat during the 2 months after completion of treatment [93–99], although not all patients return to pretreatment energy levels. Cancer patients receiving radiation therapy who have older age, advanced disease, and combination-modality therapy [100] are at increased risk for fatigue.

7.3.1.3 Comorbidities

Anemia

It has been reported that over 50% of cancer patients are diagnosed with anemia which has consistently been associated with CRF [101–104] impacting quality of life in cancer patients. Rapid induction of proinflammatory cytokines seen in cancer patient populations with cancer diagnosis as well as during treatment have been hypothesized to suppress the formation of red blood cells, leading to mild or moderate anemia [105]. Most anemia in cancer patients is treated with recombinant human erythropoietin α with patients reporting increased energy and improved QOL [101, 106, 107]. Studies have demonstrated that treatment of chemotherapy-induced anemia in this patient population results in improvement of other symptom clusters leading to improved quality of life. A recent review of 18 clinical trials found statistically and clinically significant improvements in both hemoglobin and health-related QOL (particularly with regard to fatigue) in cancer patients receiving anemia treatment as compared with those receiving placebo or standard of care [81, 108]. Predictive factors include rapidity of onset, patient age, plasma-volume status, and the number and severity of comorbidities [16, 109]. In a retrospective review to understand the problem of anemia in patients receiving radiation therapy, researchers observed that anemia was prevalent in 48% of the patients initially and increased to 57% of the patients during therapy. Anemia was also more common in women than in men. However, men with prostate cancer experienced the greatest increase in anemia during radiation therapy [110, 111]. In a pilot study to investigate the levels of fatigue and cytokines during radiation therapy and determine whether there was a correlation between anemia, proinflammatory cytokines, and fatigue, the relationships among hemoglobin values, cytokines, and fatigue were examined in women diagnosed with uterine cancer. Fatigue was assessed by a self-report instrument (Multidimensional Fatigue Inventory [MFI-20]), and hemoglobin and cytokines (Il-1, Il-6, and TNF-α) were measured before, during, and after radiotherapy. Results demonstrated that the degree of fatigue increased during radiotherapy without a significant change in IL-1, IL-6, or TNF-α levels. There was no significant correlation between changes in general fatigue and the changes in IL-1 and TNF-α or hemoglobin levels. There was a significant negative correlation between the change in IL-6 and general fatigue. Researchers concluded that although pelvic radiotherapy in women with uterine cancer is associated with increased fatigue, there were no significant relationships between anemia or cytokine levels [112]. It has also been hypothesized that cancer-associated anemia may be due to a blunted erythropoietin response and/or cytokines (interleukin-1 [IL-1], IL-6, tumor necrosis factor-α [TNF-α]), which suppress erythropoiesis. With significant increases in cytokines during cancer diagnosis as well as during treatment, it may be difficult to demonstrate any significant decreases in cytokines as well as in markers of anemia in intervention trials, especially in studies during treatment in this patient population. The pathogenesis of fatigue related to anemia during cancer treatment continues to be explored and remains to be elucidated.

Hypothyroidism

It is well established that patients treated for hyperthyroidism, neck irradiation, postpartum thyroiditis, and certain autoimmune disorders are at increased risk of hypothyroidism [113]. However, the potential for the existence of mild or subclinical hypothyroidism in breast cancer patients prior to treatment and the progression of this mild hypothyroidism to potentially overt hypothyroidism during chemotherapy have never been studied. We and others have observed that breast cancer patients who undergo adjuvant chemotherapy or autologous bone marrow transplantation experience clinically significant levels of fatigue for months or even years following the completion of active treatment. Fatigue is also widely reported in the literature in patients diagnosed with hypothyroidism. As reported previously by Huntington and others [22], we observed a significant decrease in physical activity as indicated in reduction in hours of employment and purposeful physical activity per week. The decrease in activity level from fatigue may contribute to the weight gain patients experience during treatment. Patients who demonstrated a general decrease in activity level since beginning treatment gained significantly more weight than those who reported no change or an increase in activity level [114–116]. Huntington also attributes weight gain of over 10 lbs. seen in 50% of patients treated with CMF (cyclophosphamide, methotrexate, and fluorouracil) or CMFVP (CMF plus vincristine and prednisone) to a decrease in activity level during chemotherapy [4]. This reduction in physical activity may in fact be related to fatigue attributed to lowered thyroid function, as thyroid hormones play a critical role in the regulation of resting metabolic rate. If chemotherapy causes a decrease in the production or function of thyroid hormones, this may further lower metabolic rate. This effect may be even more exaggerated in women with preexisting subclinical hypothyroidism. The decrease in resting metabolic rate may contribute to lowered activity level from fatigue leading to weight gain that patients experience during treatment. Obesity, progressive weight gain, low resting energy expenditure (REE), and increased body fat percentage have been reported in hypothyroidism, including subclinical hypothyroidism [117]. Similarly, in our study, we observed a progressive significant increase in weight of 6.7 lb, even 6 months postchemotherapy. Thus, progressive weight gain, in addition to fatigue and lowered physical activity, is a common phenomenon observed both in hypothyroidism and in breast cancer patients receiving chemotherapy. Chemotherapeutic agents have been shown to cause fibrotic changes and follicular destruction in the ovaries, and pre and perimenopausal women have been observed to have reduced serum estradiol levels during chemotherapy [118–120]. Even though not clearly established, it is questionable if the abrupt menopause induced by chemotherapy can aggravate a latent predisposition toward developing thyroid dysfunction. Especially with increasing doses in adjuvant and neoadjuvant chemotherapy and combination therapies including radiation therapy, induction of subclinical hypothyroidism is a possibility. Reports have shown that women treated with thyroxine for hypothyroidism may require a higher dose of levothyroxine if they are on estrogen therapy because estrogen increases hepatic production of thyroxine-binding globulin [117, 121, 122]. Women receiving androgen therapy for breast cancer may require a reduction in levothyroxine because androgens may have the opposite effect of estrogen in the liver and decrease the hepatic production of thyroxine-binding globulin [121, 122]. More recently [123], Hamnvik et al. comprehensively reviewed the effects of newer antineoplastic agents such as targeted therapies and immunotherapies which are associated with thyroid dysfunction. These include tyrosine kinase inhibitors, bexarotene, radioiodine-based cancer therapies, denileukin diftitox, alemtuzumab, interferon-α, interleukin-2, ipilimumab, tremelimumab, thalidomide, and lenalidomide. Although higher rates are reported, most agents contribute to primary hypothyroidism on 20–50% of patients. In addition, thyrotoxicosis and effects on thyroid-stimulating hormone secretion and thyroid hormone metabolism have also been reported. Underdiagnosis of thyroid dysfunction can have important consequences for cancer patient management. Symptoms of hypothyroidism, such as fatigue, weakness, depression, memory loss, cold intolerance, and cardiovascular effects, may be incorrectly attributed to the primary disease or to the antineoplastic agent. In addition to adversely affecting the patient's quality of life, these symptoms can lead to dose reductions of potentially life-saving therapies. Hypothyroidism can also alter the kinetics and clearance of medications, which may lead to undesirable side effects. Thyrotoxicosis can be mistaken for sepsis or a nonendocrinologic drug side effect. In some patients, thyroid disease may indicate a higher likelihood of tumor response to the agent [123]. In spite of the magnitude of this problem, physicians may overlook thyroid dysfunction because of the complexity of the clinical picture in the cancer patient [123]. Both hypothyroidism and thyrotoxicosis are easily diagnosed with inexpensive and specific tests, and in many patients, particularly those with hypothyroidism, the treatment is straightforward.

Sleep Disorders
Several sleep disorders, such as difficulty falling asleep, problems maintaining sleep, poor sleep efficiency, early awakening, and excessive daytime sleepiness, are prevalent in patients with cancer (Roscoe J) contributing to CRF. Sandadi et al. reported that sleep disturbances reduce QOL, a prognostic indicator for survival, in ovarian cancer patients. Although symptoms of fatigue and sleep disorders are distinct, several studies report these symptoms as appearing in a symptom cluster in cancer patient populations and demonstrating a strong correlation between cancer-related fatigue and various sleep parameters [124–127]. Sleep disorders have been shown to clearly contribute to fatigue [126, 127] although the timing of onset of fatigue has been varied. Although the correlation between sleep patterns and fatigue are well documented, cancer-related fatigue is generally regarded as a form of tiredness that does not improve following rest or sleep, although most cancer patients may in fact not be getting a good night's sleep or report disturbed sleep. The difference in cancer-related fatigue experienced during the day may relate to sleep/wake cycles or to the quality and quantity of sleep obtained at night. Fatigue and function during treatment and posttreatment may potentially be associated to disrupted sleep and desynchronized sleep/wake rhythms. Sleep disorders in cancer patient populations are major contributors not only of fatigue but also to the cancer patients' quality of life [126, 127]. An increasing number of studies have examined circadian variation in the excretion of hormones, the sleep/wake cycle, the core body temperature rhythm, the tone of the autonomic nervous system, and the activity rhythm are important both in health and in disease processes [128] (Gögenur I). A study of patients with metastatic colorectal cancer revealed significant correlations among serum levels of IL-6, circadian patterns of activity, serum cortisol, and tumor-related symptoms, including fatigue, supporting the hypothesis that some cancer symptoms

are related to tumor- or host-generated cytokines and could reflect cytokine effects on the circadian timing system [129] explaining insomnia related to fatigue as a symptom cluster. These patients should undergo routine screening and would benefit from interventions that aim to promote restful sleep. Sandadi et al. and others have also reported that sleep disorders (SD) are associated with increased frequency of pain, depression, anxiety, and a worse sense of well-being [125–127, 129, 130].

Nutritional Status

CC is a pathological loss of striated muscle (skeletal and cardiac) and fat stores, manifesting in the cardinal features of hypermetabolism, anorexia, emaciation, weakness affecting functional status, impaired immune system, metabolic dysfunction, and poor quality of life [131–137]. Although the etiopathogenesis of CC is not fully understood, experimental and clinical studies have demonstrated that cachexia is mediated or modulated by a highly complex interplay of multiple biologic pathways, including pathological levels of proinflammatory cytokines (IL-1, IL-6, and TNF-α) [138–143], neuroendocrine hormones [135, 144], positive and negative growth factors (IGFs, PIF, myostatin) [132, 145–148], transcription factors (NF- B, STATs) [146–151], lipolytic and proteolytic enzymes (adipose triglyceride lipase, caspases, proteasome subunits) [152–155], and other signaling pathways. Loss of skeletal muscle in CC is the result of imbalance between protein synthesis and degradation [156]. Pathologic levels of proinflammatory cytokines [138–143, 157] are associated with muscle wasting, exerted through inhibition of myosin expression and myogenic differentiation and stimulation of apoptosis [141–143]. Patients with CC often describe their fatigue as a lack of energy, which could indicate that fatigue is caused by changes in metabolism and energy production, specifically in skeletal muscles [157–161]. The reduced caloric intake compounded by increased metabolic rate accompanied by loss of skeletal muscle mass contributes to fatigue in this patient population. The most prominent feature of wasting from cachexia versus starvation or anorexia is refractoriness to treatment by dietary consumption alone demonstrating a metabolic etiology. Other nutritional intake of caffeine and alcohol consumption [162, 163] have also been related to affecting sleep ultimately resulting in insomnia and fatigue in this patient population.

Physical Inactivity

Similar to metabolic changes seen in nutrition, significant changes in physical inactivity is commonly associated with cancer therapy and cachexia, contributing to fatigue. Lack of energy and feeling of tiredness are reported consistently in this patient population. Elderly cancer patients report significant levels of fatigue [164, 165] that prevents many patients from following physical activity regimens. These symptoms are accelerated in the elderly who have relatively lower steroid hormone levels as a result of "hormonal aging," lowered physical activity, as a result of treatment-related fatigue that has been demonstrated to contribute to lowered bone mineral density and muscle mass. These age-related conditions may thus be exacerbated, resulting in falls, fractures, and general muscle weakness. Muscle wasting seen in cancer cachexia is compounded by lack of physical activity observed in this patient population.

7.3.2 Medications

Apart from chemotherapeutic regimens, specific medications such as opioid analgesics, tricyclic antidepressants, neuroleptics, beta blockers, benzodiazepines, and antihistamines that produce side effects of sedation can contribute to fatigue in cancer patients. Opioid analgesics are a cornerstone of pain therapy in the hospice and palliative care of cancer patient population [13, 127, 166]. Although the degree of sedation associated with opioids used in the treatment of cancer-related pain is varied, sedated patients often report associated symptom of fatigue. Opioids have been shown to alter the normal function of the hypothalamic secretion of gonadotropin-releasing hormone [167]. Fatigue is observed in advanced cancer patients who report greater incidence of hypogonadism that may contribute to fatigue during cancer treatment [168]. In a case-control study to examine the effects of chronic oral opioid administration in survivors of cancer, consistent with the research on intrathecal administration, researchers observed marked central hypogonadism among the opioid users with significant symptoms of sexual dysfunction, depression, and fatigue [169]. Additionally, concurrent use of other medications such as analgesics, hypnotics, antidepressants, antiemetics, steroids, or anticonvulsants – many of which act on the central nervous system – can significantly exacerbate symptoms of fatigue.

7.3.3 Psychological Factors

7.3.3.1 Depression

As the concept of distress as the sixth vital sign gains strength in cancer care, more interesting evaluation, characterizing, and treating this symptom have become critical [28]. Depression has continued to be identified as a strong predictor of fatigue in cancer patients, including those whose fatigue persists long after treatment [170, 171]. Psychologic and symptom distress have also been found to be significant predictors of fatigue [170–173]. Depression can be a comorbid, disabling syndrome that affects approximately 15–25% of persons with cancer [174]. Others have reported continued clinical levels of distress (29%), pain (19%), and fatigue (40%) 12 months postdiagnosis in cancer patients [28]. Anxiety and depression are the most common comorbid psychiatric disorders of CRF [175]. Often, fatigue is the final common pathway for a range of physical and emotional etiologies. It is believed that since depression is manifested by loss of interest, difficulty concentrating, lethargy, and feelings of hopelessness, this can compound the physical causes for fatigue in these individuals and persist long past the time when physical causes have resolved [37]. Anxiety, fear, and distress related to cancer diagnosis, treatment, long-term effects in addition to recurrence of disease are identified sources of depression in this patient population that contribute to physical and psychological fatigue [176–178]. In testicular cancer survivors, anxiety and depression were predictive of fatigue, suggesting a possible role for psychiatric intervention in fatigue management [179].

In a large population–based study of the prevalence of depressive symptoms and major depression 3–4 months following surgery for breast cancer and to identify clinical risk factors while adjusting for precancer sociodemographic factors, comorbidity, and psychiatric history [180], Christensen et al. reported an increased prevalence of depressive symptoms and major depression (13.7%) compared to population-based samples. The precancer variables: social status, net wealth, ethnicity, comorbidity, psychiatric history, and age were all independent risk factors for depressive symptoms. Of the clinical variables, only nodal status carried additional prognostic information. Physical functioning, smoking, alcohol use, and BMI were also independently associated with depressive symptoms. Inflammatory cytokines have been linked to serotonin dysregulation, fatigue, and depression [180, 181]. For example, administration of the cytokine interferon-α as a cancer chemotherapeutic agent causes anorexia and fatigue that are not easily controlled with antidepressant medication [42, 182, 183]. A weighted meta-analysis of cancer studies measuring inflammatory markers and fatigue showed significant positive correlation between fatigue and circulating levels of IL-6, IL-1 receptor antagonist, and neopterin but not IL-1β or TNF-α [184]. Level of depression at radiation therapy initiation predicted the level of morning fatigue during the course of radiation therapy [94]. In a study to prospectively examine cancer patients' physical and psychosocial concerns over the year following diagnosis, levels of distress, pain, fatigue, depression, and anxiety were monitored over a year. A total of 877 patients provided baseline data with 620, 589, and 505 retained at 3, 6, and 12 months, respectively. Although the overall levels of distress, depression, and anxiety decreased significantly over the study period, no significant changes were found in levels of pain or fatigue. Some of the factors that predicted increased depression and fatigue were demographics (being unmarried), and medical interventions (particularly having radiation therapy) predicted persistent distress, anxiety, and depression, whereas receiving psychosocial support predicted decreased levels of distress, anxiety, and depression [28]. Depression is a major contributing factor of fatigue in breast cancer population, irrespective of disease stage. Time since diagnosis and treatment modalities attributed to body image impairment from mastectomy and sexuality aftermath generate higher rates of mood disorders leading to impaired quality of life such as fatigue, cognitive attitudes of helplessness/hopelessness, and resignation [175]. However, it is also clear that the prevalence of depression appears to be especially elevated in patients with advanced cancer [185]. In a study of 101 women about to undergo surgery for breast cancer, younger age, presurgery distress, and expectations about fatigue significantly predicted fatigue levels 1 week after surgery. In the regression model, age, distress, and expectancy each uniquely contributed to fatigue, with distress and expectancy accounting for 25% of the variance [172]. In a longitudinal study with women who had gynecologic cancer, symptom, and psychologic distress significantly predicted fatigue before, during, and after treatment with chemotherapy, explaining up to 80% of the variance in fatigue scores after chemotherapy treatment [173]. Research to examine the prevalence and correlates of fatigue and depression and their relevance to health-related quality of life in 1,933 breast cancer survivors recruited from five large hospitals in Korea demonstrated that 66.1%

reported moderate to severe fatigue and 24.9% reported moderate to severe depression. Risk factors common to both fatigue and depression were lower income, dyspnea, insomnia, appetite loss, constipation, and arm symptoms. Risk factors for fatigue only included younger age, employment, presence of gastrointestinal disease, and pain, and having a musculoskeletal disease was identified as a risk factor for depression only. It was also observed that both fatigue and depression were influenced by sociodemographic factors, comorbidity, and symptom characteristics rather than cancer- or treatment-related factors. Kim [39] CRF is common in cancer of outpatients with colorectal, breast, gynecological, genitourinary, sarcoma, melanoma, and miscellaneous tumors and is associated with type of disease and treatment, as well as with emotional distress. The association between CRF and emotional distress is strong, but they are not equivalent conditions Storey [38]. It has also been observed that patients who survive cancer eventually experience less interaction with a medical team, decreased emotional support, and perhaps fear of cancer recurrence; such factors have been linked to increased depression and fatigue [186–192]. Based on these studies, it is clear that both fatigue and depression may co-occur in cancer patient populations and have a significant impact on health-related quality of life well beyond completion of treatment for cancer [40].

7.3.4   Environmental Factors

Environmental factors such as hospitalization, change in environment, and patient burden with regard to serial treatment burden have also been observed clinically to increase fatigue in the cancer patient.

7.4   Current Treatment Approaches

Since CRF has a multifactorial psychopathological etiology, intervention strategies are provided by collaborative, interdisciplinary teams of medical oncologists, psychologists, nutritionists, exercise physiologist/physical therapists, and psychosocial workers. In patients with brain tumors, additional team members would include physiatrists, in interdisciplinary collaboration with the pertinent oncology-related services, managing specific symptoms including fatigue, headache, and sleep disturbance and medical complications including depression, seizures, and thromboembolic disease [44]. The National Comprehensive Cancer Network guidelines recommend that integrative nonpharmacologic behavioral interventions be implemented for the effective management of CRF. These types of interventions may include exercise, psychosocial support, stress management, energy conservation, nutritional therapy, sleep therapy, and restorative therapy [1, 193, 194]. Pharmacological as well as nonpharmacological approaches or a combination of both approaches have been used to treat symptoms of fatigue by systematically assessing etiology of fatigue and first treating the treatable conditions that may be contributing to this symptom. Although several multidisciplinary approaches have been evaluated, no "gold standard" treatment presently exists for CRF.

7.4.1   Assessment of Etiology of Fatigue

Fatigue and the symptoms of fatigue may be assessed comprehensively in the clinical setting using fatigue symptom inventories that help clinicians characterize these symptoms and identify the etiology of fatigue. Upon identifying fatigue in the cancer patient population, continuous and periodic reassessment is recommended, especially with changing treatment regimens and patient status [193]. Since advanced fatigue is difficult to treat, the early recognition and formal assessment of this symptom is important in order to be able to treat it, before it negatively impacts the patient's quality of life [195]. Several tools to measure fatigue in cancer patient populations have been validated by international groups of scientists and clinicians, although none are diagnostic. A thorough diagnosis of fatigue can be made by thoroughly interviewing patient and family members in clinical settings along with the use of instruments to specifically characterize fatigue. These tools range from quick and simple scales such as the Visual Analog Scale (VAS) and Brief Fatigue Inventory (BFI) [196–198] (4,16,30 of Campos), a three-item fatigue scale taken from the European Organization for Research and Treatment of Cancer Core Quality of Life Questionnaire [199], to others such as the Piper Fatigue Scale (PFS) and the Brief Fatigue Inventory (BFI) [40], M. D. Anderson Symptom Inventory-Brain Tumor Module [41], Multidimensional Fatigue Inventory (MFI-20) [112] and Short Form 36 version 2 [200].to evaluate fatigue in cancer patient populations. The diagnosis of fatigue is made after eliminating comorbidities that are treatable such as hypothyroidism, pain, anemia, sleep disturbance, depression or emotional distress, and other organ dysfunctions such as myopathy, heart failure, or pulmonary fibrosis [201, 202]. Once comorbidities are addressed and none are present and patients are identified to be experiencing fatigue, patients can be screened using the tools available such as the Visual Analog Scale (VAS) or the Brief Fatigue Inventory (BFI) for assessment of fatigue in a clinical setting, or the Multidimensional Fatigue Inventory (MFI-20) has been validated as a comprehensive tool for evaluation of fatigue in cancer patient populations. If patient has no fatigue or has mild fatigue or is anticipated to become fatigued, based on treatments planned, nonpharmacological interventions and prophylactic measures to prevent onset may be considered. If patient is diagnosed with moderate and severe fatigue, both pharmacological and nonpharmacological approaches may be beneficial to ameliorate CRF. Continuous and periodic reassessment is recommended for all patients, especially with changing treatment regimens and patient status [194].

7.4.2   Pharmacological Approaches/Treating Comorbidities

Today, there are no single pharmacological approaches to treat CRF. Based on initial screening, identification and treatment of comorbidities contributing to fatigue, such as anemia, hypothyroidism, pain, emotional distress, insomnia, malnutrition, and other comorbid conditions has been recommended as the first step prior to evaluating cancer patients for fatigue. However, even with treatment of clinical comorbidities, several patients continue to experience fatigue for which additional therapeutic strategies may be required [193]. In addition, although depression, cancer cachexia, hypothyroidism, and insomnia are associated with numerous negative consequences including fatigue, these disorders remain underdiagnosed and undertreated [175, 185]. The best evidence for the treatment of fatigue is for pharmacologic measures that have been studied in cancer patients with fatigue include hematopoietics such as erythropoietin (EPA) and darbepoetin to treat anemic patients on chemotherapy [16, 101–103, 107, 199] and stimulants such as donepezil, modafinil, methylphenidate, and agents to improve sleep [195, 202–204]. Although EPA has shown promise in treating anemia, several concerns for use, such as risk of thromboembolic events, especially in patients diagnosed with multiple myeloma treated with thalidomide or lenalidomide, have led to specific guidelines for use in cancer patient populations. EPA use is to be avoided in patients with anemia not related to chemotherapy, and that they be instituted only in those patients with a hemoglobin <10 g/dL with a target level not to exceed 12 g/dL [205–207].

Among traditional psychostimulants, methylphenidate has been studied the most and is effective and well tolerated among patients with cancer despite common side effects. Modafinil, a novel psychostimulant commonly referred to as wakefulness-promoting agents as a group, has also been studied and seems to be well tolerated among patients with cancer. Some preliminary data support using modafinil for patients with CRF. Bupropion sustained release may have psychostimulant-like effects and, therefore, may be beneficial in treating fatigue. Donepezil, a cholinesterase inhibitor, has shown benefit only in open-label trials. Randomized, placebo-controlled trials with specific agents are needed to further assess the efficacy and tolerability of psychotropic medications in CRF treatment [8]. Although these approaches demonstrate promise, further evaluation in large-scale randomized clinical trials is needed to further assess the efficacy and tolerability of psychostimulants in the treatment of cancer-related fatigue [8, 199, 208]. Similarly, both hypothyroidism and thyrotoxicosis are easily diagnosed with inexpensive and specific tests. In many patients, particularly those with hypothyroidism, the treatment is straightforward. Routine testing for thyroid abnormalities in patients receiving these antineoplastic agents is therefore recommended [115, 123].

It is clear that both fatigue and depression may co-occur in cancer patient populations and have a significant impact on health-related quality of life well beyond completion of treatment for cancer, although the severity of fatigue may differ [188]. This concurrent examination of risk factors for fatigue and depression may be helpful in the development of clinical management strategies in disease-free breast cancer survivors [40]. For some patients, distress, depression, and anxiety may be transient and decrease over time, but for others, they may be sustained. Pain and fatigue may remain present in many cancer patients. It has also been recognized that both fatigue and depression may improve in response to the same therapy [28]. For example, psychologic and educational intervention focused on coping with common fears improved fatigue, energy, cancer-specific distress, fatigue and depression in cancer survivors [209]. Similar potential treatment for both depression and fatigue is light therapy, which both strengthens diurnal rhythms and improves mood [210].

Treatment of depression in breast cancer women improves their quality of life and may increase longevity. Antidepressant medications remain the cornerstone of depression treatment. The hypothetical link between their prescription and increased breast cancer risk is not supported by literature's data [175]. Risk factors for depressive symptoms were primarily restricted to precancer conditions rather than disease-specific conditions. Special attention should be given to socioeconomically deprived women with a history of somatic and psychiatric disease and poor health behaviors [180]. In a study to examine self-regulatory fatigue in a cancer population, Solberg et al. [211] demonstrated that controlling for pain severity, physical fatigue, and depression, self-regulatory fatigue scores were incrementally associated with decreased quality of life, use of avoidance coping strategies, and decreased adherence to physicians' recommendations. These results emphasize the potential role of self-regulatory capacity in coping with and adjusting to hematologic cancers [211]. Antidepressants to treat depression have been used to treat depression successfully in cancer patients. However, antidepressants for the treatment of fatigue have shown mixed results. Paroxetine shows benefit for fatigue, primarily when it is a symptom of clinical depression [199].

7.4.3   Nonpharmacological Approaches

The National Comprehensive Cancer Network guidelines recommend that integrative nonpharmacologic behavioral interventions be implemented for the effective management of CRF based on best practice standards. These types of interventions may include exercise, psychosocial support, stress management, energy conservation, nutritional therapy, sleep therapy, and restorative therapy [1].

7.4.3.1   Physical Activity Regimens/Rehabilitative Services
Since cancer patients often demonstrate diminished physical and functional well-being as compared with patients not receiving treatment [30, 212], it is logical to plan intervention programs that are targeted to improve strength and cardiovascular conditioning and reduce pain and fatigue after treatment [213]. Several interventional programs using exercise program of moderate intensity, individualized to the patient's specific needs, have been shown to reduced fatigue significantly both during and after cancer treatment [214].

In a comprehensive combined systematic and meta-analytic review of the literature to date on nonpharmacological (psychosocial and exercise) interventions to ameliorate CRF and associated symptoms (vigor/vitality) in adults with cancer, based on 119 randomized controlled trials (RCTs) and non-RCT studies, Kangas et al. [6] observed that multimodal exercise and walking programs, restorative approaches, supportive-expressive, and cognitive-behavioral psychosocial interventions show promising potential for ameliorating CRF. The results also suggest that vigor and vitality are distinct phenomena from CRF with regard to responsiveness to intervention [6]. Although exercise programs during adjuvant treatment for breast cancer can be regarded as a supportive self-care intervention which results in improved physical fitness and thus the capacity for performing activities of daily life, which may otherwise be impaired due to inactivity during treatment, studies have been ambiguous as they related to improvements in fatigue. Although the investigator argued for incorporating strategies for behavior change in future studies [212, 215], they should, in addition, take into account underlying metabolic abnormalities seen in this patient population and co-occurring symptoms of cancer.

Benign or low-grade brain tumors can cause significant disability, and since brain tumors occur over the life span, patient demonstrate progressively higher incidence of fatigue and disability with advancing age. Evidence for effectiveness of rehabilitation is favorable. Brain tumor patients treated in acute rehabilitation settings improve comparably with individuals with stroke or traumatic brain injury. Although patients with primary brain tumors have been better studied than those with metastatic disease, significant gains with inpatient rehabilitation have been reported in the latter group also. Although better screening methods need to be identified to screen this patient population over the course of the disease process, outpatient programs to address cognitive deficits in brain tumor survivors, including cognitive therapy and pharmacologic strategies, have been beneficial. While the patient is receiving rehabilitation care, physiatrists, in interdisciplinary collaboration with the pertinent oncology-related services, assist with managing symptoms including fatigue, headache, and sleep disturbance and medical complications including depression, seizures, and thromboembolic disease [44].

Patients treated with hematopoietic SCT (HSCT) exhibit various side effects that have a profound impact on a patient's life both physically and psychologically. To examine if a controlled exercise program right from the beginning of the conditioning phase could help contribute to a patient's physical and psychological recovery, Baumann et al. [216] reported significant differences in favor of the training group regarding strength, endurance, lung function, and quality of life. Baumann et al. [216] further evaluated the influence of a controlled moderate exercise program starting parallel to chemotherapeutic conditioning and total body irradiation on the patient's physical and psychological constitution. Results indicated significant differences, and/or trends in favor of the exercise group were observed regarding the primary endpoint endurance performance, muscular strength, fatigue, and emotional state without posing an additional risk for the individual. In a comprehensive review evaluating the evidence of randomized controlled studies which examined exercise during medical treatment and in the aftercare of a prostate cancer disease, Baumann et al. [216] also observed that incontinence, fitness, fatigue, body constitution, and also quality of life can be improved by clinical exercise in patients during and after prostate cancer and that "supervised exercise" is more effective than "nonsupervised exercise." Similar results were reported by other investigators based on a systematic review to evaluate exercise in reducing symptoms of fatigue in prostate cancer patients [217, 218]. Although evidence on the effectiveness of progressive exercise training on muscle strength is promising as the basis to improve symptoms of fatigue, the effects on fatigue and functioning continue to be ambiguous. However, the overall benefit is to improve functional capacity and overall quality of life, especially if initiated at the start of therapy rather than later during therapy.

7.4.3.2 Sleep Therapy

Disrupted sleep, poor sleep hygiene, decreased nighttime sleep or excessive daytime sleep, and inactivity may be causative or contributing factors in CRF [31, 127, 162]. Several studies have examined whether CRF experienced during the day relates to sleep/wake cycles or to the quality and quantity of sleep obtained at night. Although CRF does not improve following rest or sleep, objectively recorded sleep and biological rhythms have not been well investigated in these patients, but it appears that most cancer patients may in fact not be getting a good night's sleep. Thus, in cancer patients, sleep that is inadequate or unrefreshing may be important not only to the expression of fatigue, but to the patients' quality of life and their tolerance to treatment, and may influence the development of mood disorders and clinical depression [31, 127]. Using the Piper Integrated Fatigue Model which describes sleep/wake, activity/rest, circadian rhythms, and fatigue and how they interrelate in women with breast cancer, Berger and Mitchell [127] evaluated the feasibility of an intervention designed to promote sleep and modify fatigue during four cycles of adjuvant breast cancer chemotherapy. Each woman developed, reinforced, and revised an individualized sleep promotion plan (ISPP) with four components: sleep hygiene, relaxation therapy, stimulus control, and sleep restriction techniques. A daily diary, the Pittsburgh Sleep Quality Index, a wrist actigraph, and the Piper Fatigue Scale were used to collect data 2 days before and 7 days after each treatment [127]. Results indicated significant relationships between subjective and objective sleep but no consistent patterns. Higher total and subscale fatigue scores were correlated with most components of poorer subjective sleep quality [127]. The intervention was feasible, adherence rates improved over time, and most sleep and wake patterns were consistent with normal values. It was clear that more research is needed to better characterize and develop nonpharmacological interventions to treat sleep disturbances in cancer patients [127, 162]. The basic principle underlying sleep therapy in ameliorating symptoms of fatigue is to contribute to energy conservation and serves a restorative function.

7.4.3.3 Psychosocial Support

Several strategies to improve fatigue using psychological approaches such as health education, enhanced problem solving skills, stress management, psychosocial support, group support to improve mood and coping response, psychotherapy and tailored behavioral interventions have shown promise in reducing symptoms of fatigue and related symptoms [219–228]. Patient education about symptoms that can be anticipated and providing strategies to manage symptoms proactively has been the single most important component of treating patients with CRF. Additionally, since the treatment of established fatigue is more complex and presents a challenge to the medical team, anticipating and prevention of significant fatigue may be a prudent approach. The goal of psychosocial support is provide support, provide tools to manage stress, and proactively educate patients with regard to anticipated symptoms that they may experience, while providing strategies to cope with these scenarios. Patients have been educated, and an open discussion about common symptoms experienced by cancer patients must be initiated. Discussions about these symptoms and any support that can be provided must be offered and continued throughout treatment and posttreatment periodically and as needed. Barriers and facilitators for managing symptoms due to fatigue and other symptoms must be discussed. Factors such as impediments due to personal, family, caregiver, or insurance issues that could interfere with symptom management must be discussed and resolved. Patients must be educated on reporting symptoms and not take for granted that these symptoms are a part of cancer treatment. If indicated, patients should be referred to a psychologist for further therapy. Interventions such as group therapy, individual counseling [219–222], relaxation training and stress reduction [223–227], cognitive behavioral therapy and supportive interventions [223–227] have demonstrated promising results in cancer patients during treatment. In a systematic review of randomized controlled trials (RCTs) included to evaluate effectiveness of psychosocial interventions in adult cancer patients during treatment, with fatigue as an outcome measure, 27 studies with a total of 3,324 participants were included. Seven studies reported significant effects of the psychosocial intervention on fatigue with three studies reporting that the effect was maintained at follow-up [228]. Most aspects of the included studies were heterogeneous, and therefore it could not be established which other types of interventions or elements were essential in reducing fatigue. Overall, there is limited evidence that psychosocial interventions during cancer treatment are effective in reducing fatigue.

7.4.3.4 Nutritional Support and Counseling

Metabolic disorders of protein, lipids, hypermetabolism, and electrolyte and mineral imbalances are commonly observed in cancer patients. Since cancer cachexia and cancer anorexia are also symptoms that can lead to skeletal muscle loss contributing to fatigue, it may be prudent to ensure that to conserve energy, meet increase nutritional needs, nutritional interventions can contribute to restorative therapy in ameliorating symptoms of CRF in clinical settings. In addition, caffeinated beverages and alcohol can interfere with sleep patterns, and patient should be instructed to vary timing of intake or avoid these beverages to improve symptoms of sleep disturbance. Our team has demonstrated success in improving functional scores and physical activity scores in cancer patients on cytotoxic therapies by treating cancer cachexia [229].

7.5   Guidelines

The evaluation of CRF is a multidisciplinary endeavor. Multiple, systematic assessment and approaches are currently followed in various institutions around the world. Although several multidisciplinary approaches have been evaluated, no "gold standard" treatment presently exists for CRF. The following guidelines are considered best practice standards. Improved management of CRF may require a *multimodal approach by multidisciplinary teams*. Since CRF has a multifactorial psychopathological etiology, interventions strategies should be provided by collaborative, interdisciplinary teams of medical oncologists, psychologists, nutritionists, exercise physiologist/physical therapists, and psychosocial workers. In patients with brain tumors, additional team members should include physiatrists, in interdisciplinary collaboration with the pertinent oncology-related services, managing specific symptoms including fatigue, headache, and sleep disturbance and medical complications including depression, seizures, and thromboembolic disease. A systematic approach to managing cancer patients with CRF should include specific and comprehensive assessment, determining the etiology of CRF, screening for and treating preexisting comorbidities, and identifying pharmacological and nonpharmacological approaches that have demonstrated evidence to reduce or ameliorate symptoms of fatigue, in addition to monitoring and closely assessing patients for change in status. All assessment and reassessment should be conducted continuously, taking into consideration change in medications and medical status of the cancer patient. Patient education about symptoms that can be anticipated and providing strategies to manage symptoms proactively has been the single most important component of treating patients with CRF.

7.5.1 Comprehensive Assessment

A comprehensive assessment by a multidisciplinary team including an MD, RD, Pharm.D, RNs, PT, psychiatrists, and psychosocial workers must include physical assessment and subjective information of CRF, including timing of fatigue. Patients as well as family members and care givers must be included in a comprehensive interview to assess fatigue. If sleep therapists are available, they should be included in initial assessment, therapy, and follow-up of the patient with fatigue.

- The first step in assessing fatigue should include screening for other comorbidities such as thyroid abnormalities, anemia in patients receiving these antineoplastic agents, pain, emotional distress, insomnia, and other comorbid conditions that can be identified and treated proactively.
- If patients are identified as having hypothyroidism, evaluate further for both hypothyroidism and thyrotoxicosis and treat for this disorder.
- If patient is anemic, evaluate further and treat with hematopoietics such as erythropoietin (EPA) and darbepoetin. For treatment of anemia. Caution: risk of thromboembolic events, especially in patients diagnosed with multiple myeloma treated with thalidomide or lenalidomide; EPA use is to be avoided in patients with anemia not related to chemotherapy, and that they be instituted only in those patients with a hemoglobin <10 g/dL with a target level not to exceed 12 g/dL.
- If patient is evaluated as being depressed, antidepressant can be used for the treatment of fatigue. Paroxetine shows benefit for fatigue, primarily when it is a symptom of clinical depression.
- If patient reports pain and is treated with opioids, this factor must be taken into consideration as a contributor of fatigue, although the opioids are provided for the treatment of pain.
- All patients must be evaluated periodically for change in status and treatment plan revised accordingly.

Once comorbidities are addressed and none are present and patients are identified to be experiencing fatigue, patients can be screened using the tools available such as the Visual Analog Scale (VAS) or the Brief Fatigue Inventory (BFI) for assessment of fatigue in a clinical setting, or the Multidimensional Fatigue Inventory (MFI-20) has been validated as a comprehensive tool for evaluation of fatigue in cancer patient populations.

If patient has no fatigue or has mild fatigue or is anticipated to become fatigued, based on treatments planned, nonpharmacological interventions and prophylactic measures to prevent onset may be considered.

If patient is diagnosed with moderate and severe fatigue, both pharmacological and nonpharmacological approaches may be beneficial to ameliorate CRF.

Continuous and periodic reassessment is recommended for all patients, especially with changing treatment regimens and patient status.

7.5.2   Pharmacological Interventions

- The best evidence for the treatment of fatigue is for pharmacologic measures that have been studied in cancer patients with fatigue.
- Screen for other comorbidities such as thyroid abnormalities, anemia in patients receiving these antineoplastic agents, pain, emotional distress, insomnia, and other comorbid conditions that can be identified and treated proactively.
- Evaluate patient for use of psychostimulants such as donepezil, modafinil, and methylphenidate.

7.5.3   Nonpharmacological Interventions

In spite of evidence demonstrating efficacy of pharmacological interventions, several patients continue to report persistent fatigue. Additionally, since the treatment of established fatigue is more complex and presents a challenge to the medical team, anticipating and prevention of significant fatigue may be a prudent approach. Nonpharmacological approaches focus on improving physical strength, energy conservation, and nutritional status with adequate proteins to ensure that fatigue is not exacerbated as a result of poor physical fitness and strength levels as well as compromised nutritional status. Nonpharmacological approach includes psychosocial support to provide support, provide tools to manage stress, and proactively educate patients with regard to anticipated symptoms that they may experience, while providing strategies to cope with these scenarios.

7.5.3.1 Physical Activity
If fatigue is diagnosed at initial assessment or anticipated to result from treatment, patients should be proactively receiving a comprehensive assessment of physical status by a licensed physical therapist and therapy initiated within 24 h

of assessment. The basic principles are to enhance activity level and energy conservation and to improve muscle strength.

1. *Godin Leisure-Time Exercise Questionnaire* weekly to monitor physical activity.
2. *Handgrip strength dynamometry assessment*: A validated tool commonly used to assess handgrip strength is the Jamar dynamometer, which is a fast, reliable, and easy-to-perform device commonly used by our team to measure improvements in functional strength [98]. The Jamar dynamometer has a lower % coefficient of variation and is thus a more precise device than other handgrip dynamometers.
3. Cardiovascular exercises as well as strength training exercises must be recommended.
4. Multidimensional Fatigue Inventory (MFI-20) may be administered on a monthly basis to monitor change in fatigue scores.
5. Patient's ability and choice of physical activity regimen must be taken into account while planning regimen.
6. Printed instructions, activity records, and monitors such as wrist actigraphy or pedometers have been found to be motivating to the patient in clinical settings.

7.5.3.2 Nutritional Guidelines

Nutritional assessment must be performed within 24 h of admission of the patient by a registered dietitian. The primary goal is to maintain adequacy of nutritional intake in a time of increased need and provide additional support during strength training. A 3-day diet record including 1 weekend day can be used to assess nutritional intake.

1. Screen patient within 24 h of admission. This order for screening has been a standard order for all cancer patient admissions to avoid delay in timing of screening.
2. Assess all symptoms. Gastrointestinal tract: Taste alterations, smell alterations, dysphagia, dyspnea, other pain, early satiety, dry mouth, too much saliva production, anorexia, diarrhea, constipation, nausea, vomiting, dehydration, fatigue, height weight, recent weight loss, and anthropometrics. Others: (mid-arm muscle circumference, body composition [DEXA]), grip strength, psychosocial and family/caregiver support, depression, and ADL.
3. Screen and assess current nutritional status and estimate caloric, protein, and multivitamin/mineral needs (refer to Chap. 2).
4. Provide adequate nutrition by including "calorie" and "protein" boosters education material and nutritional supplements to ensure intake of proteins (recommended 0.8 g–1.0 g/kg/day). Provide dense caloric supplements up to 400 cal/day containing 1.5 kcal/mL; if intake is insufficient in protein intake, supplement with modular protein supplements, adding this to favorite beverage. (http://www.nestle-nutrition.com/Products/Default.aspx; http://abbottnutrition.com/) The choice of nutritional supplements can be based on the personal choice of the patient, patient needs, tolerance to product as well as other comorbidities.
5. Include a standard multivitamin/mineral supplementation to prevent any further deficits and meet increased needs.

6. Assess adequacy of intake and provide an appetite stimulant (megestrol acetate 20 mg–800 mg/day or alternate) if patient has cancer anorexia to ensure adequate intake and prevent further weight loss.
7. Provide each patient with nutritional guidelines to ensure adequate intake of calories and proteins and a list of suggested high-caloric and high-protein nutritional supplements to choose from, taking into consideration taste alterations, early satiety, nausea, and vomiting that are common symptoms observed in this patient population.
8. Proactive measures to provide alternate mode of nutritional support must be planned during acute phase of treatment when it would be a greater risk to feed patient via the oral route. Selection of route of feeding may be informed based on general guidelines and criteria provided in Table 2.6.
9. Other tips to better nutritional intake:
   (a) To avoid disturbances in sleep patterns, refrain from caffeinated beverages like coffee, tea, or sodas.
   (b) Avoid alcoholic beverages which also may contribute to sleep disturbances.

7.5.3.3 Psychosocial Support

A psychosocial assessment must be performed within 24 h of admission of the patient by a licensed psychosocial worker. The goal of psychosocial support is to provide support, provide tools to manage stress, and proactively educate patients with regard to anticipated symptoms that they may experience, while providing strategies to cope with these scenarios.

1. An assessment of psychosocial needs of the patient must be completed in addition to the assessment for depression.
2. Patients should be educated and an open discussion about common symptoms experienced by cancer patients must be initiated.
3. Discussions about these symptoms and any support that can be provided must be offered and continued throughout treatment and posttreatment periodically and as needed.
4. Barriers and facilitators for managing symptoms due to fatigue and other symptoms must be discussed.
5. Factors such as impediments due to personal, family, caregiver, or insurance issues that could interfere with symptom management must be discussed and resolved.
6. Patients must be educated on reporting symptoms and not take for granted that these symptoms are a part of cancer treatment.
7. If indicated, patients should be referred to a psychologist for further therapy.

7.5.3.4 Sleep Therapy

- Patients should be assessed for sleep disturbances.
- If patient has insomnia, patients should be treated with agents to improve sleep.
- Behaviors to improve sleep hygiene, relaxation therapy, stimulus control, and sleep restriction techniques have been found to have some success in improving sleep.

7.5.3.5 Markers and Instruments for Patient Monitoring and Assessment of Response to Treatment by the Interdisciplinary Medical Team

1. *Anthropometric measurements* such as participant's height, weight, and body mass index will be performed at baseline, 6 and 12 weeks, using methods previously described and validated by our group [81, 82]. Skeletal muscle function is a central determinant of functional capacity in humans. Loss of muscle as seen in CC results in poor function and decreased survival rate following critical illness [83]. Muscle size is therefore considered an important marker of functional status in studies of sarcopenia/cachexia [80].

2. *Body composition by DXA scan*: DXA should be used to assess both total lean body mass (LBM), fat mass (FM), and total bone mineral density (BMD).Total bone mineral density (BMD) is a valid indirect measure of skeletal muscle and patient activity. Total LBM is sometimes called total fat-free mass (FFM) depending upon specific DXA manufacturer. DXA instruments use an X-ray source that generates or is split into two energies to measure bone mineral mass and soft tissue from which fat and fat-free mass are estimated. The exam is quick (1–2 min), precise (0.5–1%) and noninvasive. DXA scanners have the precision required to detect changes in muscle mass as small as 5%. Radiation exposure from DXA scans is minimal. The National Council of Radiation Protection and Measurements (NCRP) has recommended that the annual effective dose limit for infrequent exposure of the general population is 5,000 μSv and that an annual effective dose of 10 μSv be considered a negligible individual dose. The effective dose of a dual-energy X-ray absorptiometry whole body scan on an adult is 2.1 μSv. Studies have shown that quality assurance is an important issue in the use of DXA scans to determine body composition including lean body mass and bone mineral density. DXA instrument manufacturer and model should remain consistent, and their calibration should be monitored throughout treatment. Use of a standardized scan acquisition protocol and appropriate and unchanging scan acquisition and analysis software is essential to achieve consist results.

3. *Dietary intake* must be assessed at baseline and monthly by conducting random weekly, 2-week days + 1 weekend day 24-h dietary recalls (gold standard for collecting dietary data) using a 5-step multipass procedure [30, 31] (which has been found to assess mean energy intake within 10% of actual intake) and using the frequently updated University of Minnesota Nutrition Data System for Research (NDS-R) version database for analysis of nutrient composition. Food portion visuals will be provided to study participants and protocols are established for training dietary interviewers and meticulous quality control.

4. *Symptom log* may be completed daily and all anticipated and unanticipated, grades of constitutional, dermatological, gastrointestinal (GI), metabolic, and pain symptoms must be obtained to continuously monitor symptoms affecting nutritional intake and utilization.

5. *Monthly* CMP and CBC to provide data on anemia, electrolytes, organ function, and immune and protein markers.

6. *Functional markers (Karnofsky performance score)*: [66] The Karnofsky Performance Scale Index allows patients to be classified as to their functional impairment. This has been used to compare effectiveness of different therapies and to assess the prognosis in individual patients and has been validated in cancer patient populations.

7. *Biochemical markers of protein status (serum albumin and transferrin)*: Assessment of protein status is critical in the identification and treatment of abnormalities in protein metabolism. There is substantial evidence of the correlation between serum hepatic proteins and inflammation, making these the most relevant biomarkers in CC. Serum transferrin, prealbumin, and albumin have been observed as intermediate endpoint biomarkers and independently associated with worse outcome in cachexia [52, 79]. Measurements of body composition combined with more objective and sensitive measure of protein nurriture is ideal for the biochemical assessment of intravascular and visceral protein stores. We have thus included the three major valid intermediate endpoint biomarkers (IEBs) that represent intravascular and visceral protein pools – transferrin, prealbumin, and albumin – as the biochemical indicators of protein status [90–92]. Although transferrin levels are affected by iron status, serum transferrin, either singly or as part of a multiparameter index, is the strongest predictor of cancer patient morbidity and mortality.

8. *Immune and inflammatory markers*: Unlike anorexia of aging, in CC, there is a range of metabolic responses triggered by inflammatory and immunological responses. It is believed that the putative mediators of CC are cytokines and increased expression of tumor necrosis factor and interleukin-6 has been observed in patients with CC. Cytokines will be measured in a panel including IL-1, IL-4, IL-6, IL-8, IL-10, GM-CSF, IFN-κ, TNF-α, and CRP (BioRad-Bioplex). All of these biomarkers have been shown to increase with disease, aging, and cytotoxic agents. Though we realize these intermediate endpoint biomarkers of cytokines cannot be reliably interpreted, as over 70% of the subjects as observed in our preliminary studies were on active treatment with cytotoxic agents, these variables are important to determine, as they may provide useful information and contribute to the better understanding of the mechanistic process.

9. *Quality of life* should be measured at baseline and monthly using the Rand Short Form (SF)-36 [93] (Medical Outcomes Study SF36) [230]. The SF-36 has been used extensively with both general, high-risk, and cancer populations and has available norms for mail and telephone versions and comparisons between group and individual scores. Scores are calculated and transformed to a 0–100 scale, with higher scores indicating increased health status. Reliability of the SF-36 scales was measured by Cronbach α coefficient, and the results ranged from 0.78 in general health perceptions to 0.91 in the physical functioning domain.

10. *The Beck Depression Inventory* which has been validated extensively in cancer patient populations should be used to monitor changes in depression symptoms.
11. *Pain* as a symptom should be evaluated periodically and treated for the same. This will ensure that lack of interest in physical activity and normal function is not related to pain.
12. *Fatigue symptom scales*: Patient's change in fatigue status should be monitored using the tools available such as the Visual Analog Scale (VAS) or the Brief Fatigue Inventory (BFI) for assessment of fatigue in a clinical setting or the Multidimensional Fatigue Inventory (MFI-20) which has been validated as a comprehensive tool for evaluation of fatigue in cancer patient populations.

7.5.3.6 Follow-up

Patients must be seen by members of the interdisciplinary team at the start of treatment as well as on a regularly scheduled basis as needed to monitor progress and to review of compliance to exercise and diet intake adequacy, functional status, symptom logs, change in concomitant medications, and any other issues related to fatigue status and response to interventions.

7.6   Future Directions

A growing body of scientific evidence supports the use of pharmacological, non-pharmacological, and combined approaches in the treatment of fatigue in cancer patient populations. Research on these interventions has yielded positive outcomes in cancer survivors with different diagnoses undergoing a variety of cancer treatments. Although fatigue is an important problem in clinical oncology, this has not translated into an increase in clinical trials for assessment and therapy of CRF in this population. Future clinical intervention trials must focus on multimodal approaches, taking into consideration the mechanistic etiology of fatigue. Symptoms such as cancer cachexia, nausea, vomiting, dehydration, loss of skeletal musculature, mucositis, and other symptoms of cancer treatment and their underlying etiology may have a significant impact on fatigue in the cancer patient. Multietiological symptoms have to be targeted with multimodal interventions using multidisciplinary teams. Future research should include evaluation of pharmacological and nonpharmacological approaches to the treatment of fatigue, taking into consideration the underlying mechanisms, moderators, and mediators of fatigue as well as other symptom clusters that confound this symptom or co-occur with this symptom. With improved methodological approaches, further research in this area may soon provide clinicians with effective strategies for reducing CRF and enhancing the lives of millions of cancer patients and survivors.

Summary for the Clinician

Since CRF has a multifactorial psychopathological etiology, intervention strategies are provided by collaborative, interdisciplinary teams of medical oncologists, psychologists, nutritionists, exercise physiologist/physical therapists, and psychosocial workers. In patients with brain tumors, additional team members would include physiatrists, in interdisciplinary collaboration with the pertinent oncology-related services, managing specific symptoms including fatigue, headache, and sleep disturbance and medical complications including depression, seizures, and thromboembolic disease.

A systematic approach to managing cancer patients with CRF should include specific and comprehensive assessment, determining the etiology of CRF, screening for and treating preexisting comorbidities and identifying pharmacological and nonpharmacological approaches that have demonstrated evidence to reduce or ameliorate symptoms of fatigue, in addition to monitoring and closely assessing patients for change in status.

All assessment and reassessment should be conducted continuously, taking into consideration change in medications and medical status of the cancer patient.

The first step in assessing fatigue should include screening for other comorbidities such as thyroid abnormalities, anemia in patients receiving these antineoplastic agents, pain, emotional distress, insomnia, and other comorbid conditions that can be identified and treated proactively. Patient education about symptoms that can be anticipated and providing strategies to manage symptoms proactively has been the single most important component of treating patients with CRF.

- If patients are identified as having hypothyroidism, evaluate further for both hypothyroidism and thyrotoxicosis and treat for this disorder.
- If patient is anemic, evaluate further and treat with hematopoietics such as erythropoietin (EPA) and darbepoetin. For treatment of anemia. Caution: risk of thromboembolic events, especially in patients diagnosed with multiple myeloma treated with thalidomide or lenalidomide; EPA use is to be avoided in patients with anemia not related to chemotherapy and that they be instituted only in those patients with a hemoglobin <10 g/dL with a target level not to exceed 12 g/dL.
- If patient is evaluated as being depressed, antidepressant can be used for the treatment of fatigue. Paroxetine shows benefit for fatigue, primarily when it is a symptom of clinical depression.
- If patient reports pain and is treated with opioids, this factor must be taken into consideration as a contributor of fatigue, although the opioids are provided for the treatment of pain.

Once comorbidities are addressed and none are present and patients are identified to be experiencing fatigue, patients can be screened using the tools available such as the Visual Analog Scale (VAS) or the Brief Fatigue Inventory

(BFI) for assessment of fatigue in a clinical setting or the Multidimensional Fatigue Inventory (MFI-20) that has been validated as a comprehensive tool for evaluation of fatigue in cancer patient populations.

If patient has no fatigue or has mild fatigue or is anticipated to become fatigued, based on treatments planned, nonpharmacological interventions and prophylactic measures to prevent onset may be considered.

If patient is diagnosed with moderate and severe fatigue, both pharmacological and nonpharmacological approaches may be beneficial to ameliorate CRF.

The best evidence for the treatment of fatigue is for pharmacologic measures that have been studied in cancer patients with fatigue. Evaluate patient for use of psychostimulants such as donepezil, modafinil, and methylphenidate.

In spite of evidence demonstrating efficacy of pharmacological interventions, several patients continue to report persistent fatigue.

Nonpharmacological approaches focus on improving physical strength, energy conservation, and nutritional status with adequate proteins to ensure that fatigue is not exacerbated as a result of poor physical fitness and strength levels as well as compromised nutritional status.

Nonpharmacological approach includes psychosocial support to provide support, provide tools to manage stress, and proactively educate patients with regard to anticipated symptoms that they may experience, while providing strategies to cope with these scenarios.

References

1. National Comprehensive Cancer Network NCCN Clinical Practice Guidelines in Oncology (2008) Cancer-related fatigue. [Internet]. Fort Washington (PA): NCCN. Available from: http://www.nccn.org/professionals/physician_gls/PDF/fatigue.pdf (accessed 6.11.2011)
2. Glaus A, Crow R, Hammond S (1996) A qualitative study to explore the concept of fatigue/tiredness in cancer patients and in healthy individuals. Eur J Cancer Care (Engl) 5:8–23
3. Wu HS, McSweeney M (2007) Cancer-related fatigue: "It's so much more than just being tired". Eur J Oncol Nurs 11:117–125
4. Harrington CB, Hansen JA, Moskowitz M, Todd BL, Feuerstein M (2010) It's not over when it's over: long-term symptoms in cancer survivors – a systematic review. Int J Psychiatry Med 40(2):163–181
5. Weigang-Köhler K (2003) Fatigue – when cancer patients are consistently without drive and energy. Determine the etiology. MMW Fortschr Med 145(11):30–34
6. Kangas M, Bovbjerg DH, Montgomery GH (2008) Cancer-related fatigue: a systematic and meta-analytic review of non-pharmacological therapies for cancer patients. Psychol Bull 134(5):700–741
7. Mitchell SA (2010) Cancer-related fatigue: state of the science. PM R 2(5):364–383
8. Breitbart W, Alici Y (2008) Pharmacologic treatment options for cancer-related fatigue: current state of clinical research. Clin J Oncol Nurs 12(suppl 5):27–36
9. Husain A, Myers J, Selby D, Thomson B, Chow E (2011) Subgroups of advanced cancer patients clustered by their symptom profiles: quality-of-life outcomes. J Palliat Med 14:1246–1253

10. Caravati-Jouvenceaux A, Launoy G, Klein D, Henry-Amar M, Abeilard E, Danzon A, Pozet A, Velten M, Mercier M (2011) Health-related quality of life among long-term survivors of colorectal cancer: a population-based study. Oncologist 16:1626–1636

11. Hofman M, Ryan JL, Figueroa-Moseley CD, Jean-Pierre P, Morrow GR (2007) Cancer-related fatigue: the scale of the problem. Oncologist 12(suppl 1):4–10

12. Gripp S, Moeller S, Bolke E, Schmitt G, Matuschek C, Asgari S, Asgharzadeh F, Roth S, Budach W, Franz M, Willers R (2007) Survival prediction in terminally ill cancer patients by clinical estimates, laboratory tests, and self-rated anxiety and depression. J Clin Oncol 25:3313–3320

13. Andrykowski MA, Curran SL, Lightner R (1998) Off-treatment fatigue in breast cancer survivors: a controlled comparison. J Behav Med 21:1–18

14. Barton-Burke M (2006) Cancer-related fatigue and sleep disturbances. Am J Nurs 106(suppl): 72–77

15. Berger AM, Farr LA, Kuhn BR, Fischer P, Agrawal S (2007) Values of sleep/wake, activity/rest, circadian rhythms, and fatigue prior to adjuvant breast cancer chemotherapy. J Pain Symptom Manage 33:398–409

16. Kimel M, Leidy NK, Mannix S, Dixon J (2008) Does epoetin α improve health-related quality of life in chronically ill patients with anemia? Summary of trials of cancer, HIV/AIDS, and chronic kidney disease. Value Health 11:57–75

17. Curt GA, Breitbart W, Cella D et al (2000) Impact of cancer-related fatigue on the lives of patients: new findings from the fatigue coalition. Oncologist 5(5):353–360

18. Abstract/FREE Full Text6. Vogelzang NJ, Breitbart W, Cella D et al (1997) Patient, caregiver, and oncologist perceptions of cancer-related fatigue: results of a tripart assessment survey. The fatigue coalition. Semin Hematol 34(3 Suppl. 2):4–12

19. MedlineWeb of Science7. Stasi R, Abriani L, Beccaglia P et al (2003) Cancer-related fatigue: evolving concepts in evaluation and treatment. Cancer 98(9):1786–1801

20. CrossRefMedline8. Flechtner H, Bottomley A (2003) Fatigue and quality of life: lessons from the real world. Oncologist 8(Suppl. 1):5–9

21. Wang XS, Giralt SA, Mendoza TR et al (2002) Clinical factors associated with cancer-related fatigue in patients being treated for leukemia and non-Hodgkin's lymphoma. J Clin Oncol 20(5):1319–1328

22. Curt GA, Breitbart W, Cella D, Groopman JE, Horning SJ, Itri LM et al (2000) Impact of cancer-related fatigue on the lives of patients: new findings from the fatigue coalition. Oncologist 5:353–360

23. Berglund G, Bolund C, Fornander T, Rutqvist LE, Sjoden PO (1991) Late effects of adjuvant chemotherapy and postoperative radiotherapy on quality of life among breast cancer patients. Eur J Cancer 27:1075–1081

24. Dimsdale JE, Ancoli-Israel S, Ayalon L, Elsmore TF, Gruen W (2007) Taking fatigue seriously. II: variability in fatigue levels in cancer patients. Psychosomatics 48:247–252

25. Jereczek-Fossa BA, Marsiglia HR, Orecchia R (2002) Radiotherapy-related fatigue. Crit Rev Oncol Hematol 41:317–325

26. Bower JE, Ganz PA, Desmond KA, Bernaards C, Rowland JH, Meyerowitz BE, Belin TR (2006) Fatigue in long-term breast carcinoma survivors: a longitudinal investigation. Cancer 106:751–758

27. Bower JE, Ganz PA, Desmond KA, Rowland JH, Meyerowitz BE, Belin TR (2000) Fatigue in breast cancer survivors: occurrence, correlates, and impact on quality of life. J Clin Oncol 18:743–753

28. Carlson LE, Waller A, Groff SL, Giese-Davis J, Bultz BD (2011) What goes up does not always come down: patterns of distress, physical and psychosocial morbidity in people with cancer over a one year period. Psychooncology. doi:10.1002/pon.2068

29. Mulrooney DA, Ness KK, Neglia JP, Whitton JA, Green DM, Zwltzer LK, Robison LL, Mertens AC (2008) Fatigue and sleep disturbance in adult survivors of childhood cancer: a report from the childhood cancer survivor study (CCSS). Sleep 31:271–281

30. Adams JM, Cory S (1991) Transgenic models of tumor development. Science 254: 1161–1167

31. Ancoli-Israel S, Liu L, Marler MR, Parker BA, Jones V, Sadler GR, Dinsdale J, Cohen-Zion M, Fiorentino L (2006) Fatigue, sleep, and circadian rhythms prior to chemotherapy for breast cancer. Support Care Cancer 14:201–209
32. Bower JE (2008) Behavioral symptoms in patients with breast cancer and survivors. J Clin Oncol 26:768–777
33. Morrow GR, Andrews PLR, Hickok JT, Roscoe JA, Matteson S (2002) Fatigue associated with cancer and its treatment. Support Care Cancer 10:389–398
34. Lee BN, Dantzer R, Langley KE, Benentt GJ, Dougherty PM, Dunn AJ, Meyers CA, Miller AH, Payne R, Reuben JM, Wang XS, Cleeland CS (2004) A cytokine-based neuroimmunologic mechanism of cancer-related symptoms. Neuroimmunomodulation 11:279–292
35. Pinto AC, de Azambuja E (2011) Improving quality of life after breast cancer: dealing with symptoms. Maturitas 70:343–348
36. Montazeri A (2008) Health-related quality of life in breast cancer patients: a bibliographic review of the literature from 1974 to 2007. Exp Clin Cancer Res 27:32
37. Cella D, Davis K, Breitbart W et al (2001) Cancer-related fatigue: prevalence of proposed diagnostic criteria in a United States sample of cancer survivors. J Clin Oncol 19(14): 3385–3391
38. Storey DJ, McLaren DB, Atkinson MA, Butcher I, Frew LC, Smyth JF, Sharpe M (2011) Clinically relevant fatigue in men with hormone-sensitive prostate cancer on long-term androgen deprivation therapy. Ann Oncol
39. Kim BR, Chun MH, Han EY, Kim DK (2011) Fatigue assessment and rehabilitation outcomes in patients with brain tumors. Support Care Cancer
40. Meeske K, Katz ER, Palmer SN, Burwinkle T, Varni JW (2004) Parent proxy-reported health-related quality of life and fatigue in pediatric patients diagnosed with brain tumors and acute lymphoblastic leukemia. Cancer 101(9):2116–2125
41. Armstrong TS, Cron SG, Bolanos EV, Gilbert MR, Kang DH (2010) Risk factors for fatigue severity in primary brain tumor patients. Cancer 116(11):2707–2715
42. Malik UR, Makower DF, Wadler S (2001) Interferon-mediated fatigue. Cancer 92(suppl 6): 1664–1668
43. Vargo M (2011) Brain tumor rehabilitation. Am J Phys Med Rehabil 90(5 suppl 1):S50–S62
44. Bower JE, Ganz PA, Aziz N et al (2002) Fatigue and proinflammatory cytokine activity in breast cancer survivors. Psychosom Med 64(4):604–611
45. Evans WJ, Lambert CP (2007) Physiological basis of fatigue. Am J Phys Med Rehabil 86(suppl 1): S29–S46
46. Bower JE, Ganz PA, Tao ML et al (2009) Inflammatory biomarkers and fatigue during radiation therapy for breast and prostate cancer. Clin Cancer Res 15(17):5534–5540
47. Dantzer R (2001) Cytokine-induced sickness behavior: mechanisms and implications. Ann N Y Acad Sci 933:222–234
48. Hart BL (1988) Biological basis of the behavior of sick animals. Neurosci Biobehav Rev 12(2):123–137
49. Eisenberger NI, Inagaki TK, Mashal NM et al (2010) Inflammation and social experience: an inflammatory challenge induces feelings of social disconnection in addition to depressed mood. Brain Behav Immun 24(4):558–563
50. Bower JE, Ganz PA, Aziz N (2005) Altered cortisol response to psychologic stress in breast cancer survivors with persistent fatigue. Psychosom Med 67(2):277–280
51. Bower JE, Ganz PA, Dickerson SS et al (2005) Diurnal cortisol rhythm and fatigue in breast cancer survivors. Psychoneuroendocrinology 30(1):92–100
52. Morrow GR, Andrews PL, Hickok JT et al (2002) Fatigue associated with cancer and its treatment. Support Care Cancer 10(5):389–398
53. Jager A, Sleijfer S, van der Rijt CC (2008) The pathogenesis of cancer related fatigue: could increased activity of pro-inflammatory cytokines be the common denominator? Eur J Cancer 44(2):175–181
54. Chow E, Fan G, Hadi S, Wong J, Kirou-Mauro A, Filipczak L (2008) Symptom clusters in cancer patients with brain metastases. Clin Oncol (R Coll Radiol) 20(1):76–82, Epub 2007 Nov 5

55. Ryu E, Kim K, Cho MS, Kwon IG, Kim HS, Fu MR (2010) Symptom clusters and quality of life in Korean patients with hepatocellular carcinoma. Cancer Nurs 33(1):3–10

56. Broeckel JA, Jacobsen PB, Horton J, Balducci L, Lyman GH (1998) Characteristics and correlates of fatigue after adjuvant chemotherapy for breast cancer. J Clin Oncol 16: 1689–1696

57. Ryan JL, Carroll JK, Ryan EP, Mustian KM, Fiscella K, Morrow GR (2007) Mechanisms of cancer-related fatigue. Oncologist 12(suppl 1):22–34

58. Ludbrook JJ, Truong PT, MacNeil MV, Lesperance M, Webber A, Joe H, Martins H, Lim J (2003) Do age and comorbidity impact treatment allocation and outcomes in limited stage small-cell lung cancer? A community-based population analysis. Int J Radiat Oncol Biol Phys 55(5):1321–1330

59. Giani C, Fierabracci P, Bonacci R et al (1996) Relationship between breast cancer and thyroid disease: relevance of autoimmune thyroid disorders in breast malignancy. J Clin Endocrinol Metab 81(3):990–994, PMID: 8772562

60. Rasmussen B, Feldt-Rasmussen U, Hegedus L, Perrild H, Bech K, Hoier-Madsen M (1987) Thyroid function in patients with breast cancer. Eur J Cancer Clin Oncol 23(5):553–556

61. Adamopoulos DA, Vassilaros S, Kapolla N, Papadiamantis J, Georgiakodis F, Michalakis A (1986) Thyroid disease in patients with benign and malignant mastopathy. Cancer 57(1): 125–128

62. Smyth PP (1997) The thyroid and breast cancer: a significant association? Ann Med 29(3): 189–191

63. Cutuli B, Quentin P, Rodier JF, Barakat P, Grob JC (2000) Severe hypothyroidism after chemotherapy and locoregional irradiation for breast cancer. Radiother Oncol 57(1):103–105

64. Shering SG, Zbar AP, Moriarty M, McDermott EW, O'Higgins NJ, Smyth PP (1996) Thyroid disorders and breast cancer. Eur J Cancer Prev 5(6):504–506

65. Brenta G, Schnitman M, Gurfinkiel M et al (1999) Variations of sex hormone-binding globulin in thyroid dysfunction. Thyroid 9(3):273–277

66. Brenta G, Bedecarras P, Schnitman M et al (2002) Characterization of sex hormone-binding globulin isoforms in hypothyroid women. Thyroid 12(2):101–105

67. Hansen D, Bennedbaek FN, Hansen LK, Hoier-Madsen M, Jacobsen BB, Hegedus L (1999) Thyroid function, morphology and autoimmunity in young patients with insulin-dependent diabetes mellitus. Eur J Endocrinol 140(6):512–518

68. Kami M, Tanaka Y, Chiba S et al (2001) Thyroid function after bone marrow transplantation: possible association between immune-mediated thyrotoxicosis and hypothyroidism. Transplantation 71(3):406–411, PMID: 11233902

69. Cooper DS (2001) Clinical practice. Subclinical hypothyroidism. N Engl J Med 345(4): 260–265

70. Fatourechi V (2001) Subclinical thyroid disease. Mayo Clin Proc 76(4):413–416; quiz 416–417. PMID: 11322357. T

71. Brown-Grant K (1957) The iodide concentrating mechanism of the mammary gland. J Physiol 135(3):644–654

72. Eskin BA (1970) Iodine metabolism and breast cancer. Trans N Y Acad Sci 32(8):911–947

73. Ghent WR, Eskin BA, Low DA, Hill LP (1993) Iodine replacement in fibrocystic disease of the breast. Can J Surg 36(5):453–460

74. Goldman MB, Monson RR, Maloof F (1990) Cancer mortality in women with thyroid disease. Cancer Res 50(8):2283–2289

75. Chlebowski RT, Weiner JM, Reynolds R, Luce J, Bulcavage L, Bateman JR (1986) Long-term survival following relapse after 5-FU but not CMF adjuvant breast cancer therapy. Breast Cancer Res Treat 7(1):23–30, PMID: 3516262

76. Balkwill F, Coussens LM (2004) Cancer: an inflammatory link. Nature 431:405–406

77. Ben-Baruch A (2006) Inflammation-associated immune suppression in cancer: the roles played by cytokines, chemokines and additional mediators. Semin Cancer Biol 16:38–52

78. Cleeland CS, Bennett GJ, Dantzer R, Dougherty PM, Dunn AJ, Meyers CA, Miller AH, Payne R, Reuben JM, Wang XS, Lee BN (2003) Are the symptoms of cancer and cancer treatment

due to a shared biologic mechanism? A cytokine-immunologic model of cancer symptoms. Cancer 97:2919–2925

79. Neta R (2000) The promise of molecular epidemiology in defining the association between radiation and cancer. Health Phys 79:77–84

80. Pusztai L, Mendoza TR, Reuben JM, Martinez MM, Willey JS, Lara J, Syed A, Fritsche HA, Bruera E, Booser D, Valero V, Arun B, Ibrahim N, Rivera E, Royce M, Cleeland CS, Hortobagyi GN (2004) Changes in plasma levels of inflammatory cytokines in response to paclitaxel chemotherapy. Cytokine 25:94–102

81. Winningham ML, Nail LM, Burke MB et al (1994) Fatigue and the cancer experience: the state of the knowledge. Oncol Nurs Forum 21(1):23–36

82. Persohn E, Canta A, Schoepfer S, Traebert M, Mueller L, Gilardini A, Galbiati S, Nicolini G, Scuteri A, Lanzani F, Giussani G, Cavaletti G (2005) Morphological and morphometric analysis of paclitaxel and docetaxel-induced peripheral neuropathy in rats. Eur J Cancer 41:1460–1466

83. Polomano RC, Mannes A, Clark US, Bennett GJ (2001) A painful peripheral neuropathy in the rat produced by the chemotherapeutic drug, paclitaxel. Pain 94:293–304

84. Chao CC, Gallagher M, Phair J, Peterson PK (1990) Serum neopterin and interleukin-6 levels in chronic fatigue syndrome. J Infect Dis 162:1412–1413

85. Patarca R, Klimas NG, Lugtendorf S, Antoni M, Fletcher MA (1994) Dysregulated expression of tumor necrosis factor in chronic fatigue syndrome: interrelations with cellular sources and patterns of soluble immune mediator expression. Clin Infect Dis 18(suppl 1):S147–S153

86. Ziefle S, Egberts F, Heinze S, Volkenandt M, Schmid-Wendtner M, Tilgen W, Linse R, Boettjer J, Vogt T, Spieth K, Eigentler T, Brockmeyer NH, Heinz A, Hauschild A, Schaefer M (2011) Health-related quality of life before and during adjuvant interferon-α treatment for patients with malignant melanoma (DeCOG-trial). J Immunother 34(4):403–408

87. Collado-Hidalgo A, Bower JE, Ganz PA, Cole SW, Irwin MR (2006) Inflammatory biomarkers for persistent fatigue in breast cancer survivors. Clin Cancer Res 12:2759–2786

88. Berger AM, Lockhart K, Agrawal S (2009) Variability of patterns of fatigue and quality of life over time based on different breast cancer adjuvant chemotherapy regimens. Oncol Nurs Forum 36(5):563–570 [PUBMED Abstract]

89. So WK, Marsh G, Ling WM et al (2009) The symptom cluster of fatigue, pain, anxiety, and depression and the effect on the quality of life of women receiving treatment for breast cancer: a multicenter study. Oncol Nurs Forum 36(4):E205–E214

90. Piper BF, Rieger PT, Brophy L et al (1989) Recent advances in the management of biotherapy-related side effects: fatigue. Oncol Nurs Forum 16(6):27–34

91. Haeuber D (1989) Recent advances in the management of biotherapy-related side effects: flu-like syndrome. Oncol Nurs Forum 16(6):35–41

92. Mattson K, Niiranen A, Iivanainen M et al (1983) Neurotoxicity of interferon. Cancer Treat Rep 67(10):958–961

93. Hickok JT, Morrow GR, McDonald S et al (1996) Frequency and correlates of fatigue in lung cancer patients receiving radiation therapy: implications for management. J Pain Symptom Manage 11(6):370–377

94. Donovan KA, Jacobsen PB, Andrykowski MA et al (2004) Course of fatigue in women receiving chemotherapy and/or radiotherapy for early stage breast cancer. J Pain Symptom Manage 28(4):373–380

95. Miaskowski C, Paul SM, Cooper BA et al (2008) Trajectories of fatigue in men with prostate cancer before, during, and after radiation therapy. J Pain Symptom Manage 35(6):632–643

96. Greenberg DB, Sawicka J, Eisenthal S et al (1992) Fatigue syndrome due to localized radiation. J Pain Symptom Manage 7(1):38–45 [PUBMED Abstract]

97. Haylock PJ, Hart LK (1979) Fatigue in patients receiving localized radiation. Cancer Nurs 2(6):461–467 [PUBMED Abstract]

98. King KB, Nail LM, Kreamer K et al (1985) Patients' descriptions of the experience of receiving radiation therapy. Oncol Nurs Forum 12(4):55–61 [PUBMED Abstract]

99. Nail LM (1993) Coping with intracavitary radiation treatment for gynecologic cancer. Cancer Pract 1(3):218–224

100. Larson PJ, Lindsey AM, Dodd MJ et al (1993) Influence of age on problems experienced by patients with lung cancer undergoing radiation therapy. Oncol Nurs Forum 20(3):473–480

101. Fobair P, Hoppe RT, Bloom J et al (1986) Psychosocial problems among survivors of Hodgkin's disease. J Clin Oncol 4(5):805–814

102. Groopman JE, Itri LM (1999) Chemotherapy-induced anemia in adults: incidence and treatment. J Natl Cancer Inst 91:1616–1634

103. Hurter B, Bush NJ (2007) Cancer-related anemia: clinical review and management update. Clin J Oncol Nurs 11:349–359

104. Knight K, Wade S, Balducci L (2004) Prevalence and outcomes of anemia in cancer: a systematic review of the literature. Am J Med 116(suppl 7A):11S–26S

105. Mercadante S, Gebbia V, Marrazzo A, Filosto S (2000) Anaemia in cancer: pathophysiology and treatment. Cancer Treat Rev 26:303–311

106. Guan Z, Vgontzas AN, Omori T, Peng X, Bixler EO, Fang J (2005) Interleukin-6 levels fluctuate with the light-dark cycle in the brain and peripheral tissues in rats. Brain Behav Immun 19:526–529

107. Demetri GD, Gabrilove JL, Blasi MV, Hill RJ, Glaspy J (2002) Benefits of epoetin α in anemic breast cancer patients receiving chemotherapy. Clin Breast Cancer 3:45–51

108. Tas F, Eralp Y, Basaran M, Sakar B, Alici S, Argon A, Bulutlar G, Camlica H, Aydiner A, Topuz E (2002) Anemia in oncology practice: relation to diseases and their therapies. Am J Clin Oncol 25(4):371–379

109. Savonije JH, van Groeningen CJ, Wormhoudt LW, Giaccone G (2006) Early Intervention with epoetin alfa during platinum-based chemotherapy: an analysis of quality-of-life results of a multicenter, randomized, controlled trial compared with population normative data. Oncologist 11(2):197–205

110. Johnston E, Crawford J (1998) The hematologic support of the cancer patient. In: Berger A, Portenoy RK, Weissman DE (eds) Principles and practice of supportive oncology. Lippincott-Raven Publishers, Philadelphia, pp 549–569

111. Samper Ots PM, Muñoz J, Biete A, Ortiz MJ, Acuña M, Cabrera J, López Carrizosa C, Bayo E, Herruzo I, Pérez MM, Domínguez MA, Morillo Macías V, Mira M, Pérez Casas AM, Sevillano MM, García Ríos I, Andreu F, Sotoca A, Álvarez A, López E, Pérez Escutia MÁ, Loayza Villaroel A (2011) PITASOR epidemiological study: prevalence, incidence and treatment of anaemia in radiation therapy oncology departments in Spain. Clin Transl Oncol 13(5):322–327

112. Bush RS (1986) The significance of anemia in clinical radiation therapy. Int J Radiat Oncol Biol Phys 12(11):2047–2050

113. Ahlberg K, Ekman T, Gaston-Johansson F (2004) Levels of fatigue compared to levels of cytokines and hemoglobin during pelvic radiotherapy: a pilot study. Biol Res Nurs 5(3):203–210

114. Voskuil DW, van Nes JG, Junggeburt JM, van de Velde CJ, van Leeuwen FE, de Haes JC (2010) Maintenance of physical activity and body weight in relation to subsequent quality of life in postmenopausal breast cancer patients. Ann Oncol 21(10):2094–2101, Epub 2010 Mar 31

115. Kumar N, Allen KA, Riccardi D, Bercu BB, Cantor A, Minton S, Balducci L, Jacobsen PB (2004) Fatigue, weight gain, lethargy and amenorrhea in breast cancer patients on chemotherapy: is subclinical hypothyroidism the culprit? Breast Cancer Res Treat 83(2):149–159. Huntington MO (1985) Weight gain in patients receiving adjuvant chemotherapy for carcinoma of the breast. Cancer 56(3):472–474. PMID: 3839160

116. Tagliaferri M, Berselli ME, Calo G et al (2001) Subclinical hypothyroidism in obese patients: relation to resting energy expenditure, serum leptin, body composition, and lipid profile. Obes Res 9(3):196–201

117. Rose DP, Davis TE (1977) Ovarian function in patients receiving adjuvant chemotherapy for breast cancer. Lancet 1(8023):1174–1176

118. Lincoln SR, Ke RW, Kutteh WH (1999) Screening for hypothyroidism in infertile women. J Reprod Med 44(5):455–457

119. Krassas GE (2000) Thyroid disease and female reproduction. Fertil Steril 74(6):1063–1070

120. Ahlberg K, Ekman T, Gaston-Johansson F (2004) Levels of fatigue compared to levels of cytokines and hemoglobin during pelvic radiotherapy: a pilot study. Biol Res Nurs 5(3):203–210

121. Sher L, Rosenthal NE, Wehr TA (1999) Free thyroxine and thyroid-stimulating hormone levels in patients with seasonal affective disorder and matched controls. J Affect Disord 56(2–3):195–199

122. Armada-Dias L, Carvalho JJ, Breitenbach MM, Franci CR, Moura EG (2001) Is the infertility in hypothyroidism mainly due to ovarian or pituitary functional changes? Braz J Med Biol Res 34(9):1209–1215

123. Hamnvik OP, Larsen PR, Marqusee E (2011) Thyroid dysfunction from antineoplastic agents. J Natl Cancer Inst 103(21):1572–1587, Epub 2011 Oct 18. Review

124. Roscoe JA, Kaufman ME, Matteson-Rusby SE, Palesh OG, Ryan JL, Kohli S, Perlis ML, Morrow GR (2007) Cancer-related fatigue and sleep disorders. Oncologist 12(suppl 1):35–42, Review

125. Vena C, Parker K, Allen R, Bliwise D, Jain S, Kimble L (2006) Sleep-wake disturbances and quality of life in patients with advanced lung cancer. Oncol Nurs Forum 33(4):761–769

126. Ancoli-Israel S, Liu L, Marler MR et al (2006) Fatigue, sleep, and circadian rhythms prior to chemotherapy for breast cancer. Support Care Cancer 14(3):201–209

127. Berger AM, Mitchell SA (2008) Modifying cancer-related fatigue by optimizing sleep quality. J Natl Compr Canc Netw 6(1):3–13

128. Gögenur I (2010) Postoperative circadian disturbances. Dan Med Bull 57(12):B4205, Review

129. Delgado-Guay M, Yennurajalingam S, Parsons H, Palmer JL, Bruera E (2011) Association between self-reported sleep disturbance and other symptoms in patients with advanced cancer. J Pain Symptom Manage 41(5):819–827, Epub 2011 Feb 9

130. Sandadi S, Frasure HE, Broderick MJ, Waggoner SE, Miller JA, von Gruenigen VE (2011) The effect of sleep disturbance on quality of life in women with ovarian cancer. Gynecol Oncol 123(2):351–355

131. Ross PJ, Ashley S, Norton A, Priest K, Waters JS, Eisen T et al (2004) Do patients with weight loss have a worse outcome when undergoing chemotherapy for lung cancers? Br J Cancer 90:1905–1911

132. Jatoi A (2008) Weight loss in patient with advanced cancer: effects, causes, and potential management. Curr Opin Support Palliat Care 2(1):45–48

133. Evans WJ, Morley JE, Argilés J, Bales C, Baracos V, Guttridge D, Jatoi A et al (2008) Cachexia: a new definition. Clin Nutr 27(6):793–799, Epub 2008 Aug 21. PMID: 18718696

134. Behl D, Jatoi A (2007) Pharmacological options for advanced cancer patients with loss of appetite and weight. Expert Opin Pharmacother 8(8):1085–1090

135. Morley JE (2002) Pathophysiology of anorexia. Clin Geriatr Med 18(4):661–673, v, Review. PMID: 12608495

136. Melstrom LG, Melstrom KA Jr, Ding XZ, Adrian TE (2007) Mechanisms of skeletal muscle degradation and its therapy in cancer cachexia. Histol Histopathol 22(7):805–814

137. Mantovani G, Macciò A, Madeddu C, Serpe R, Massa E, Dessì M, Panzone F, Contu P (2010) Randomized phase III clinical trial of five different arms of treatment in 332 patients with cancer cachexia. Oncologist 15(2):200–211, Epub 2010 Feb 15

138. Barton BE (2001) IL-6-like cytokines and CC: consequences of chronic inflammation. Immunol Res 23(1):41–58, Review. PMID: 11417859

139. Mantovani G, Madeddu C, Gramignano G, Ferreli L, Massa E, Contu P, Serpe R (2004) Association of serum IL-6 levels with comprehensive geriatric assessment variables in a population of elderly cancer patients. Oncol Rep 11(1):197–206

140. Barber MD, Wigmore SJ, Ross JA, Fearon KC, Tisdale MJ (1998) Proinflammatory cytokines, nutritional support, and the cachexia syndrome: interactions and therapeutic options. Cancer 82(5):1000

141. Evans WJ (2010) Skeletal muscle loss: cachexia, sarcopenia, and inactivity. Am J Clin Nutr 91(4):1123S–1127S, Epub 2010 Feb 17

142. Pickering WP, Price SR, Bircher G, Marinovic AC, Mitch WE, Walls J (2002) Nutrition in CAPD: serum bicarbonate and the ubiquitin-proteasome system in muscle. Kidney Int 61:1286–1292

143. Du J, Wang X, Miereles C et al (2004) Activation of caspase-3 is an initial step triggering accelerated muscle proteolysis in catabolic conditions. J Clin Invest 113:115–123, 23 12

144. Mantovani G, Maccio A, Mura L, Massa E, Mudu MC, Mulas C et al (2000) Serum levels of leptin and proinflammatory cytokines in patients with advanced-stage cancer at different sites. J Mol Med 78(10):554–561

145. Deans DA, Wigmore SJ, Gilmour H, Tisdale MJ, Fearon KC, Ross JA (2008) Expression of the proteolysis-inducing factor core peptide mRNA is upregulated in both tumour and adjacent normal tissue in gastro-esophageal malignancy. Br J Cancer 98(1):242; author reply 243. PMCID: PMC2361198

146. Wigmore SJ, Todorov PT, Barber MD, Ross JA, Tisdale MJ, Fearon KC (2000) Characteristics of patients with pancreatic cancer expressing a novel cancer cachectic factor. Br J Surg 87(1):53–58

147. Whitehouse AS, Tisdale MJ (2003) Increased expression of the ubiquitin-proteasome pathway in murine myotubes by proteolysis-inducing factor (PIF) is associated with activation of the transcription factor NF-kappaB. Br J Cancer 89(6):1116–1122

148. Melstrom LG, Melstrom KA Jr, Ding XZ, Adrian TE (2007) Mechanisms of skeletal muscle degradation and its therapy in cancer cachexia. Histol Histopathol 22(7):805–814. Mitch WE, Price SR (2001) Transcription factors and muscle cachexia: is there a therapeutic target? Lancet 357(9258):734–735. PMID: 11253960

149. Ciechanover A, Orian A, Schwartz AL (2000) The ubiquitin-mediated proteolytic pathway: mode of action and clinical implications. J Cell Biochem Suppl 34:40–51

150. Voges D, Zwickl P, Baumeister W (1999) The 26S proteasome: a molecular machine designed for controlled proteolysis. Annu Rev Biochem 68:1015–1068

151. Ghosh S, Karin M (2002) Missing pieces in the NF-kappaB puzzle. Cell 109(suppl): S81–S96

152. Maltoni M, Fabbri L, Nanni O, Scarpi E, Pezzi L, Flamini E et al (1997) Serum levels of tumor necrosis factor alpha and other cytokines do not correlate with weight loss and anorexia in cancer patients. Support Care Cancer 5(2):130–135; comments in Support Care Cancer. 1997;5(5):422–423. PMID: 9069613

153. Blum B, Omlin A, Fearon K, Baracos V, Radbruch L, Kaasa S, Strasser F, European Palliative Care Research Collaborative (2010) Evolving classification systems for CC: ready for clinical practice? Support Care Cancer 18(3):273–279, PMID: 20076976

154. Whitehouse AS, Khal J, Tisdale MJ (2003) Induction of protein catabolism in myotubes by 15(S)-hydroxyeicosatetraenoic acid through increased expression of the ubiquitin-proteasome pathway. Br J Cancer 89(4):737–745

155. Das SK, Eder S, Schauer S, Diwoky C, Temmel H, Guertl B, Gorkiewicz G, Tamilarasan KP, Kumari P, Trauner M, Zimmermann R, Vesely P, Haemmerle G, Zechner R, Hoefler G (2011) Adipose triglyceride lipase contributes to cancer-associated cachexia. Science 333(6039):233–238, Epub 2011 Jun 16

156. Fearon KC (2011) Cancer cachexia and fat-muscle physiology. N Engl J Med 365(6): 565–567

157. Kirkova J, Aktas A, Walsh D, Davis MP (2011) Cancer symptom clusters: clinical and research methodology. J Palliat Med 14(10):1149–1166, Epub 2011 Aug 23

158. Laird BJ, Scott AC, Colvin LA, McKeon AL, Murray GD, Fearon KC, Fallon MT (2011) Pain, depression, and fatigue as a symptom cluster in advanced cancer. J Pain Symptom Manage 42(1):1–11, Epub 2011 Mar 12

159. Barsevick AM (2007) The elusive concept of the symptom cluster. Oncol Nurs Forum 34(5): 971–980

160. Kirkova J, Walsh D, Aktas A, Davis MP (2010) Cancer symptom clusters: old concept but new data. Am J Hosp Palliat Care 27(4):282–288, Epub 2010 Mar 29

161. Walsh D, Nelson KA, Mahmoud FA (2003) Established and potential therapeutic applications of cannabinoids in oncology. Support Care Cancer 11(3):137–143, Epub 2002 Aug 21. Review. PMID: 12618922

162. Berger AM, Parker KP, Young-McCaughan S, Mallory GA, Barsevick AM, Bck SL, Carpenter JS, Carter PA, Farr LA, Hinds PS, Lee KA, Miaskowski C, Mock V, Payne JK, Hall M (2005) Sleep wake disturbances in people with cancer and their caregivers: state of the science. Oncol Nurs Forum 32:E98–E126

163. Mystakidou K, Parpa E, Tsilika E, Pathiaki M, Patiraki E, Galanos A, Vlahos L (2007) Sleep quality in advanced cancer patients. J Psychosom Res 62:527–533

164. Everson CA (1993) Sustained sleep deprivation impairs host defense. Am J Physiol 265:R1148–R1154

165. Everson CA (2005) Clinical assessment of blood leukocytes, serum cytokines, and serum immunoglobulins as responses to sleep deprivation in laboratory rats. Am J Physiol Regul Integr Comp Physiol 289:R1054–R1063

166. Anisimov VN, Ukraintseva SV, Yashin AI (2005) Cancer in rodents: does it tell us about cancer in humans? Nat Rev Cancer 5:807–819

167. Katz N, Mazer NA (2009) The impact of opioids on the endocrine system. Clin J Pain 25(2):170–175 [PUBMED Abstract]

168. Strasser F, Palmer JL, Schover LR et al (2006) The impact of hypogonadism and autonomic dysfunction on fatigue, emotional function, and sexual desire in male patients with advanced cancer: a pilot study. Cancer 107(12):2949–2957, [PUBMED Abstract]

169. Rajagopal A, Vassilopoulou-Sellin R, Palmer JL et al (2004) Symptomatic hypogonadism in male survivors of cancer with chronic exposure to opioids. Cancer 100(4):851–858 [PUBMED Abstract]

170. Matthews EE, Schmiege SJ, Cook PF, Sousa KH (2011) Breast cancer and symptom clusters during radiotherapy. Cancer Nurs

171. de Vries U, Reif K, Petermann F (2011) Cancer-related fatigue and its psychosocial burden. Internist (Berl) 52:1317–1323

172. Montgomery GH, Schnur JB, Erblich J et al (2010) Presurgery psychological factors predict pain, nausea, and fatigue one week after breast cancer surgery. J Pain Symptom Manage 39(6):1043–1052

173. Prue G, Allen J, Gracey J et al (2010) Fatigue in gynecological cancer patients during and after anticancer treatment. J Pain Symptom Manage 39(2):197–210

174. Henriksson MM, Isometsä ET, Hietanen PS et al (1995) Mental disorders in cancer suicides. J Affect Disord 36(1–2):11–20

175. Reich SG (1986) The tired patient: psychological versus organic causes. Hosp Med 22(7):142–154

176. Cimprich B (1999) Pretreatment symptom distress in women newly diagnosed with breast cancer. Cancer Nurs 22(3):185–194; quiz 195

177. Sugawara Y, Akechi T, Okuyama T et al (2005) Occurrence of fatigue and associated factors in disease-free breast cancer patients without depression. Support Care Cancer 13(8):628–636

178. Bower JE, Ganz PA, Desmond KA et al (2006) Fatigue in long-term breast carcinoma survivors: a longitudinal investigation. Cancer 106(4):751–758

179. Fosså SD, Dahl AA, Loge JH (2003) Fatigue, anxiety, and depression in long-term survivors of testicular cancer. J Clin Oncol 21(7):1249–1254

180. Christensen S, Zachariae R, Jensen AB, Vaeth M, Møller S, Ravnsbaek J, von der Maase H (2009) Prevalence and risk of depressive symptoms 3–4 months post-surgery in a nationwide cohort study of Danish women treated for early stage breast-cancer. Breast Cancer Res Treat 113(2):339–355, Epub 2008 Feb 16

181. Wichers M, Maes M (2002) The psychoneuroimmuno-pathophysiology of cytokine-induced depression in humans. Int J Neuropsychopharmacol 5:375–388

182. Capuron L, Gumnick JF, Musselman DL, Lawson DH, Reemsnyder A, Nemeroff CB, Miller AH (2002) Neurobehavioral effects of interferon-α in cancer patients: phenomenology and paroxetine responsiveness of symptom dimensions. Neuropsychopharmacology 26:643–652

183. Raison CL, Demetrashvili M, Capuron L, Miller AH (2005) Neuropsychiatric adverse effects of interferon-α: recognition and management. CNS Drugs 19:105–123
184. Schubert C, Hong S, Natarajan L, Mills PJ, Dimsdale JE (2007) The association between fatigue and inflammatory marker levels in cancer patients: a quantitative review. Brain Behav Immun 21:413–427
185. Caplette-Gingras A, Savard J (2008) Depression in women with metastatic breast cancer: a review of the literature. Palliat Support Care 6(4):377–387
186. Arnold EM (1999) The cessation of cancer treatment as a crisis. Soc Work Health Care 29:21–38
187. McKinley ED (2000) Under Toad days: surviving the uncertainty of cancer recurrence. Ann Intern Med 133:479–480
188. Stanton AL, Ganz PA, Kwan L, Meyerowitz BE, Bower JE, Krupnick JL, Rowland JH, Leedham B, Belin TR (2005) Outcomes from the moving beyond cancer psychoeducational, randomized, controlled trial with breast cancer patients. J Clin Oncol 23:6009–6018
189. Vickberg SM (2003) The concerns about recurrence scale (CARS): a systematic measure of women's fears about the possibility of breast cancer recurrence. Ann Behav Med 25:16–24
190. Thewes B, Butow P, Zachariae R, Christensen S, Simard S, Gotay C (2011) Fear of cancer recurrence: a systematic literature review of self-report measures. Psychooncology. doi:10.1002/pon.2070
191. Vickberg SMJ (2001) Fears about breast cancer recurrence. Cancer Pract 9:237–243
192. Waldrop DP, O'Connor TL, Trabold N (2011) "Waiting for the other shoe to drop:" distress and coping during and after treatment for breast cancer. J Psychosoc Oncol 29(4):450–473
193. Mustian KM, Morrow GR, Carroll JK, Figueroa-Moseley CD, Jean-Pierre P, Williams GC (2007) Integrative nonpharmacologic behavioral interventions for the management of cancer-related fatigue. Oncologist 12(suppl 1):52–67
194. Campos MP, Hassan BJ, Riechelmann R, Del Giglio A (2011) Cancer-related fatigue: a practical review. Ann Oncol 22(6):1273–1279, Epub 2011 Feb 16
195. Rao AV, Cohen HJ (2008) Fatigue in older cancer patients: etiology, assessment, and treatment. Semin Oncol 35(6):633–642
196. Mock V, Atkinson A, Barsevick A et al (2000) NCCN practice guidelines for cancer-related fatigue. Oncology (Williston Park) 14(11A):151–161
197. Fan HG, Houédé-Tchen N, Yi QL et al (2005) Fatigue, menopausal symptoms, and cognitive function in women after adjuvant chemotherapy for breast cancer: 1- and 2-year follow-up of a prospective controlled study. J Clin Oncol 23(31):8025–8032
198. Mendoza TR, Wang XS, Cleeland CS et al (1999) The rapid assessment of fatigue severity in cancer patients: use of the brief fatigue inventory. Cancer 85(5):1186–1196
199. Minton O, Stone P, Richardson A, Sharpe M, Hotopf M (2008) Drug therapy for the management of cancer related fatigue. Cochrane Database Syst Rev 1:CD006704
200. Davenport TE, Stevens SR, Baroni K, Mark Van Ness J, Snell CR (2011) Reliability and validity of short form 36 version 2 to measure health perceptions in a sub-group of individuals with fatigue. Disabil Rehabil 33:2596–2604
201. Knobel H, Håvard Loge J, Brit Lund M et al (2001) Late medical complications and fatigue in Hodgkin's disease survivors. J Clin Oncol 19(13):3226–3233
202. Escalante CP, Kallen MA, Valdres RU et al (2010) Outcomes of a cancer-related fatigue clinic in a comprehensive cancer center. J Pain Symptom Manage 39(4):691–701
203. Minton O, Richardson A, Sharpe M, Hotopf M, Stone P (2008) A systematic review and meta-analysis of the pharmacological treatment of cancer-related fatigue. J Natl Cancer Inst 100(16):1155–1166, Epub 2008 Aug 11. Review
204. Jedlicka F, Elbl L, Vásová I, Tomásková I, Vorlícek J, Spinar J (2007) Chronic fatigue syndrome in cancer patients. Diagnostic and treatment options. Vnitr Lek 53(9):979–985, Review. Czech
205. National Comprehensive Cancer Network (NCCN) Clinical Practice Guidelines in Oncology (2010) Cancer- and treatment-related anemia. [cited 24 April 2010; Version 2. 2010]. Published by the National Comprehensive Cancer Network online at www.nccn.org

206. Rizzo JD, Somerfield MR, Hagerty KL et al (2008) Use of epoetin and darbepoetin in patients with cancer: 2007 American Society of Clinical Oncology/American Society of Hematology clinical practice guideline update. J Clin Oncol 26(1):132–149

207. Tazi el M, Errihani H (2011) Evaluation and management of fatigue in oncology: a multidimensional approach. Indian J Palliat Care 17(2):92–97

208. Breitbart W, Alici Y (2010) Psychostimulants for cancer-related fatigue. J Natl Compr Canc Netw 8(8):933–942

209. Bremberg ER, Brandberg Y, Hising C, Friesland S, Eksborg S (2007) Anemia and quality of life including anemia-related symptoms in patients with solid tumors in clinical practice. Med Oncol 24:95–102

210. Liu L, Marler MR, Parker BA, Jones V, Johnson S, Cohen-Zion M, Fiorentino L, Sadler GR, Ancoli-Israel S (2005) The relationship between fatigue and light exposure during chemotherapy. Support Care Cancer 13:1010–1017

211. Solberg Nes L, Ehlers SL, Patten CA, Gastineau DA (2011) Self-regulatory fatigue in hematologic malignancies: impact on quality of life, coping, and adherence to medical recommendations. Int J Behav Med

212. Cramp F, Daniel J (2008) Exercise for the management of cancer-related fatigue in adults. Cochrane Database Syst Rev 2:CD006145

213. Silver JK (2007) Rehabilitation in women with breast cancer. Phys Med Rehabil Clin N Am 18:521–537

214. Schneider CM, Hsieh CC, Sprod LK, Carter SD, Hayward R (2007) Effects of supervised exercise training on cardiopulmonary function and fatigue in breast cancer survivors during and after treatment. Cancer 110:918–925

215. Markes M, Brockow T, Resch KL (2006) Exercise for women receiving adjuvant therapy for breast cancer. Cochrane Database Syst Rev 4:CD005001

216. Baumann FT, Kraut L, Schüle K, Bloch W, Fauser AA (2010) A controlled randomized study examining the effects of exercise therapy on patients undergoing haematopoietic stem cell transplantation. Bone Marrow Transplant 45(2):355–362, Epub 2009 Jul 13

217. Keogh JW, Macleod RD (2012) Body composition, physical fitness, functional performance, quality of life, and fatigue benefits of exercise for prostate cancer patients: a systematic review. J Pain Symptom Manage 43(1):96–110, Epub 2011 Jun 2

218. van Weerta E, Hoekstra-Weebers J, Renée Ottera, Klaas Postem, Robbert Sandermanc, Cees van der Schansa (2006) Cancer-related fatigue: predictors and effects of rehabilitation. Oncologist 11(2):184–196

219. Luebbert K, Dahme B, Hasenbring M (2001) The effectiveness of relaxation training in reducing treatment-related symptoms and improving emotional adjustment in acute nonsurgical cancer treatment: a meta-analytical review. Psychooncology 10(6):490–502

220. Jacobsen PB, Meade CD, Stein KD et al (2002) Efficacy and costs of two forms of stress management training for cancer patients undergoing chemotherapy. J Clin Oncol 20(12):2851–2862

221. Carlson LE, Speca M, Patel KD, Goodey E (2004) Mindfulness-based stress reduction in relation to quality of life, mood, symptoms of stress and levels of cortisol, dehydroepiandrosterone sulfate (DHEAS) and melatonin in breast and prostate cancer outpatients. Psychoneuroendocrinology 29(4):448–474

222. Decker TW, Cline-Elsen J, Gallagher M (1992) Relaxation therapy as an adjunct in radiation oncology. J Clin Psychol 48(3):388–393

223. Given C, Given B, Rahbar M et al (2004) Effect of a cognitive behavioral intervention on reducing symptom severity during chemotherapy. J Clin Oncol 22(3):507–516

224. Gaston-Johansson F, Fall-Dickson JM, Nanda J et al (2000) The effectiveness of the comprehensive coping strategy program on clinical outcomes in breast cancer autologous bone marrow transplantation. Cancer Nurs 23(4):277–285

225. Gielissen MF, Verhagen S, Witjes F, Bleijenberg G (2006) Effects of cognitive behavior therapy in severely fatigued disease-free cancer patients compared with patients waiting for cognitive behavior therapy: a randomized controlled trial. J Clin Oncol 24(30):4882–4887

226. Stanton AL, Ganz PA, Kwan L et al (2005) Outcomes from the moving beyond cancer psychoeducational, randomized, controlled trial with breast cancer patients. J Clin Oncol 23(25):6009–6018
227. Yates P, Aranda S, Hargraves M et al (2005) Randomized controlled trial of an educational intervention for managing fatigue in women receiving adjuvant chemotherapy for early-stage breast cancer. J Clin Oncol 23(25):6027–6036
228. Goedendorp MM, Gielissen MF, Verhagen CA, Bleijenberg G (2009) Psychosocial interventions for reducing fatigue during cancer treatment in adults. Cochrane Database Syst Rev. Gutstein HB (2001) The biologic basis of fatigue. Cancer 9(Suppl. 6):1678–1683
229. Kumar NB, Kazi A, Smith T, Crocker T, Yu D, Reich RR, Reddy K, Hastings S, Exterman M, Balducci L, Dalton K, Bepler G (2010) Cancer cachexia: traditional therapies and novel molecular mechanism-based approaches to treatment. Curr Treat Options Oncol 11(3–4): 107–117, Review
230. Garratt AM, Ruta DA, Abdalla MI, Buckingham JK, Russell IT (1993) The SF36 health survey questionnaire: an outcome measure suitable for routine use within the NHS? BMJ 306(6890):1440–1444

Treatment-Induced Enteritis (Radiation- or Combination Therapy–Induced Enteropathies)

8

Core Messages

Combination cancer therapies, specifically radiation therapy, increase locoregional control and survival in patients, but significantly increase clinical toxicity in thoracic, abdominal, and pelvic cancers, specifically including cervical, ovarian, prostate, bladder, testicular, sigmoid, or colorectal cancer malignancies.

Radiation enteritis specifically refers to a functional disorder of the large and small bowel that occurs during or after a course of radiation therapy to the abdomen, pelvis, or rectum. Since this definition limits only to enteritis associated to radiation therapy, the term alimentary tract mucositis is also used to define this symptom that may result from both radiation and chemotherapy or combination therapies.

Alimentary tract enteritis involves inflammation and mucosal ulceration of this tract, resulting in symptoms including pain, abdominal bloating, vomiting, diarrhea, and malabsorption of fat, lactose, bile salts, and vitamin B_{12}. Symptoms of proctitis include mucoid rectal discharge, rectal pain, rectal urgency or tenesmus, and rectal bleeding contributing to radiation damage to the anus or rectum.

It is reported that cancer treatment regimens that include radiation therapy to the abdominal region for cervical, ovarian, prostate, sigmoid, or colorectal cancer contributed to RT-induced diarrhea, enteritis, and colitis in more than 80% of patients with cancer. Symptoms may be acute or chronic.

Etiology of radiation enteritis is mostly treatment-induced and can be exacerbated within any one patient by several factors and other cancer or treatment-related symptom clusters. Patient-related factors include age, previous abdominal or pelvic surgery, low body mass index, malnutrition, previous abdominal surgery, and presence of other comorbid conditions, such as hypertension, diabetes mellitus, pelvic inflammatory disease, or inadequate nutrition.

Radiation therapy exerts a cytotoxic effect mainly on rapidly proliferating epithelial cells, like those lining the large and small bowel. Crypt cell-wall necrosis can be observed 12–24 h after a daily dose of 1.5–3 Gy with progressive loss of cells, villous atrophy, and cystic crypt dilation occur in the ensuing days and weeks as treatment progresses.

Proinflammatory markers are elevated in the gastrointestinal epithelia of radiated animal as well as in human studies. These initial molecular mechanisms contributing to the etiology of radiation enteritis continue to evolve and may have significant implications for clinically identifying agents that can target these pathways implicated in the development of fibrosis related to radiation enteritis.

8.1   Definition

Radiation therapy in combination with other treatments, such as surgery and chemotherapy, has been demonstrated to increase locoregional control and survival in patients with thoracic, abdominal, and pelvic cancers, specifically including cervical, ovarian, prostate, bladder, testicular, sigmoid, or colorectal cancer malignancies. Nevertheless, significant clinical toxicity with combined treatments may be seen in these patient populations [1–3]. Radiation enteritis specifically refers to a functional disorder of the large and small bowel that occurs during or after a course of radiation therapy to the abdomen, pelvis, or rectum. Since this definition limits only to enteritis associated to radiation therapy, the term alimentary tract mucositis is also used to define this symptom that may result from both radiation, chemotherapy, and combination therapies. Clinical features of chronic radiation enteritis are multiple as the disease can affect any part of the gastrointestinal tract (GI). GI tract enteritis involves inflammation and mucosal ulceration of this tract, resulting in symptoms including pain, abdominal bloating, vomiting, and diarrhea [2, 3]. With disruption or loss of the gastrointestinal tract function, malabsorption of fat, lactose, bile salts, and vitamin B_{12} is common. Symptoms of proctitis as a result of radiation damage to the anus or rectum can cause symptoms such as mucoid rectal discharge, rectal pain, rectal urgency or tenesmus, and rectal bleeding (if mucosal ulceration is present).

Symptoms can be immediate or delayed, chronic or transient. Acute-phase symptoms may persist for a short time, yet long-term complications can represent significant clinical conditions with high morbidity [4]. Acute radiation injury to the rectum generally occurs within 6 weeks of therapy and includes symptoms such as diarrhea, rectal urgency, or tenesmus, and, uncommonly, bleeding. Acute enteritis symptoms usually resolve 2–3 weeks after the completion of treatment, and the mucosa may appear nearly normal [5]. Injuries clinically evident during the first course of radiation and up to 8 weeks later are considered acute [6]. These symptoms usually resolve without specific therapy within 2–6 months [6, 7]. However, chronic radiation proctosigmoiditis has a more delayed onset, and first signs often occur about 9–14 months following radiation exposure but may develop after more than 2 years in some patients [8–11], or it may begin as acute enteritis and persist after the cessation of treatment. With disruption or loss of the gastrointestinal tract function, malabsorption of fat, lactose, bile salts, and vitamin B_{12} is common. Acute enteritis symptoms usually resolve 2–3 weeks after the completion of treatment, and the mucosa may appear nearly normal [5].

8.2 Prevalence

It is reported that cancer treatment regimens that include radiation therapy to the abdominal region for cervical, ovarian, prostate, sigmoid, or colorectal cancer contributed to RT-induced diarrhea, enteritis, and colitis in more than 80% of patients with cancer [12]. Other studies suggest that 50% of people may suffer from chronic radiation enteritis (CRE) [13, 14]. Using a score of 0 to indicate no symptoms, 47% of women gained scores indicative of CRE (>0), range 20–85 (mean 34, SD 14.4). Younger women ($p < 0.001$) and women with cervical cancer ($p < 0.05$) were more likely to score for CRE. No significant relationship was observed between score and either radiotherapy dose or stage of cancer [15]. Five percent to 15% of persons treated with radiation to the abdomen will develop chronic problems [7]. It has also been reported that the prevalence of radiation enteritis may be underestimated, as not all patients with gastrointestinal symptoms after radiotherapy will seek medical attention [16]. However, novel approaches in radiation therapy (RT) techniques to minimize radiation injury have contributed significantly to prevent this complication.

8.3 Etiology

Several factors have been associated to contribute to the etiology of alimentary mucositis or radiation enteritis. Additionally, symptom etiology within any one patient may be multifactorial and contributed by several factors and other cancer or treatment-related symptom clusters [6, 16–18]. Patient-related factors include age, previous abdominal or pelvic surgery, low body mass index, and presence of other comorbid conditions [16]such as hypertension, diabetes mellitus, pelvic inflammatory disease, or inadequate nutrition [17, 18].

Treatment-related factors including radiation dose, fractionation and technique, tumor size and extent, volume of normal bowel treated, concomitant use of chemotherapy, and radiation intracavitary implants contribute to occurrence and severity of radiation enteritis [12, 17, 18]. The small bowel and colorectum are sensitive to ionizing radiation, and acute side effects to the intestines occur at approximately 10 Gy. Since curative doses for many abdominal or pelvic tumors range between 50 and 75 Gy, use of higher doses is common, and radiation-induced enteritis is inevitable in this cancer patient population [5]. Additionally, comorbid conditions can also decrease vascular flow to the bowel wall and impair bowel motility, increasing the chance of radiation injury [17, 18]. Radiation therapy exerts a cytotoxic effect mainly on rapidly proliferating epithelial cells, like those lining the large and small bowel. Crypt cell-wall necrosis can be observed 12–24 h after a daily dose of 1.5–3 Gy with progressive loss of cells, villous atrophy, and cystic crypt dilation occur in the ensuing days and weeks as treatment progresses [5].

Others have observed that for cervical, ovarian, prostate, sigmoid, or colorectal cancer, radiation therapy potentially disturb the colonization resistance of the indigenous gut flora, causing RT-induced diarrhea, enteritis, and colitis in majority of the patients [12], providing an opportunity to identify agents that restore the microbial flora of the gastrointestinal tract.

Recent progress in molecular biology has shed some light on the pathogenesis of CRE, which is characterized by fibrosis, involving several molecular cascades in radiation-induced intestinal fibrosis [19]. The development of fibrosis was reported to be correlated with transforming growth factor $\beta1$ (TGF-$\beta1$) and its downstream effector Smad3, which stimulates fibrogenic downstream mediators, such as connective tissue growth factor (CTGF). The inhibition of Ras homologue (Rho) and Rho-associated kinase (ROCK) signaling pathway was demonstrated to ameliorate radiation-induced intestinal fibrosis in vitro and in animal studies. Proinflammatory cytokines have previously been implicated in the pathophysiology of chemotherapy-induced gastrointestinal mucositis. To understand the role of proinflammatory cytokines in radiation-induced gastrointestinal mucositis, Zhu et al. [19] characterized the expression of proinflammatory cytokines in the gastrointestinal tract using a rat model of fractionated radiotherapy-induced toxicity and demonstrated that radiotherapy-induced subacute damage was associated with significantly upregulated IL-1β, IL-6, and TNF mRNA levels in the jejunum and colon. The majority of proinflammatory cytokine protein expression in the jejunum and colon exhibited minimal change following fractionated radiotherapy. Proinflammatory cytokines may thus play a key role in radiotherapy-induced gastrointestinal mucositis in the subacute onset setting [2]. Erbil et al. [20] observed that irradiation significantly increased the intestinal and pancreatic myeloperoxidase (MPO) activities and caspase-3 activities and malondialdehyde (MDA) levels in comparison to sham group. Glutamine treatment significantly decreased this elevation. Histopathological examination revealed that the intestinal mucosal structure was preserved and pancreatic inflammation decreased in the glutamine-treated group. In irradiation group, NF-kB overexpression was detected. To date, the implication and connection between these pathways have not been elucidated [19]. These initial molecular mechanisms contributing to the etiology of radiation enteritis continue to evolve and may have significant implications for clinically identifying agents that can target these pathways implicated in the development of fibrosis related to radiation enteritis (Fig. 8.1).

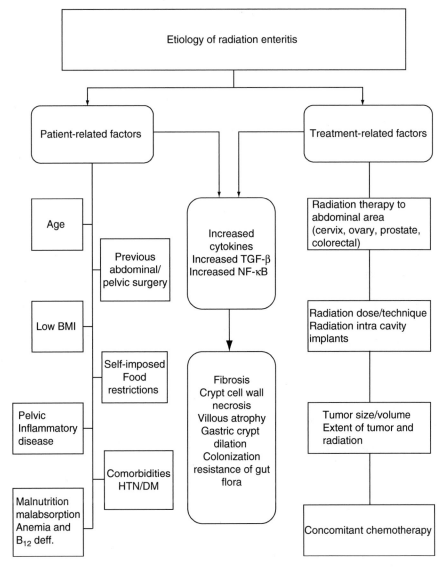

Fig. 8.1 Etiology of radiation enteritis

8.4   Current Therapies for Treatment of Alimentary Tract Enteritis

The evidence base for therapeutic and preventative strategies in treating chronic radiation enteritis is limited. However, it has been shown that adopting a structured, comprehensive approach to assessing gastrointestinal symptoms after radiotherapy should allow better targeting of current symptoms related to treatment. It has been shown that close collaboration between oncologists, surgeons, nutritionists, and gastroenterologists will facilitate a more structured approach, not only in managing individual patients, but also in establishing clinical and research networks for this expanding disease, in order to improve the evidence base for its management [16].

Although the evidence base for current therapies is limited, tissue-/organ-sparing radiation therapy techniques, surgical management, and pharmaceutical and nutritional approaches have been shown to be effective in managing symptoms of enteritis. In addition, modification of treatment sequencing of radiation, chemotherapy, and surgery to modulate the severity of enteritis remains key to management of treatment-related symptoms in this target population.

8.4.1   Screening and Comprehensive Evaluation

Comprehensive screening must include usual pattern of elimination and pattern of diarrhea, including the onset, duration, frequency, amount, and characteristics of stools. In addition, presence of other symptoms such as flatus, cramping, nausea, abdominal distension, tenesmus, bleeding, and rectal excoriation should be assessed [21]. To increase the diagnostic yield of radiation enteritis, capsule endoscopy (CE) has been proven to be a sensitive and safe tool for the examination of the small bowel and has been evaluated in other patient populations having anemia or chronic abdominal pain after chemoradiotherapy. Although capsule endoscopy may safely and effectively diagnose radiation enteritis in patients previously treated with chemoradiotherapy on the upper abdomen [22], careful patient selection is required to avoid complications, primarily capsule retention. In a study to evaluate the rate of capsule retention in patients with suspected chronic small bowel obstruction and to analyze the role and the impact of subsequent surgical intervention, it was observed that capsule retention is a frequent complication of CE in patients with symptoms of chronic small bowel obstruction. Surgery, with the removal of the retained capsule, is proven to be beneficial in identifying the location of, and treating, the underlying disease in these patients [23]. A thorough nutritional assessment of the patients including determining anthropometric measurements, comorbidities, other symptom clusters, nutritional intake patterns and analysis, anemia, electrolyte levels, liver function, level of function, fatigue and symptoms of enteritis, and usual lifestyle patterns is essential to plan nutritional strategies. Since in most cases, the radiation-induced enteritis may be predictable, initial screening and evaluation must include educating patients and warning them of potential symptoms and duration may be critical as studies have shown that often quality of life is affected due to lack of warning signs of these symptoms [24].

8.4.2   Radiation Techniques

Given the significant morbidity and mortality associated with chronic radiation enteritis, current available preventative strategies have included tissue-sparing radiotherapy techniques [16]. With the advent of tridimensional conformal radiotherapy (3D-CRT), dose-volume histograms (DVH) can be generated to assess the dose received by the organs at risk [1]. These techniques include the use of a three- or four-field technique (as opposed to a two-field technique) to minimize the amount of small bowel exposed to treatment; treatment of the patient in a physical position that will aid in removing as much small bowel from the treatment field as possible (e.g., treating a patient with a full bladder each day to aid in pushing the small bowel up and out of the pelvis when pelvic radiation is given); daily treatment of all fields, resulting in a lower integral dose and more homogenous dose distribution and use of computerized radiation dosimetry to best design the treatment plan; and the use of high-energy treatment machines such as linear accelerators that deliver a high dose-to-tumor volume while sparing the normal structures [25]. Others have shown that intensity-modulated radiotherapy (IMRT) can reduce dose to small bowel, bladder, and bone marrow compared with three-field conventional radiotherapy (CRT) technique in the treatment of rectal cancer. IMRT is associated with a clinically significant reduction in lower GI toxicity compared with CRT [26]. Concurrent chemoradiotherapy (CCRT) is the mainstay treatment for locally advanced cervical cancer. In a study to investigate the treatment outcomes and toxicity of definitive intensity-modulated radiotherapy (IMRT) with concurrent chemotherapy for patients with locally advanced carcinoma of the cervix in a single institution, Chen et al. [27] demonstrated positive outcomes that were well tolerated with favorable acute and late toxicity. Similarly, compared with 3D-CRT, IMRT significantly decreased the acute and late GI toxicity in patients treated with androgen deprivation therapy for prostate cancer [28]. Despite dosimetric differences in the volume of bowel, bladder, and rectum irradiated in the low-dose and median-dose regions, whole pelvic IMRT results only in a clinically significant increase in acute GI toxicity, in comparison to prostate only IMRT, with no difference in GU or late GI toxicity [29]. Thompson et al. [30] reported that patients developing short bowel syndrome (SBS) are at risk for hepatobiliary complications and that radiation enteritis and radiation-induced liver disease are potential complications of radiation therapy (XRT). Short bowel syndrome (SBS) patients with a history of XRT were more likely to develop cirrhosis and portal hypertension than SBS patients with malignancy alone [30]. Future improvement in radiation therapy technology such as IMRT and modifying sequencing of multiple treatment strategies promises to ensure targeted treatment of tumors while reducing gastrointestinal toxicities.

8.4.3   Surgical Management

Surgical interventions are undertaken only after careful assessment of the patient's clinical condition and extent of radiation damage since wound healing is often delayed. Patients assessed with severe damage are medically managed with surgical interventions [31]. It is estimated that fewer than 2% of the 5–15% of patients who received abdominal or pelvic radiation will require surgical intervention [32]. Although there is no consensus regarding timing and choice of surgical techniques, it is clear that removal of diseased bowel decreases the mortality rate for resection and is comparable to the bypass procedure [33]. The consensus that simple lysis of adhesions is inadequate and that fistulas require bypass [33, 34] remains somewhat controversial. More recently, a lower operative mortality (21% vs. 10%) and a lower incidence of anatomic dehiscence (36% vs. 6%) have been reported with intestinal bypass as compared with resection [33]. Ruiz-Tovar et al. [35] observed that the most frequent location of radiation injury is ileum (71%), followed by rectum (28%). Of these patients, 36% were medically managed and 64% required surgical treatment. Surgical mortality was 4%; complication rate, 9%, and 16% presented recurrence of radiation-related illness. However, the 5-year survival rate was 90% and the 10-year survival rate 83%, indicating that surgical treatment should not be delayed fearing postoperative complications and pursued as an option in those cases where damage is noted and when there is no response to medical management. Late effects are more susceptible to appear in deteriorated patients and in damaged locations when not resected [35]. Similarly, morbidity (75% for early complications and 100% for late complications) and mortality in the early postoperative period (25%) were higher in the patients undergoing bridectomy than in the patients undergoing other surgical methods. The rate of early and late complications (71.4% and 66.6%, respectively) was lower in the patients undergoing resection-anastomosis with a higher of quality life [36]. These results demonstrated that as the postoperative complication rate, overall and operative mortality of patients treated for radiation enteropathies as emergent surgery is high; specialists following this group of patients may favor removal of the pathologic tissue to avoid complications in the early and late postoperative period. In spite of surgical interventions, symptoms may persist in a significant proportion of patients [37, 38].

8.4.4 Pharmaceutical Management

The principle of pharmaceutical management includes control of diarrhea, infections, enzyme deficiency, malabsorption, inflammation, dehydration, spasms, abdominal and rectal discomfort, and treatment of pain. Medications to serve as antidiarrheals include natural or synthetic agents such as Kaopectate and Imodium (loperamide hydrochloride), taken orally after each loose bowel movement; agents such as Lomotil (diphenoxylate hydrochloride with atropine sulfate) or paregoric and cholestyramine, a bile salt sequestering agent, have also been found effective [39]. Four double-blind and placebo-controlled studies used 5-aminosalicilates in the prevention of acute radiation enteritis. Only for sulfasalazine 2 g/day was a positive effect proven. If acute radiation enteritis was present, octreotide ameliorated radiation-induced diarrhea in a randomized study. Two investigations, only one of them randomized, described the effectiveness of loperamide in the treatment of acute radiation enteritis. If diarrhea was also the main symptom of chronic radiation enteritis, loperamide reduced stool frequency in a double-blind and placebo-controlled study [40]. Donnatal, an anticholinergic antispasmodic agent to alleviate bowel cramping is used as needed. In addition, opioids may offer relief from abdominal pain. If proctitis is present, a steroid foam given rectally may offer relief from symptoms. In patients with pancreatic cancer experiencing diarrhea during radiation therapy, oral pancreatic enzyme replacement has been shown to ameliorate diarrheal symptoms. There is some evidence that the combined treatment with pentoxifylline and tocopherol might alter the pathogenesis of radiation-induced fibrosis. In a retrospective analysis, Hille et al. [41] examined the clinical benefit of the treatment with pentoxifylline/tocopherol on radiation-induced proctitis/enteritis compared to supportive care and demonstrated that combination treatment for at least 6–12 months with pentoxifylline and tocopherol seems to have a benefit in patients with grade I–II radiation-induced proctitis/enteritis [41].

8.4.5   Nutritional Management

Cancer treatment regimens that include radiation therapy (RT) to the abdominal region for cervical, ovarian, prostate, sigmoid, or colorectal cancer potentially disturb the colonization resistance of the indigenous gut flora, causing RT-induced diarrhea, enteritis, and colitis in more than 80% of patients with cancer. In addition to disturbing the colonization in the natural gut flora, it is well documented that ionizing radiation can impact living systems that are ascribed to free-radical production [4]. It has been observed that acute-phase symptoms may persist for a short time, yet long-term complications can represent significant clinical conditions with high morbidity. Several groups have investigated the efficacy of a high-potency probiotic preparation on prevention of radiation-induced diarrhea in experimental and cancer patient populations for ameliorating symptoms of radiation-induced enteritis and colitis [4, 42]. Probiotic supplementation showed beneficial effect in the prevention and treatment of radiation-induced diarrhea in experimental animal studies [4, 42]. Randomized clinical trials have demonstrated efficacy of probiotic preparations VSL #3 and *Lactobacillus casei* DN-114 001 in decreasing the incidence and grade of RT-induced diarrhea [12] since damage to the intestinal villi from radiation therapy results in a reduction or loss of enzymes, one of the most important of these being lactase [31]. Probiotic lactic acid-producing bacteria are an easy, safe, and feasible approach to protect cancer patients against the risk of radiation-induced diarrhea [43]. In a study performed to determine the ability of a probiotic containing live *Lactobacillus acidophilus* plus *Bifidobacterium bifidum* to reduce the incidence of radiation-induced diarrhea in locally advanced cervical cancer patients, patients in the study drug group had a significantly improved stool consistency ($p < 0.001$) [44]. With early results appearing promising in animal [45] and human studies, probiotic therapies continue to be investigated to ameliorate symptoms of radiation-induced enteritis in well-performed, randomized, placebo-controlled studies [42–45].

Total parenteral nutrition (TPN) is widely used in the management of intestinal fistulas resulting from radiation [46]. Short-term parenteral nutrition is however commonly accepted in patients with acute gastrointestinal complications from chemotherapy and radiotherapy, and long-term (home) parenteral nutrition will sometimes be a life-saving maneuver in patients with subacute/chronic radiation enteropathy [47]. In spite of favorable intestinal anatomy, patients with SBS who underwent radiation therapy were less likely to wean from PN [30] due to other factors such as the occurrence of bacterial overgrowth [48] and increasing their dependence to TPN. The presence of nutrients within the intestinal lumen and certain gastrointestinal hormones has an influence on a successful transition [48].

Over the past decade, several preclinical studies have been undertaken to investigate the possible protective effect of glutamine and arginine-enriched diets against radiation-induced intestinal, hepatic, and pancreatic toxicity [20, 49, 50] in animal models. These studies demonstrated beneficial effects with these agents targeting modulation of the inflammatory pathway. Erbil et al. [20] observed that irradiation significantly increased the intestinal and pancreatic myeloperoxidase (MPO) and caspase-3 activities and malondialdehyde (MDA) levels in comparison to sham group. Glutamine treatment significantly decreased this elevation. Histopathological examination revealed that the intestinal mucosal structure was preserved and pancreatic inflammation decreased in the glutamine-treated group. In irradiation group, NF-κB overexpression was detected. These early trials appear promising and provide an opportunity to validate these studies in clinical trials.

There is no recent evidence to demonstrate that specific dietary regimens or restricted diets are effective to control symptoms of radiation enteritis, although malnutrition as a result of diarrhea, reduced intake, and malabsorption are common in this patient population. Most patients with chronic radiation enteritis manage their diets as tolerated, and it is recommended that health professionals dissuade them from unnecessarily restricting their diet, which may result in malnutrition [24].

8.5   Guidelines for Treatment of Gastrointestinal Mucositis/Radiation Enteritis

There are no single standard therapies that have been proven to be effective in the prevention and management of radiation enteritis. The evidence base for therapeutic and preventative strategies in treating chronic radiation enteritis is limited. Since it is clear that several similarities and differences exist between radiation therapy- and chemotherapy- or combination therapy–induced enteritis, with each having specific time to occurrence and location, there is a need for targeting management strategies for risk prediction, prevention, and treatment. From the vast body of literature, it is clear that the basic principles of treatments that have been evaluated for the prevention and management of radiation enteritis have been to screen proactively and predict/detect organ injury early and assess nutritional status and nature of enteritis, taking into consideration specific patient-related factors while targeting the biological basis of the manifestation of the symptoms. Although the evidence base for current therapies is limited, tissue-/organ-sparing radiation therapy techniques, surgical management, and pharmaceutical and nutritional approaches have been shown to be effective in managing symptoms of enteritis. In addition, modification of treatment sequencing of radiation, chemotherapy, and surgery to modulate the severity of enteritis remains key to management of treatment-related toxicities in this target population.

The following guidelines are thus best practice standards based on the current research literature.

8.5.1   Assessment and Medical/Surgical Management

1. Symptoms can be immediate or delayed, chronic or transient. Acute-phase symptoms may persist for a short time, yet long-term complications can represent significant clinical conditions with high morbidity:
   (a) Acute radiation injury to the rectum generally occurs within 6 weeks of therapy and include symptoms such as diarrhea, rectal urgency or tenesmus, and, uncommonly, bleeding. Acute enteritis symptoms usually resolve 2–3 weeks after the completion of treatment, and the mucosa may appear nearly normal. Injuries clinically evident during the first course of radiation and up to 8 weeks later are considered acute. These symptoms usually resolve without specific therapy within 2–6 months
   (b) Chronic radiation proctosigmoiditis has a more delayed onset, and first signs often occur about 9–14 months following radiation exposure but may develop after more than 2 years in some patients, or it may begin as acute enteritis and persist after the cessation of treatment.
2. Institutions providing radiation therapy for these patient populations should adopt a structured, comprehensive approach to assessing gastrointestinal symptoms after radiotherapy and base their treatment plan based on the specific symptoms identified.
3. The assessment and plan of care should be led by a multidisciplinary group of oncologists, surgeons, clinical nutritionists, clinical pharmacists, and gastroenterologists The basic goal of this screening is to obtain a collective measurement of gastrointestinal symptoms and signs including pain and functional disturbances. Based on initial screening and course of treatment, frequent review of symptoms during treatment should be planned.
4. Whenever possible, clinicians should utilize tissue-sparing radiotherapy techniques [1] such as intensity-modulated radiotherapy and modify sequencing of multiple treatment strategies to ensure targeted treatment of tumors while reducing gastrointestinal toxicities.
5. Other techniques such as tridimensional conformal radiotherapy (3D-CRT) have been shown to minimize the amount of small bowel exposed to treatment.
6. It is predictable that certain patient populations are more vulnerable than others for the development of radiation enteritis. These patients must be considered high risk, and thus a proactive mucositis assessment must be incorporated as standard of care.
7. Several toxicity evaluation scales are available, although no radiation enteritis scales were available or validated. The most commonly used scale is the National Cancer Institute Common Toxicity Criteria (NCI-CTC) and has been shown to

be accurate in recording symptoms associated with mucositis and continues to be used in clinical settings.

8. Surgical treatment (removal of diseased bowel) should not be delayed fearing postoperative complications and pursued as an option in those cases where damage is noted and when there is no response to medical management. Late effects are more susceptible to appear in deteriorated patients and in damaged locations when not resected.

9. Symptoms of proctitis – including mucoid rectal discharge, rectal pain, and rectal bleeding (if mucosal ulceration is present) – may result from radiation damage to the anus or rectum. Patients at risk for these symptoms may be proactively cautioned and treated for pain.

8.5.2 Nutritional Assessment and Therapy

Nutritional assessment must be performed within 24 h of admission of the patient by a registered dietitian/nutritionist.

1. Screen patient within 24 h of admission. This order for screening has been a standard order for all cancer patient admissions to avoid delay in timing of screening.

2. Assess all symptoms: gastrointestinal tract: taste alterations, smell alterations, dysphagia, dyspnea, other pain, early satiety, dry mouth, too much saliva production, anorexia, diarrhea, constipation, nausea, vomiting, dehydration, fatigue, height weight, recent weight loss, anthropometrics, (mid-arm muscle circumference, body composition [DEXA], grip strength); psychosocial: family/caregiver support, depression, ADL.

3. Assess current nutritional status and estimate caloric, protein, and multivitamin/mineral needs.

4. Provide adequate nutrition by including "calorie" and "protein" boosters, education material, and nutritional supplements to ensure intake of proteins (recommended 0.8–1.0 g/kg/day). Provide dense caloric supplements up to 400 cal/day containing 1.5 kcal/mL; if intake is insufficient in proteins intake, supplement with modular protein supplements, adding this to favorite beverage (http://www.nestle-nutrition.com/Products/Default.aspx; http://abbottnutrition.com/). The choice of nutritional supplements can be based in the personal choice of the patient, patient needs, tolerance to product, as well as other comorbidities.

5. Include a standard multivitamin mineral supplementation to prevent any further deficits and meet increased needs.

6. Assess adequacy of intake and provide an appetite stimulant (megestrol acetate 320–800 mg/day or alternate) if patient has cancer anorexia to ensure adequate intake and prevent further weight loss.

7. Provide each patient with nutritional guidelines to ensure adequate intake of calories and proteins and a list of suggested high-caloric and high-protein nutritional supplements to choose from, taking into consideration taste alterations, early satiety, nausea, and vomiting that are common symptoms observed in this patient population.

8. Proactive measures to provide alternate mode of nutritional support must be planned during acute phase of treatment when it would be a greater risk to feed patient via the oral route.

9. Selection of route of feeding may be informed based on general guidelines and criteria provided in Table 2.7.

10. With disruption or loss of the gastrointestinal tract function, malabsorption of fat, lactose, bile salts, and vitamin B_{12} is common. A clinical dietitian should perform a thorough assessment and follow patient periodically through therapy and postcompletion of therapy and ensure that repletion of deficiencies is accomplished as they become evident.

11. In the absence of obstruction, diets as tolerated without major restriction, management with antidiarrheals and antispasmodics is recommended.

12. The regular use of probiotics has been shown to be effective in reducing symptoms of radiation enteritis.

13. Short-term parenteral nutrition may be indicated in patients with short bowel syndrome and acute gastrointestinal complications from chemotherapy and radiotherapy, and long-term parenteral nutrition has been shown to improve clinical outcomes in patients with subacute/chronic radiation enteropathy.

14. Although several amino acids and immunomodulators have shown promise in vitro and in animal models, there is only weak evidence of benefit at this time. Well-powered clinical trials are needed to confirm safety and efficacy for the management of cancer treatment related radiation enteritis.

15. There is no recent evidence to demonstrate that specific dietary regimens or restricted diets are effective to control symptoms of radiation enteritis, although malnutrition as a result of diarrhea, reduced intake, and malabsorption are common in this patient population. Most patients with chronic radiation enteritis manage their diets as tolerated, and it is recommended that health professionals dissuade them from unnecessarily restricting their diet, which may result in malnutrition.

16. Other specific guidelines for patients with radiation enteritis:
    - An intake of 6–8 cups of room-temperature liquids must be consumed to help prevent dehydration. These may include nonacidic fruit juices, Gatorade®, ginger ale, nectars, water, or weak teas. Juice may be better tolerated if diluted with water.
    - Caffeinated beverages must be limited or avoided.
    - Carbonated beverages should be allowed to lose their fizz or stirred briskly before consumption.
    - Electrolyte loss must be replaced by increasing the intake of beverages containing potassium and sodium, such as broths and electrolyte solutions.
    - BRATT diets – bananas, rice, applesauce, tea, and toast – have been demonstrated to be effective in reducing symptoms.
    - Pectin from applesauce, amylase-resistant starch from green bananas, or other hydrophilic fiber may help control diarrhea.
    - Frequent, small meals (5–6/day) have been effective.

- Greasy foods and highly spiced foods such as cajun, curry, or pepper must be avoided.
- Specific foods high in fibers such as high-fiber bran cereals, nuts, seeds, popcorn, coconut, beans, and peas may not be well tolerated and may be avoided.
- Breads made from refined flour without seeds or nuts may be better tolerated than those made with whole grains during the acute phase.
- Raw vegetables and the skins, seeds, and stringy fibers of unpeeled fruits may not be well tolerated and may be avoided.
- Patients can resume consumption of higher fiber-containing foods, fruits, and vegetables once the diarrhea subsides by starting with foods rich in carbohydrates first, then proteins, and lastly fats.
- Dairy products may not be well tolerated secondary to lactose intolerance and can be substituted with Lactaid-treated milk, cultured yogurt, or soymilk.
- If steatorrhea (fatty stools and malabsorption) is present, recommend a low-fat, high-protein, and high-carbohydrate diet. Medium-chain triglyceride-based oils (MCT) may be recommended as they are hydrolyzed rapidly and better absorbed than other oils. MCT oil is best absorbed when ingested with food than when administered by spoonfuls.
- Normally divided doses of 15 mg of oil per feeding used in salad dressings or sandwich spreads are best tolerated.

8.5.3   Pharmacotherapy

- *Bulk-producing agents*
  - Polycarbophil calcium (FiberCon®)
  - Psyllium hydrophilic mucilloid (Metamucil®)
- *Probiotics*
  - *Lactobacillus* sp. (Lactinex®)
  - Dairy Ease®
- *Antidiarrheal agents*
  - Diphenoxylate HCl and atropine sulfate (Lomotil®)
  - Kaolin (Kaopectate®)
  - Loperamide HCl (Imodium®)
  - Tincture of opium
  - Camphorated tincture of opium (paregoric)
  - Cholestyramine
  - Lipisorb® for steatorrhea
- *Fluid and electrolytes*
  - Oral hydration solution (Rehydralyte®)
- *Pain*
  - Patients must be evaluated for pain and treated to manage pain.
  - Infusion method with opiates has demonstrated relief and must be evaluated and considered for pain management.
    Donnatal, an anticholinergic antispasmodic agent to alleviate bowel cramping

- *Radiation-induced fibrosis*
  - Pentoxifylline and tocopherol

8.5.4 Markers and Instruments for Patient Monitoring and Assessment of Response to Treatment by the Interdisciplinary Medical Team

- *Anthropometric measurements* such as participant's height, weight, and body mass index can be performed at admission and at regular intervals established by the medical team. Skeletal muscle function is a central determinant of functional capacity in humans. Loss of muscle as seen in CC results in poor function and decreased survival rate following critical illness. Muscle size is therefore considered an important marker of functional status in studies of sarcopenia/cachexia.
- *Body composition by DXA scan*: DXA should be used to assess both total lean body mass (LBM), fat mass (FM), and total bone mineral density (BMD). Total bone mineral density (BMD) is a valid indirect measure of skeletal muscle and patient activity. Total LBM is sometimes called total fat-free mass (FFM), depending upon specific DXA manufacturer. DXA instruments use an X-ray source that generates or is split into two energies to measure bone mineral mass and soft tissue from which fat and fat-free mass are estimated. The exam is quick (1–2 min), precise (0.5–1%), and noninvasive. DXA scanners have the precision required to detect changes in muscle mass as small as 5%. Radiation exposure from DXA scans is minimal. The National Council of Radiation Protection and Measurements (NCRP) has recommended that the annual effective dose limit for infrequent exposure of the general population is 5,000 μSv and that an annual effective dose of 10 μSv be considered a negligible individual dose. The effective dose of a dual-energy X-ray absorptiometry whole-body scan on an adult is 2.1 μSv. Studies have shown that quality assurance is an important issue in the use of DXA scans to determine body composition including lean body mass and bone mineral density. DXA instrument manufacturer and model should remain consistent, and their calibration should be monitored throughout treatment. Use of a standardized scan acquisition protocol and appropriate and unchanging scan acquisition and analysis software is essential to achieve consist results.
- *Dietary intake* must be assessed at baseline and at regularly scheduled intervals by conducting random weekly, 2 weekdays + 1 weekend day, 24-h dietary recalls (gold standard for collecting dietary data) using a 5-step multipass procedure [33, 34] (which has been found to assess mean energy intake within 10% of actual intake) and using the frequently updated University of Minnesota Nutrition Data System for Research (NDSR) version database for analysis of nutrient composition. Food portion visuals can be provided to patients to estimate portion sizes of foods while monitoring intake.
- *Symptom log* may be completed daily and collected from patients on a monthly basis. Based on these symptoms, all anticipated and unanticipated, grades of

constitutional, dermatological, gastrointestinal (GI), metabolic, and pain symptoms can be continuously monitored including those symptoms affecting nutritional intake and utilization.

- *Monthly* CMP and CBC should be monitored to assess electrolytes and organ function. Evaluate for anemia and B_{12} deficiency.
- *Functional markers (Karnofsky performance score)*: Evaluation of patients' functional status and barriers to obtaining adequate nutrients is also necessary. A physical exam combined with personal interview should include the evaluation of functional status such as the ability to chew and swallow, dental or oral problems causing odynophagia or dysphagia, signs of muscle wasting or anasarca, presence of edema, presence of skin or mouth lesion, and ability to perform instrumental activities of daily living (IADLs) such as cooking, shopping, and self-feeding. It is critical to assess activities of daily living, physical activity, exercise, sleep, and ability to work and perform other functional roles. Limitations in the activities of daily living have been identified secondary to and as a cause of weight loss in cancer patients. Cancer and other chronic diseases pose difficulties specifically for the cancer patient receiving treatment and the elderly in carrying out activities of daily living. A loss of postural and locomotive muscle mass has been observed within 7 days of inactivity. The Karnofsky Performance Scale Index allows patients to be classified as to their functional impairment. This has been used to compare effectiveness of different therapies and to assess the prognosis in individual patients and has been validated in cancer patient populations.
- *Biochemical markers of protein status (serum albumin and transferrin)*: Assessment of protein status is critical in the identification and treatment of abnormalities in protein metabolism. There is substantial evidence of the correlation between serum hepatic proteins and inflammation, making these the most relevant biomarkers in cancer patient populations. Serum transferrin, prealbumin, and albumin have been observed as intermediate endpoint biomarkers and independently associated with clinical outcomes. Measurements of body composition combined with a more objective and sensitive measure of protein nutriture are ideal for the biochemical assessment of intravascular and visceral protein stores. We have thus included the three major valid intermediate endpoint biomarkers (IEBs) that represent intravascular and visceral protein pools – transferrin, prealbumin, and albumin – as the biochemical indicators of protein status. Although transferrin levels are affected by iron status, serum transferrin, either singly or as part of a multiparameter index, is the strongest predictor of cancer patient morbidity and mortality.
- *Immune and inflammatory markers*: A range of metabolic responses triggered by inflammatory and immunological responses in cancer patient with radiation enteritis. Cytokines can be measured in a panel including IL-1, IL-4, IL-6, IL-8, IL-10, GM-CSF, IFN-κ, TNF-α, and CRP (BioRad-Bioplex). All of these biomarkers have been shown to increase with disease, aging, and cytotoxic agents. Though we realize these intermediate endpoint biomarkers of cytokines cannot

be reliably interpreted, as over 70% of the subjects as observed in our studies were on active treatment with cytotoxic agents, these variables are important to determine as they may provide useful information and contribute to the better understanding of the mechanistic process.

- *Quality of life* should be measured at baseline and monthly using the Rand Short Form SF-36 (Medical Outcomes Study SF36). The SF-36 has been used extensively with both general, high-risk, and cancer populations and has available norms for mail and telephone versions and comparisons between group and individual scores. Scores are calculated and transformed to a 0–100 scale, with higher scores indicating increased health status. Reliability of the SF-36 scales was measured by Cronbach α coefficient, and the results ranged from 0.78 in general health perceptions to 0.91 in the physical functioning domain.

8.5.5   Follow-up

Patients must be seen by the multidisciplinary team on a monthly basis to monitor progress and to review compliance to intervention including diet intake adequacy, symptom logs, change in concomitant medications, and any other issues related to treatment. Improved management of malnutrition with nutritional therapy may require a multimodal intervention by multidisciplinary teams using a comprehensive and integrated approach. Initial screening and knowledge of treatment trajectory of the cancer patient should guide a plan for reassessment of the cancer patient at regularly planned intervals. Subjective and objective data on progress and response to nutritional therapy may be assessed using the indicators used in the comprehensive nutritional assessment. Newly developed symptoms resulting from treatment or progression of disease may require additional monitoring or revision of nutritional therapy. Reassessment/reevaluation for monitoring and evaluation of nutritional therapy must include monitoring of clinical, functional, dietary, and behavioral outcomes that were identified by the comprehensive nutritional assessment.

8.6   Future Directions

Significant progress has been made in developing novel techniques to reduce dose, intensity, and frequency of radiation to reduce gastrointestinal toxicities. To date, the implication and connection between several mechanistic pathways contributing to the incidence and severity of radiation enteritis have not been elucidated. Initial studies on potential molecular mechanism contributing to the etiology of radiation enteritis continues to evolve and may have significant implications for clinically identifying agents that can target these pathways implicated in the development of fibrosis related to radiation enteritis. Agents and treatment modalities targeting these pathways must be developed in the future. Over the past decade, several preclinical studies have been undertaken to investigate the possible protective effect of glutamine and arginine-enriched diets against radiation-induced intestinal, hepatic, and pancreatic toxicity in animal models. These studies demonstrated beneficial effects with these agents targeting modulation of the inflammatory pathway. These early studies appear promising and need to be evaluated for safety and effectiveness in ameliorating symptoms of radiation enteritis in well-powered clinical trials targeting specific cancer and treatment groups.

Summary for the Clinician

There are no single standard therapies that have been proven to be effective in the prevention and management of radiation enteritis. However, multimodal therapies have shown effectiveness in ameliorating symptoms of radiation enteritis.

Although the evidence base for current therapies is limited, tissue-/organ-sparing radiation therapy techniques, surgical management, and pharmaceutical and nutritional approaches have been shown to be effective in managing symptoms of enteritis.

In addition, modification of treatment sequencing of radiation, chemotherapy, and surgery to modulate the severity of enteritis remains key to management of treatment-related toxicities in this target population.

Assessment and treatment of radiation enteritis should be performed and implemented using a multiprofessional approach to clinical care, research, and education associated with enteral injury in cancer patients.

Proactive, systematic screening, assessment, and early identification of high-risk populations for specific treatments should be part of standard of care. The basic goal of this screening is to obtain a collective measurement of gastrointestinal symptoms, signs, and functional disturbances, including pain.

Screening and follow-up evaluation can be made utilizing the National Cancer Institute Common Toxicity Criteria (NCI-CTC).

Surgical treatment should not be delayed fearing postoperative complications and pursued as an option in those cases where damage is noted and when there is no response to medical management. Late effects are more susceptible to appear in deteriorated patients and in damaged locations when not resected.

Although several amino acids and immunomodulators have shown promise in vitro and in animal models, there is only weak evidence of benefit at this time. Well-powered clinical trials are needed to confirm safety and efficacy for the management of cancer treatment–related radiation enteritis.

In the absence of obstruction, diets as tolerated without major restriction, managed with antidiarrheals and antispasmodics is recommended. The regular use of probiotics has been shown to be effective in reducing symptoms of radiation enteritis.

Short-term parenteral nutrition may be indicated in patients with short bowel syndrome and acute gastrointestinal complications from chemotherapy and radiotherapy, and long-term parenteral nutrition has been shown to improve clinical outcomes in patients with subacute/chronic radiation enteropathy.

To date, the implication and connection between several mechanistic pathways contributing the incidence and severity of radiation enteritis have not been elucidated. Initial studies on potential molecular mechanism contributing to the etiology of radiation enteritis continues to evolve and may have significant implications for clinically identifying agents that can target these pathways implicated in the development of fibrosis related to radiation enteritis. Agents and treatment modalities targeting these pathways must be developed in the future.

Over the past decade, several preclinical studies have been undertaken to investigate the possible protective effect of glutamine and arginine-enriched diets against radiation-induced intestinal, hepatic and pancreatic toxicity in animal models. These studies demonstrated beneficial effects with these agents targeting modulation of the inflammatory pathway. These early studies appear promising and need to be evaluated for safety and effectiveness in ameliorating symptoms of radiation enteritis in well-powered clinical trials targeting specific cancer and treatment groups.

References

1. Rodríguez ML, Martín MM, Padellano LC, Palomo AM, Puebla YI (2010) Gastrointestinal toxicity associated to radiation therapy. Clin Transl Oncol 12(8):554–561, Review. PubMed PMID: 20709653
2. Ong ZY, Gibson RJ, Bowen JM, Stringer AM, Darby JM, Logan RM, Yeoh AS, Keefe DM (2010) Pro-inflammatory cytokines play a key role in the development of radiotherapy-induced gastrointestinal mucositis. Radiat Oncol 5:22
3. Stringer AM, Gibson RJ, Bowen JM, Keefe DM (2009) Chemotherapy-induced modifications to gastrointestinal microflora: evidence and implications of change. Curr Drug Metab 10(1): 79–83, Review
4. Spyropoulos BG, Misiakos EP, Fotiadis C, Stoidis CN (2011) Antioxidant properties of probiotics and their protective effects in the pathogenesis of radiation-induced enteritis and colitis. Dig Dis Sci 56(2):285–294, Epub 2010 Jul 15. Review. PubMed PMID: 20632107
5. Fajardo LF (1982) Alimentary tract. In: Fajardo LF (ed) Pathology of radiation injury. Masson Publishers, New York, pp 47–76
6. Yeoh EK, Horowitz M (1987) Radiation enteritis. Surg Gynecol Obstet 165(4):373–379 [PUBMED Abstract]
7. Schultheiss TE, Lee WR, Hunt MA et al (1997) Late GI and GU complications in the treatment of prostate cancer. Int J Radiat Oncol Biol Phys 37:3
8. O'Brien PH, Jenrette JM JM 3rd, Garvin AJ (1987) Radiation enteritis. Am Surg 53(9): 501–504 [PUBMED Abstract]
9. Babb RR (1996) Radiation proctitis: a review. Am J Gastroenterol 91:1309
10. Gilinsky NH, Burns DG, Barbezat GO et al (1983) The natural history of radiation-induced proctosigmoiditis: an analysis of 88 patients. Q J Med 52:40

11. Lucarotti ME, Mountford RA, Bartolo DC (1991) Surgical management of intestinal radiation injury. Dis Colon Rectum 34:865
12. Visich KL, Yeo TP (2010) The prophylactic use of probiotics in the prevention of radiation therapy-induced diarrhea. Clin J Oncol Nurs 14(4):467–473
13. Andreyev J (2005) Gastrointestinal complications of pelvic radiotherapy: are they of any importance? Gut 54(8):1051–1054
14. Gami B, Harrington K, Blake P, Dearnaley D, Tait D, Davies J, Norman AR, Andreyev HJ (2003) How patients manage gastrointestinal symptoms after pelvic radiotherapy. Aliment Pharmacol Ther 18(10):987–994
15. Abayomi JC, Kirwan J, Hackett AF (2009) Coping mechanisms used by women in an attempt to avoid symptoms of chronic radiation enteritis. J Hum Nutr Diet 22(4):310–316, Epub 2009 Jun 10
16. Theis VS, Sripadam R, Ramani V, Lal S (2010) Chronic radiation enteritis. Clin Oncol (R Coll Radiol) 22(1):70–83, Epub 2009 Nov 7. Review. PubMed PMID: 19897345
17. Gallagher MJ, Brereton HD, Rostock RA et al (1986) A prospective study of treatment techniques to minimize the volume of pelvic small bowel with reduction of acute and late effects associated with pelvic irradiation. Int J Radiat Oncol Biol Phys 12(9):1565–1573 [PUBMED Abstract]
18. Haddad GK, Grodsinsky C, Allen H (1983) The spectrum of radiation enteritis. Surgical considerations. Dis Colon Rectum 26(9):590–594 [PUBMED Abstract]
19. Zhu Y, Zhou J, Tao G (2011) Molecular aspects of chronic radiation enteritis. Clin Invest Med 34(3):E119–E124
20. Erbil Y, Oztezcan S, Giri M, Barbaros U, Olgaç V, Bilge H, Küçücük H, Toker G (2005) The effect of glutamine on radiation-induced organ damage. Life Sci 78(4):376–382, Epub 2005 Aug 29
21. Yasko JM (1982) Care of the client receiving external radiation therapy. Reston Publishing Company, Inc., Reston
22. Kim HM, Kim YJ, Kim HJ, Park SW, Bang S, Song SY (2011) A pilot study of capsule endoscopy for the diagnosis of radiation enteritis. Hepatogastroenterology 58(106):459–464, PubMed PMID: 21661413
23. Singeap AM, Trifan A, Cojocariu C, Sfarti C, Stanciu C (2011) Outcomes after symptomatic capsule retention in suspected small bowel obstruction. Eur J Gastroenterol Hepatol 23(10):886–890
24. Abayomi J, Kirwan J, Hackett A (2009) The prevalence of chronic radiation enteritis following radiotherapy for cervical or endometrial cancer and its impact on quality of life. Eur J Oncol Nurs 13(4):262–267, Epub 2009 Jul 28
25. Minsky BD, Cohen AM (1988) Minimizing the toxicity of pelvic radiation therapy in rectal cancer. Oncology (Huntingt) 2(8):21–25, 28–9, [PUBMED Abstract]
26. Samuelian JM, Callister MD, Ashman JB, Young-Fadok TM, Borad MJ, Gunderson LL (2011) Reduced acute bowel toxicity in patients treated with intensity-modulated radiotherapy for rectal cancer. Int J Radiat Oncol Biol Phys. [Epub ahead of print]
27. Chen CC, Lin JC, Jan JS, Ho SC, Wang L (2011) Definitive intensity-modulated radiation therapy with concurrent chemotherapy for patients with locally advanced cervical cancer. Gynecol Oncol 122(1):9–13, Epub 2011 Apr 22
28. Sharma NK, Li T, Chen DY, Pollack A, Horwitz EM, Buyyounouski MK (2011) Intensity-modulated radiotherapy reduces gastrointestinal toxicity in patients treated with androgen deprivation therapy for prostate cancer. Int J Radiat Oncol Biol Phys 80(2):437–444, Epub 2010 Nov 2
29. Deville C, Both S, Hwang WT, Tochner Z, Vapiwala N (2010) Clinical toxicities and dosimetric parameters after whole-pelvis versus prostate-only intensity-modulated radiation therapy for prostate cancer. Int J Radiat Oncol Biol Phys 78(3):763–772, Epub 2010 Feb 18
30. Thompson JS, Weseman R, Rochling F, Grant W, Botha J, Langnas A, Mercer D (2011) Radiation therapy increases the risk of hepatobiliary complications in short bowel syndrome. Nutr Clin Pract 26(4):474–478

31. Stryker JA, Bartholomew M (1986) Failure of lactose-restricted diets to prevent radiation-induced diarrhea in patients undergoing whole pelvis irradiation. Int J Radiat Oncol Biol Phys 12(5):789–792 [PUBMED Abstract]
32. Galland RB, Spencer J (1986) Surgical management of radiation enteritis. Surgery 99(2): 133–139 [PUBMED Abstract]
33. Lillemoe KD, Brigham RA, Harmon JW et al (1983) Surgical management of small-bowel radiation enteritis. Arch Surg 118(8):905–907 [PUBMED Abstract]
34. Wobbes T, Verschueren RC, Lubbers EJ et al (1984) Surgical aspects of radiation enteritis of the small bowel. Dis Colon Rectum 27(2):89–92 [PUBMED Abstract]
35. Ruiz-Tovar J, Morales V, Hervás A, Sanjuanbenito A, Lobo E, Martínez-Molina E (2009) Late gastrointestinal complications after pelvic radiotherapy: radiationenteritis. Clin Transl Oncol 11(8):539–543
36. Parlakgumus A, Caliskan K, Parlakgumus HA, Kayaselcuk F, Ezer A, Colakoglu T, Belli S, Yildirim S (2011) Emergent surgical treatment of radiation-inducedenteropathies for patients with urogynecological and colorectal carcinomas. Clin Exp Obstet Gynecol 38(1):63–66
37. Wellwood JM, Jackson BT (1973) The intestinal complications of radiotherapy. Br J Surg 60(10):814–818 [PUBMED Abstract]
38. Boland E, Thompson J, Rochling F, Sudan D (2010) A 25-year experience with postresection short-bowel syndrome secondary to radiation therapy. Am J Surg 200(6):690–693; discussion 693. PubMed PMID: 21146003
39. Tuchmann L, Engelking C (2001) Cancer-related diarrhea. In: Gates RA, Fink RM (eds) Oncology nursing secrets, 2nd edn. Hanley and Belfus, Philadelphia, pp 310–322
40. Zimmerer T, Böcker U, Wenz F, Singer MV (2008) Medical prevention and treatment of acute and chronic radiation induced enteritis–is there any proven therapy? A short review. Gastroenterology 46(5):441–448
41. Hille A, Christiansen H, Pradier O, Hermann RM, Siekmeyer B, Weiss E, Hilgers R, Hess CF, Schmidberger H (2005) Effect of pentoxifylline and tocopherol on radiation proctitis/enteritis. Strahlenther Onkol 181(9):606–614
42. Fuccio L, Guido A, Eusebi LH, Laterza L, Grilli D, Cennamo V, Ceroni L, Barbieri E, Bazzoli F (2009) Effects of probiotics for the prevention and treatment of radiation-induced diarrhea. J Clin Gastroenterol 43(6):506–513
43. Delia P, Sansotta G, Donato V, Frosina P, Messina G, De Renzis C, Famularo G (2007) Use of probiotics for prevention of radiation-induced diarrhea. World J Gastroenterol 13(6):912–915
44. Chitapanarux I, Chitapanarux T, Traisathit P, Kudumpee S, Tharavichitkul E, Lorvidhaya V (2010) Randomized controlled trial of live *Lactobacillus acidophilus* plus *Bifidobacterium bifidum* in prophylaxis of diarrhea during radiotherapy in cervical cancer patients. Radiat Oncol 5:31
45. Seal M, Naito Y, Barreto R, Lorenzetti A, Safran P, Marotta F (2007) Experimental radiotherapy-induced enteritis: a probiotic interventional study. J Dig Dis 8(3):143–147
46. Sepehripour S, Papagrigoriadis S (2010) A systematic review of the benefit of total parenteral nutrition in the management of enterocutaneous fistulas. Minerva Chir 65(5):577–585
47. Bozzetti F, Arends J, Lundholm K, Micklewright A, Zurcher G, Muscaritoli M, ESPEN (2009) ESPEN guidelines on parenteral nutrition: non-surgical oncology. Clin Nutr 28(4):445–54, Epub 2009 May 23
48. Ballesteros Pomar MD, Vidal Casariego A (2007) Short bowel syndrome: definition, causes, intestinal adaptation and bacterial overgrowth. Nutr Hosp 22(Suppl 2):74–85
49. Ersin S, Tuncyurek P, Esassolak M, Alkanat M, Buke C, Yilmaz M, Telefoncu A, Kose T (2000) The prophylactic and therapeutic effects of glutamine- and arginine-enriched diets on radiation-induced enteritis in rats. J Surg Res 89(2):121–125
50. Gurbuz AT, Kunzelman J, Ratzer EE (1998) Supplemental dietary arginine accelerates intestinal mucosal regeneration and enhances bacterial clearance following radiation enteritis in rats. J Surg Res 74(2):149–154

Neurocognitive Impairment (NI)

9

Core Messages

Survivors of breast, colon, and gynecological cancer are increasingly concerned about the possible cognitive sequelae (called chemo brain or chemo fog) associated with chemotherapy and radiation treatment regimens.

Neurocognitive impairment (NI) is observed in childhood cancer patients, both related to CNS malignancies as well as those related to treatment in adult survivors of brain tumors, head and neck sarcomas, as well as acute lymphoblastic leukemia (ALL).

Symptoms in cancer patients are characterized by subtle or severe alterations across a variety of cognitive domains, including verbal memory, nonverbal memory, information processing speed, and visuospatial function. Children treated for a brain tumor (BT) and ALL demonstrate neurocognitive impairment that are more numerous and has more severe manifestations.

Although it was first thought that NI, that is, chemotherapy-induced, is acute and reversible, suggesting a transient nature of this phenomenon, more recent studies have revealed neurocognitive impairment (NI) to be progressive and lasting anywhere from 6 months to 10 years posttreatment in cancer survivors, especially in breast and adult survivors of childhood cancers.

The etiology of NI may be multifactorial in breast cancer survivors and contributed by one or more of the following mechanisms: age, vascular injury, oxidative damage, inflammation, direct injury to neuron, autoimmune responses, chemotherapy-induced anemia, amyloid-β (Aβ) peptide accumulation, abrupt steroid hormone deficit, hypothyroidism, and genetic polymorphisms. In childhood cancers, NI can be attributed to CNS malignancies, tumor-related deficits due to direct invasion of the brain, seizures, hydrocephalus, systemic chemotherapy with methotrexate at high doses and combined intrathecal (IT) cytarabine and corticosteroid, and in chemoradiation therapies that lead to leukoencephalopathy.

Recent prospective studies show that ~20% of cancer patients experience cognitive dysfunction even before commencement of chemotherapy as cancer

N.B. Kumar, *Nutritional Management of Cancer Treatment Effects*,
DOI 10.1007/978-3-642-27233-2_9, © Springer-Verlag Berlin Heidelberg 2012

patients exhibit increased circulating levels of cytokines and inflammation that can produce systemic effects and have been shown to be associated with impairment of cognition. Other psychosocial factors such as stress, anxiety, depression, fatigue, age, social support, education level, and intelligence have been shown to contribute to NI.

Other than subjective reports of NI using cognitive function tools in this population, studies have reported more objective chemotherapy-related decreases in the integrity of white matter in the brain area associated with changes in electrophysiological indexes of processing speed using imaging techniques.

Current interventions for the treatment of NI include treatment of anemia, having studied the pharmacological interventions to treat anemia with recombinant human erythropoietin; treatment of fatigue with dexmethylphenidate (d-MPH), physical activity, fluoxetine (a selective serotonin reuptake inhibitor [SSRI]), donepezil, and modafinil (a central nervous system stimulant); cognitive training; nutrients; and nutrient-derived agents with antioxidant and anti-inflammatory properties.

9.1   Definition

Cognitive function is a multidimensional concept that describes the domains resulting from healthy brain performance, namely, attention and concentration, executive function, information processing speed, language, visuospatial skill, psychomotor ability, learning, and memory [1]. In the past decade, survivors of breast [2–15], colon [16], and gynecological cancer [16] are increasingly concerned about the possible cognitive sequelae (called chemo brain or chemo fog) associated with chemotherapy and radiation treatment regimens [2–16]. Symptoms are characterized by subtle or severe alterations across a variety of cognitive domains, including verbal memory, nonverbal memory, information processing speed, and visuospatial function [17]. Children treated for a brain tumor (BT) or acute lymphoblastic leukemia (ALL) also demonstrate neurocognitive impairment (NI) that has more severe manifestations. Survivors of childhood cancers of the central nervous system (CNS), ALL, and head and neck tumors continue to be at risk for NI well into adulthood, and that impairment is related to social outcomes [18–21]. Deficits occur in a variety of domains such as general intelligence, age-appropriate developmental disorders, academic achievement, visual and perceptual motor skills, nonverbal and verbal memory, receptive and expressive language, and attention and involve impairment of executive function and global cognitive abilities. Fortunately, the cancer survivor population – both pediatric and adult – is increasing. However, the neurocognitive late effects appear relatively common and have been demonstrated to exacerbate long-term physiological and psychological health leading to premature mortality and morbidity. Consequently, the public health consequences are substantial.

9.2 Prevalence

Neurocognitive impairment is observed in childhood cancer patients, both related to CNS malignancies as well as those related to treatment in adult survivors of brain tumors, head and neck sarcomas as well as ALL [18–21]. Treatment-related neurocognitive impairment related to cancer treatment is most frequently reported in breast cancer patient population who comprise 22% of the 11 million survivors today in the USA. One of the most common adverse effects reported by breast cancer patients after treatment is "chemo brain," the phenomenon of cognitive impairment (CI) described by 30–75% of patients treated with chemotherapy for breast cancer and lasting anywhere from 6 months to 10 years [7–12]. In a recent study of cognitive impairment in older adults over 65, females with gynecological cancers were significantly at higher risk of CI, lasting up to 3 years after treatment [15]. Although most standard chemotherapy regimens at standardized doses appear to not cross the blood–brain barrier, even mild toxicity to the central nervous system (CNS) has been shown to produce significant changes to cognitive function (CF) [6–12, 22, 23]. Additionally, although it was first thought that NI, that is, chemotherapy-induced, is acute and reversible, suggesting a transient nature of this phenomenon, more recent studies have revealed cognitive impairment (CI) to be progressive and lasting anywhere from 6 months to 10 years posttreatment in breast cancer survivors [6–12]. More recently, our team at the Moffitt Cancer Center [12] examined the extent to which cognitive functioning continues to change in the post-treatment period and examined residualized CI in breast cancer survivors from 6 months to 3 years posttreatment compared to an age- and education-matched sample of women without cancer assessed over a comparable time period. Our findings suggest that adjuvant treatment for breast cancer, particularly chemotherapy, is associated with long-term deficits across a number of cognitive domains. Similarly, others have observed that patients treated for colorectal cancer experience cognitive impairment up to 6 months after the completion of treatment [16]. Irrespective of type and duration of chemotherapy, there is consistent evidence of CI in patients receiving cytotoxic drugs for cancer treatment.

Adults treated for a childhood cancer in the 1970s and 1980s were three times more likely than their siblings to have developed a later, chronic health condition, according to a large study of childhood cancer survivors [24, 25]. More than 11 million cancer survivors are alive in the USA, at least 270,000 of whom were originally diagnosed when they were under the age of 21. Advances in cancer treatment have meant that today, almost 80% of children diagnosed with cancer are alive at least 5 years after diagnosis. Many ultimately will be considered cured [18–21]. Neurocognitive late effects most commonly follow treatment of malignancies that require CNS-directed therapies such as cranial radiation intraventricular/intrathecal chemotherapy, affecting children with CNS tumors, head and neck sarcomas, and

ALL [18–21]. For both CNS tumors and ALL, younger age at time of treatment is associated with an increase in neurocognitive deficits [18]. Leukemia is the most common form of pediatric cancer, accounting for 25% of all cancers occurring before 20 years of age [26]. Acute lymphoblastic leukemia (ALL) accounts for roughly 75% of all leukemia diagnoses, with over 3,000 new cases diagnosed annually [27, 28]. Improvements in the treatment of ALL have led to a remarkable increase in the survival rate for children younger than 15 years, which currently exceeds 80% [1]. With this decreased mortality, it is estimated that 1 out of every 640 young adults will be a pediatric cancer survivor, and approximately half of them will have history of ALL [29, 30]. The "late effects" that commonly occur in survivors of pediatric ALL include neurocognitive impairment [4], estimated to occur in roughly 40% of long-term survivors [27].

9.3   Etiology

9.3.1   Etiology of NI in All Cancers

As discussed, CI is most prevalent and reported in breast cancer survivors, pediatric cancer patients with CNS malignancies, and adult survivors of childhood cancers, especially brain tumors, head and neck cancers, and ALL. In considering the etiological basis of NI that is observed postchemotherapy in breast cancer patients, several studies [8–12, 31–34] have hypothesized that this phenomenon may be multifactorial and may be contributed by one or more of the following mechanisms: age, vascular injury, oxidative damage, inflammation, direct injury to neuron, autoimmune responses, chemotherapy-induced anemia, amyloid-β (Aβ) peptide accumulation, abrupt steroid hormone deficit, hypothyroidism, and genetic polymorphisms [31–35]. Chemotherapeutic agents reduce trophic factors such as brain-derived neurotrophic factor (BDNF) and neurogenesis, and this may be another factor that leads to CI [36, 37]. We have reported prevalence of chemotherapy-induced loss of thyroid function [31] which has been associated to decrements in working memory and intentional and executive disturbances similar to those observed in breast cancer survivors. Others have examined the relationship of epsilon 4 allele of APOE genotype which may be a potential genetic marker for the increased vulnerability to chemotherapy-induced cognitive decline seen in breast cancer and lymphoma survivors [2]. However, recent studies in twins from a large database demonstrated female survivors (not males) were significantly more likely to exhibit cognitive impairments or more years after treatment as their co-twin without cancer. This was more evident for gynecological cancers such as ovarian cancer [15].

9.3.2   Etiology of NI in Adult Cancers

Oxidative stress and inflammation contribute to several organ toxicities, including neurotoxicities, after common cancer chemotherapy regimen. In breast cancer patient populations, doxorubicin and other platinum-based therapies have been documented to cause the generation of free radicals and the induction of oxidative stress associated with cellular injury [22]. Adriamycin (ADR) is a chemotherapeutic for the treatment of solid tumors. This quinone-containing anthracycline is well known to produce large amounts of reactive oxygen species (ROS) in vivo. A common complaint of patients undergoing long-term treatment with ADR is somnolence, often referred to as "chemo brain." While ADR itself does not cross the blood–brain barrier (BBB) [3], it was recently shown in a preclinical model that ADR administration causes a peripheral increase in tumor necrosis factor-α (TNF-α), which migrates across the BBB and leads to inflammation and oxidative stress in brain, most likely contributing to the observed decline in cognition, supporting the rationale for interventions with antioxidants to prevent ADR-induced cognitive dysfunction. An increased activity of glutathione peroxidase (GPx) and a significant reduction in GST and GR activity in mice brains, 72 h post–i.p. injection of ADR, was observed. As chemotherapeutics have been shown to reduce neurogenesis, this treatment regimen can directly impact this negative action of cytotoxic agents [36, 37]. Some of the contributing factors could be vascular injury and oxidative damage, inflammation, and direct injury to neurons [7]. The basis for the use of nutritional supplements as a moderator of age-related cognitive decline is the age-related increase in oxidative stress [38, 39], similar to those observed during cytotoxic therapies for cancer. The principle is to not only scavenge reactive oxygen species (ROS) [23, 40] but modify protein kinases, apoptosis signaling, and regulate signal transduction via modification of cellular redox reactions [16, 41–44]. Several imaging studies completed have found evidence of structural and functional changes in brain regions that are believed to be involved in the cognitive deficits experienced by cancer survivors who received chemotherapy. Recently, several reports have focused on brain-imaging studies and have reported chemotherapy-related decreases in the integrity of white matter in the brain area associated with changes in electrophysiological indexes of processing speed [42, 43]. Inagaki et al. [44]. discovered structural brain changes in cancer survivors associated with reduced superior frontal gyri and parahippocampal gyrus volume being correlated with poor attention/concentration and impaired memory performance, respectively, 4 months after completion of treatment. Corresponding functional brain changes have also been reported by de Ruiter et al. [41]. who observed hyporesponsiveness in both the prefrontal cortex and parahippocampal gyrus during executive functioning and episodic memory tasks in cancer survivors who had received chemotherapy almost 10 years previously.

9.3.3 Etiology of NI in Childhood Cancers and Adult Survivors of Childhood Cancers

In childhood cancer involving CNS malignancies, tumor-related deficits have been attributed to direct invasion of the brain, seizures, and hydrocephalus. Additionally, systemic methotrexate in high doses and combined with radiation therapy can lead to a well-described leukoencephalopathy, in which severe neurocognitive deficits are obvious [45]. In addition, treatment-related neurocognitive problems in childhood ALL are often attributed to intrathecal or high-dose intravenous methotrexate [46]. Dexamethasone has been shown to be a potent cytotoxic agent, with higher rates of CNS penetrance than prednisone [47] and increased memory impairment [48]. Because of its penetrance capability into the CNS, systemic methotrexate has been used in a variety of low-dose and high-dose regimens for leukemia CNS prophylaxis. However, the deleterious effects of systemic methotrexate, especially at doses above 1 g/m^2, may be no different or worse than those of 18 Gy of cranial radiation therapy [49]. In a large epidemiological study of adult survivors of childhood cancer, we recently demonstrated elevated rates of neurocognitive impairment among survivors of ALL [50]. Studies at St. Jude's Children's hospital compared 5,937 adult survivors to 382 siblings on attention/processing speed, emotional regulation, organization, and memory. The rate of impairment in survivors was 50% higher than that for siblings. Survivors treated with dexamethasone were 40% more likely to report impairment compared to survivors treated with surgery or other chemotherapy agents (RR = 1.4, 95% CI 1.1–1.8). Survivors who reported significant emotional distress were more likely to report impaired attention/processing speed (RR = 3.9, 3.4–4.4), organization (RR = 2.9, 2.5–3.4), memory (RR = 5.8, 5.2–6.6), and emotional regulation (RR = 3.5, 3.2–3.8). These results document higher rates of problems with neurocognitive functions in adult survivors of childhood ALL, with contribution to these problems from dexamethasone. Recent research has questioned the higher neurotoxicity associated with dexamethasone. When comparing survivors of childhood ALL treated with dexamethasone (n = 51) or prednisone (n = 41), no group differences were found on neurocognitive assessments [51]. However, this study compared exposures that occurred during induction therapy with outcomes in early adolescence, prior to adult maturation of brain and physical functions. We have recently reported results linking dexamethasone exposure to memory and executive function deficits in adult survivors of ALL. Corticosteroids, which are administered with methotrexate in ALL chemotherapy regimens, have also been reported to impact neurocognitive skills [48]. Corticosteroids inhibit glucose utilization by neurons and glia, increasing concentration of glutamate, which can lead to excitotoxic neuronal death as a result of overstimulation [52]. Reduced synaptic plasticity in hippocampal neurons and reduced CNS development following use of corticosteroids, particularly during early periods of brain development, have been reported [53]. On the other hand, lower doses of methotrexate do not produce consistent patterns of cognitive deficits [54]. In a prospective trial of infants who received high-dose systemic methotrexate combined with intrathecal (IT) cytarabine and methotrexate for CNS leukemia prophylaxis and who were tested 3–9 years posttreatment showed that cognitive function was in the average range [55]. ALL patients who receive IT chemotherapy with no cranial radiation have reportedly milder CI with limited decline in the number of cognitive domains, especially in girls at a younger age, demonstrating the contribution of gender, dose, and age of patient [56, 57]. Although using lower doses and more targeted volumes of craniospinal radiation in children have demonstrated improved results, in general, studies of children treated with cranial or craniospinal radiation therapy for CNS tumors demonstrated

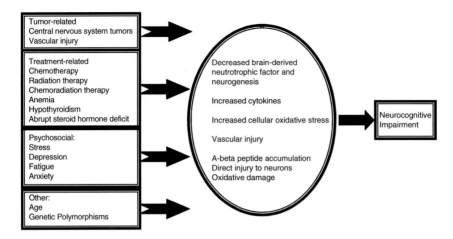

Fig. 9.1 Etiology of cognitive impairment and potential mechanism contributing to neurocognitive deficits in cancer patient population

a significant adverse neurocognitive effect [19]. Patient characteristics such as younger age at diagnosis, epilepsy, and shunt placement, history of stroke, paralysis, or auditory difficulties were associated CI [19, 58].

Complicating the issue somewhat, recent prospective studies show that ~20% of cancer patients experience cognitive dysfunction even before commencement of chemotherapy. Patients with cancer in general exhibit increased circulating levels of cytokines; in both preclinical and clinical studies, increased levels of cytokines and inflammation can produce systemic effects and have been shown to be associated with impairment of cognition [59–61]. In addition to the biological plausibility, others have proposed psychosocial factors such as stress, anxiety, depression, fatigue, age, social support, education level, and intelligence as other influential factors to CI. Stress, anxiety, and depression may in part be attributed to recent diagnosis and the trepidation regarding treatment. These studies clearly demonstrate the multifactorial nature of the etiology of this phenomenon and *establish the need for multifaceted approaches to the treatment* (Fig. 9.1).

9.4   Current Interventions for the Treatments for Chemotherapy-Induced Cognitive Impairment

9.4.1   Treatment of Anemia

Studies that hypothesize that CI may be attributed to symptoms of anemia have studied pharmacological interventions to treat anemia with recombinant human erythropoietin [62]. Erythropoietin (EPO), originally discovered as hematopoietic growth factor, has direct effects on cells of the nervous system that make it a highly attractive candidate drug for neuroprotection/neuroregeneration [63]. Several preclinical and clinical studies have examined the usefulness of intervention with EPO for modulating cognitive impairment and provide support for the hypothesis that significant increases in hemoglobin over the course of chemotherapy supplemented with rHuEPO administration would be accompanied by significant improvement in cognitive performance [64]. Epoetin alfa therapy was well tolerated and shown to have attenuated the cognitive impairment and fatigue that occurred during adjuvant breast cancer chemotherapy [32]. In elderly cancer patients, treating anemia could be useful to preserve cognitive abilities [63, 65]. Although these studies have demonstrated an increase in hemoglobin levels and provide some evidence that EPO may be effective in improving cognition in the short term [32, 65–67] and decrease fatigue in those cancer patients with anemia, the small sample sizes, lack of control arms, use of cohorts with various cancers and treatment regimens (heterogenous populations), thrombic events, lack of information with regard to long-term use, and short duration of interventions fail to provide meaningful data as to the efficacy of this as an intervention strategy to prevent cognitive impairment.

9.4.2 Treatment of Fatigue

Since fatigue is a cardinal symptom recognized in most cancer patient populations, with 99% of breast cancer patients reporting fatigue during treatment and 61% of patients receiving chemotherapy or radiation therapy report that their fatigue lasts well past treatment, it is hypothesized that "chemo fog" may be related to fatigue, and these symptoms may not be independent of each other [16, 22, 23, 31–42, 68–70]. Based on this principle, drugs in the class of CNS stimulants are being tested in this population. In a phase II clinical trial of the safety and efficacy of dexmethylphenidate (d-MPH), patients with ovarian and breast cancer were treated for a period of 8 weeks [67]. Although the primary aim of the study was to treat fatigue, symptoms of chemo brain was also examined. Although fatigue scores improved in this patient population, cognitive function was not significantly improved. Similarly, two recent randomized, placebo-controlled studies failed to find a clear benefit of MPH on cognition in cancer patients receiving chemotherapy [67, 71]. However, the long-term safety of these agents, including impact on neurochemistry and the amphetamine-like effects, continues to be a concern. Most promising is a study of a single-arm pilot study of a brief cognitive-behavioral treatment aimed at managing cognitive dysfunction associated with adjuvant chemotherapy (Memory and Attention Adaptation Training; MAAT) [72], which reported that participants reported high treatment satisfaction and rated MAAT as helpful in improving ability to compensate for memory problems. Based on the available evidence, MPH has not been found useful for the prevention or treatment of chemotherapy-induced cognitive deficits. Well-powered clinical trials using homogenous target populations need to be completed for these preliminary observations to be implemented in clinical practice. Since physical activity is a symptom cluster associated with fatigue, improvement in physical activity has been hypothesized to improve cognitive performance. Several preclinical and early clinical trials have been initiated and demonstrated improvement in cognitive function in chemotherapy-administered rat models [61, 73–75]. Research in the general population has consistently demonstrated slower cognitive decline with higher lifetime physical activity compared to those with lower lifetime PA [73, 76]. Specifically, aerobic exercise in elderly individuals has been shown to improve executive functioning and memory [73], which are the cognitive domains affected by chemotherapy, individuals with higher levels of physical activity have larger hippocampal volume in later life [77]. On the other hand, individuals with low levels of activity have greater levels of systemic inflammation [73]. Although there are no systematic clinical trials to demonstrate these principles in improving chemotherapy-induced NI, physical activity has shown to have neuroprotective effects and may lessen the adverse impact of chemotherapy on cognition [4].

Other agents currently under evaluation in preclinical trials are fluoxetine, a selective serotonin reuptake inhibitor (SSRI) that is used primarily in the treatment of depression; donepezil, a cholinesterase inhibitor that is widely used to treat cognitive impairment in cancer-free populations to slow the progression of dementia and act as a neuroprotectant through reduction of inflammation, regulation of catecholamines, and enhancement of neuroplastic activity [78]; modafinil, a central nervous system stimulant that appears to exert its effects through the release of the catecholamines norepinephrine and dopamine; and histamine [79]. In healthy adults, modafinil acts as an enhancer of cognition, primarily improving attention [80]; in cancer patients, it has been shown to reduce fatigue [81]. However, to date, effectiveness of these treatments have not proven efficacy in ameliorating NI or safety in cancer patient populations.

9.4.3   Cognitive Training (CT)

With the recent understanding of the multifactorial etiology of NI, similar to those observed in NI related to aging and associated diseases, structured CT strategies that have already demonstrated efficacy in aging and diseases related to NI appear to offer promise for the treatment of chemotherapy-induced NI. Over the past 25 years, several studies have demonstrated that among relatively healthy, older adults without dementia, cognitive abilities can be enhanced through a variety of cognitive intervention techniques [38, 82–86]. In the current proposal, we utilize a commercially available cognitive training system, InSight™ that was based upon the original useful field of view (UFOV) training protocol that was evaluated in the NIH-sponsored ACTIVE cognitive intervention trial [87]. We have adopted this method of cognitive training intervention for several reasons. First, research using this methodology indicates that relatively healthy older adults in general improve on the cognitive ability training [38, 87, 88] and that transfer to improvement on everyday abilities is more likely when those who have experienced some subtle cognitive decline at baseline are included in training [87]. Further, this cognitive training technique is particularly promising in that transfer of training has been demonstrated to performance of timed instrumental activities of daily living (TIADL) [89, 90], safer on-road driving performance [91], and maintained health-related quality of life [92, 93]. Research has indicated that individuals, who exhibit slowed cognitive speed of processing as measured by UFOV, are most likely to benefit from and experience transfer of speed of processing training to functional outcomes [87]. There are several cognitive training protocols currently available for use similar to the one described and used by treatment centers around the world which are valid and useful tools for training patients with cognitive deficits or those populations in which NI is anticipated.

9.4.3.1 Nutrients and Nutrient-Derived Agents to Ameliorate Symptoms of NI

Oxidative stress and inflammation contribute to several organ toxicities, including neurotoxicities, after common breast cancer chemotherapy regimen. Doxorubicin and other platinum-based therapies have been documented to cause the generation of free radicals and the induction of oxidative stress, associated with cellular injury [22]. Although the debate continues as to the safety of antioxidant use during chemotherapy to reduce oxidative stress, the utility of these agents to ameliorate treatment-induced consequences postcancer treatment, including NI, has not been examined. Much of the work using antioxidant agents in treating NI comes from the aging literature. The basis for the use of nutritional supplements as a moderator of age-related cognitive decline is the age-related increase in oxidative stress [39], similar to those observed during cytotoxic therapies for cancer. Antioxidants, such as polyphenols, not only scavenge reactive oxygen species (ROS) [23, 40] but are also involved in modification of protein kinases, apoptosis signaling, and regulating signal transduction via modification of cellular redox reactions [37, 68]. It is generally well accepted that dietary supplementation of antioxidants can prevent ROS accumulation and contribute to healthy aging, including cognitive functioning. Interventions to treat CI using antioxidant therapies with Vitamins A, C, and E have been disappointing to treat markers of CI in cancer survivors, similar to those observed in the aging literature [71, 94–98]. Nonvitamin phytochemicals such as polyphenols, which are the most abundant antioxidants in our diets, have been shown to possess strong anti-inflammatory properties, as well as stronger antioxidant activity [71, 94–125], as compared to traditional antioxidant vitamins, which have never been tested before to improve NI in this cohort. Our group has considerable experience and demonstrated the safety of polyphenolic [108–113] and $n - 3$ fatty acids [125–127] supplementation in cancer patient cohorts and the effectiveness of these nonvitamin nutritional supplementation [99, 103–105, 128] in preclinical studies to improve cognitive function. Single and combination polyphenolic compounds have demonstrated improvements on cognitive tasks such as the Morris water maze, radial arm maze (water and land), t-maze passive and active avoidance tasks, as well as classical eyeblink conditioning tasks. Dr. Bickford [23] established the precedent for cognitive improvement in normal aging rats with dietary supplementation of foods high in ORAC (oxygen radical absorbance capacity). In addition, Bickford et al. demonstrated the synergistic effects of components (NT-020) to increase actions on the progenitor cell populations and to reduce inflammation and oxidative stress to protect primary neuronal cultures as well as microglial cell cultures from oxidative stress, in addition to neuroprotective and neurogenic effects [104].

Additionally, combination approaches due to synergistic effects demonstrated greater effects in improvement on CF, as seen by our group and that of others as we have proposed in this trial. Finally, in a recent experiment, we examined the impact of NT-020 on Morris water maze performance among young animals ($n = 10$), as well as older animals who received treatment of NT-020 ($n = 13$) or a control diet ($n = 13$) for 3 weeks prior to behavioral testing. All animals were tested on the Morris water maze test, four trials per day for 5 days. The animals in the NT-020 arm of study exhibited lower cumulative distance, as compared to the older control animals ($p < 0.05$). Further, there was much less variability among the treated old animals, as compared to the control animals. The brains of these rats were then examined for neurogenesis and markers of inflammation using unbiased serological measures. There was a significant increase in the numbers of Ki67 and DCX labeled cells in the dentate gyrus of the NT-020 rats that was accompanied by a decrease in OX6 (MHC Class II) positive microglia indicating that there was a reduction in inflammatory mediators. As chemotherapeutics have been shown to reduce neurogenesis, this treatment regimen can directly impact this negative action of cytotoxic agents [37, 129, 139].

More recent trials have demonstrated that NT-020 components can be measured in serum and plasma, found to cross the blood–brain barrier and are found in measurable levels within the brain [114]. For example, NT-020 contains blueberry anthocyanins which are considered to be one of the major active fractions and can be found in the brain of several mammalian animal models [115–117]. Catechins, which are components of green tea, have also been found to cross the blood–brain barrier [118–120]. In summary, our team and others have demonstrated that the components of NT-020 can be detected in human serum/plasma, shown to cross the blood–brain barrier and localize in various brain regions important for learning and memory such as cerebellum, striatum, and hippocampus in measurable quantities. Studies have correlated peripheral markers of inflammation, immune function, and oxidative stress in serum/plasma with central inflammation and central nervous system functioning.

9.4.3.2   Anti-inflammatory Agents (n – 3 Fatty Acids) and Cognitive Function

In view of the high omega-3 polyunsaturated fatty acid content of the brain, it is evident that these fats are involved in brain biochemistry, physiology, and functioning and thus in some neuropsychiatric diseases and in the cognitive decline of aging [126, 127, 130–133]. DHA (docosahexaenoic acid) is one for the major building structures of membrane phospholipids of the brain and is absolutely necessary for neuronal function. Deficiency of DHA alters the course of brain development and perturbs the composition of brain cell membranes, neurons, oligodendrocytes, and astrocytes, as well as subcellular particles such as myelin, nerve endings (synaptosomes), and mitochondria. These alterations induce physicochemical modifications in membranes, lead to biochemical and physiological perturbations, and result in neurosensory and behavioral upset [130–133]. The literature reveals growing mechanistic evidence that cognitive function of the aging brain can be preserved or loss of function can be diminished with docosahexaenoic acid, a long-chain $(n - 3)$ PUFA. In addition, omega-3 polyunsaturated fatty acids $(n - 3$ PUFAs) [127, 134] have been shown to modulate levels of proinflammatory cytokines, hepatic acute-phase proteins, eicosanoids, and tumor-derived factors in animal models of cancer. Omega-3 fatty acids can be detected in human serum/plasma, shown to cross the blood–brain barrier, and are the primary component of membranes of the nerve cells in the brain. Deficits in omega-3 fatty acids are associated with damage to brain biochemistry, structure, and cognitive function [130, 131]. In contrast, a diet high in $n - 3$ fatty acids reduced beta-amyloid (Abeta) and reduced the amount of plaque in the brain, especially in the hippocampus and parietal cortex, and reduced the amount of APP, the beta-amyloid precursor protein [132, 133], improving NI. Thus, based on the etiologies of cognitive changes, animal and early clinical trial evidence of safety, bioavailability in blood and brain tissue, and preliminary evidence of efficacy to improve CF, it is logical to supplement combination nutrition supplements that can provide antioxidant, anti-inflammatory nutrients critical to the physiochemical composition and functioning of the neurological system to "rescue" tissues from the effects of the oxidative damage and inflammation and reverse chemotherapy-induced cognitive impairment. Our preclinical work and early clinical trials demonstrate that the components of antioxidant/anti-inflammatory agents are potentially ideal components that can be detected in human serum/plasma, shown to cross the blood–brain barrier and localize in various brain regions important for learning and memory, suggesting that these components may deliver its signal modifying capabilities centrally, producing improvements in cognitive function. However, these early studies have to be validated further in well-powered clinical trials.

9.4.4 Timing of Intervention

It is clear that tissue injury due to oxidative stress and inflammation has been demonstrated to occur during active treatment [7–12, 96]. Although it is logical to initiate interventions with antioxidants and anti-inflammatory agents during chemotherapy, in theory, these agents, especially antioxidants, may decrease the efficacy of these cytotoxic agents by quenching free radicals. There is thus a concern that antioxidants might counteract the effect of cytotoxic agents especially those which mediate their action by generating free radicals such as alkylating agents and antimetabolites [96]. On the other hand, studies in the aging literature have shown that supplementing with antioxidants and anti-inflammatory agents posttreatment may serve to "rescue" tissues from the effects of the oxidative damage in addition to replenishing depleted status of these critical nutrients and reversing cognitive impairment. More recently [12], our group at Moffitt examined the extent to which cognitive functioning continues to change in the posttreatment period and examined residualized CI in breast cancer survivors from 6 months to 3 years posttreatment compared to an age- and education-matched sample of women without cancer assessed over a comparable time period. Our findings suggest that adjuvant treatment for breast cancer, particularly chemotherapy, is associated with long-term deficits across a number of cognitive domains. It may be ideal to select the timing of intervention to be initiated posttreatment based on this potential nutrient-cytotoxic agent interaction if administered during treatment [71, 96, 129] and our recent findings of the residual NI seen also posttreatment [12].

9.5   Guidelines

In spite of the large body of literature demonstrating CI to be a significant and distressing problem for patients with cancer and posttreatment for cancer, currently there are no proven treatments or preventive measures for this side effect. Thus, the current recommendations are best practice guidelines, based on available evidence, and in general considered safe and may not cause harm to this patient population.

9.5.1   Neuropsycho-Oncology Referral

Patients receiving cytotoxic therapies for treatment of breast or prostate cancer or cranial radiotherapy are currently candidates at high risk for NI. Intervention for the treatment of cognitive deficits must include the following:

- Evaluate extent of cognitive deficit using using standardized neuropsychological assessments along with a comprehensive symptom assessment scale for other related symptoms.
- Patient should be first screened to be evaluated for anemia and treated if anemia is present.
- Patient should be screened for fatigue, and interventions to treat fatigue should be initiated if fatigue is present.
- Patient should also be evaluated for depression and, if diagnosed, must be treated for depression.
- Refer to a neuropsychologist for screening and cognitive training:
  - There are several readily available reliable and valid software available for cognitive training. We utilize InSight™ for training. This intervention is designed to improve the efficiency and accuracy of visual and information processing, visual memory, and the ability to perform complex visual attention tasks. This program is an expanded version of the original UFOV training program that was evaluated in the ACTIVE clinical trial [85]. Over time, the difficulty and complexity of each task is systematically increased as users successfully attain specified performance criteria. We will be testing the latest version of this training program named InSight™. In developing the present version Posit Science™ retained the tasks used in previous efficacy trials, but modified the delivery platform so that it is user-friendly and can be easily self-administered. At the same time, more challenging and varying training tasks were added to the program. These modifications dramatically improve the potential cognitive benefits from the program as well as the ease with which the intervention can be distributed and implemented across a variety of settings

and contexts. Furthermore, the addition of certain game elements will improve user engagement and is likely to enhance compliance. This training program involves only adaptive training sessions. This type of training has been found to produce larger training effects that more broadly transfer to everyday outcomes than the results from the ACTIVE trial, which included five standard training sessions and five adaptive training sessions. The efficacy of the original UFOV speed of processing intervention at enhancing information processing speed and improving the useful field of view has been demonstrated in several prior studies. Recent data validates the new program as effective in enhancing UFOV performance [87, 88].

Timing: Although there are no clinical trials available, it is prudent that the CT training intervention begin soon after the patient completes treatment regimen. Participants should be trained two times per week to introduce them to the training using the software for four sessions over 2 weeks. Patients will then be provided the software to take home with them along with extra technical support instructions including how to troubleshoot problems at home. Patients who have no access to a computer should be offered the opportunity to return to the lab for biweekly sessions. Follow-up calls by phone should be made to check in with them every 4 weeks. Use can be monitored online for each patient. The program records the time and performance as they use it. The duration for the CT intervention should be 6 months. Each training session lasts 1 h. Prior studies involving ten sessions of adaptive training found improved cognitive performance, as well as transfer to everyday functional performance outcomes, including enhanced health-related quality of life and protection against depressive symptoms. Patients can be screened at regular intervals to assess response to CT.

9.5.2 Nutrition Screening, Assessment, and Therapy

Nutritional assessment must be performed within 24 h of admission of the patient by a registered dietitian.

The goals of nutrition care in this patient population is to:

1. Assess current nutritional status and estimate caloric, protein, and multivitamin/ mineral needs.
2. Provide adequate nutrition by including "calorie" and "protein" boosters education material and nutritional supplements to ensure intake of proteins 0.8 g–1.0 g/kg/day and dense caloric supplements up to 400 cal/day containing 1.5 kcal/mL (Ensure Plus or alternate). The choice of nutritional supplements will be based in the personal choice of the patient. Supplement diet if inadequate with smoothies, instant breakfast powders, Scandishake®, Ensure Plus®, Boost Plus®, or Resource®.
3. Include a standard multivitamin/mineral supplementation to prevent any further deficits and meet increased needs.
4. Assess adequacy of intake and provide an appetite stimulant (megestrol acetate 800 mg/day or alternate) if patient has cancer anorexia to ensure adequate intake and prevent further weight loss.

5. Provide each patient with nutritional guidelines to ensure adequate intake of calories and proteins and a list of suggested high-caloric and high-protein nutritional supplements to choose from, taking into consideration taste alterations, early satiety, nausea, and vomiting that are common symptoms observed in this patient population.
6. Other tips to enhance nutritional intake:

Although the preclinical evidence demonstrating the effectiveness of nutrient-derived polyphenolic and other compounds appear promising, these have not been evaluated in clinical trials targeting cancer patients *during cancer treatment* for improvement of symptoms related to NI. Thus, the current evidence does not support any commercial use of supplements to improve cognitive function. Similarly, although there are no systematic clinical trials to demonstrate these principles in improving chemotherapy or radiation-induced NI, supplementing with diet-derived antioxidants and anti-inflammatory agents posttreatment may serve to "rescue" tissues from the effects of the oxidative damage. In addition, as demonstrated in these early preclinical and pilot trials, these nutrient-derived substances may replenish depleted status of these critical nutrients and reverse cognitive impairment posttreatment. The most prudent strategy would be to include foods rich in antioxidants and anti-inflammatory properties after cancer treatment. Examples include:

Anthocyanins (fleshy berry fruits such as wild blueberry, bilberry, cranberry, elderberry, raspberry seeds, and strawberry),

Resveratrol (grapes, peanuts, and certain berries and products made from these sources),

Green tea polyphenols (green tea and products),

Isoflavones (fermented soy, flax seed), and

Omega-3 fatty acids (fish such as salmon, cod, and halibut and a few uncommon plant sources, such as flax seed, walnut, and pumpkin seed and oils).

9.5.3 Physical Activity

Fatigue is a common symptom that co-occurs with NI. Patients should be proactively receiving a comprehensive assessment of physical status by a licensed physical therapist and therapy initiated postchemotherapy or radiation therapy. The basic principle is to enhance activity level, conserve energy, and improve muscle strength.

1. Godin Leisure-Time Exercise Questionnaire weekly to monitor physical activity.
2. Handgrip strength dynamometry assessment: A validated tool commonly used to assess handgrip strength is the Jamar dynamometer, which is a fast, reliable, and easy-to-perform device commonly used by our team to measure improvements in functional strength. The Jamar dynamometer has a lower % coefficient of variation and is thus a more precise device than other handgrip dynamometers.
3. Cardiovascular exercises as well as strength training exercises must be recommended.

4. Multidimensional Fatigue Inventory (MFI-20) may be administered on a monthly basis to monitor change in fatigue scores.
5. Patient's ability and choice of physical activity regimen must be taken into account while planning regimen.
6. Printed instructions, activity records, and monitors such as wrist actigraphy or pedometers have been found to be motivating to the patient in clinical settings.

9.5.4   Markers and Instruments for Patient Monitoring and Assessment of Response to Treatment by the Interdisciplinary Medical Team

1. *Anthropometric measurements* such as participant's height, weight, and body mass index can be performed at admission and at regular intervals established by the medical team.
2. *Body composition by DXA scan*: DXA should be used to assess both total lean body mass (LBM) and fat mass (FM) and total bone mineral density (BMD). Total bone mineral density (BMD) is a valid indirect measure of skeletal muscle and patient activity. Total LBM is sometimes called total fat-free mass (FFM) depending upon specific DXA manufacturer. DXA instruments use an X-ray source that generates or is split into two energies to measure bone mineral mass and soft tissue from which fat and fat-free mass are estimated. The exam is quick (1–2 min), precise (0.5–1%), and noninvasive. DXA scanners have the precision required to detect changes in muscle mass as small as 5%. Radiation exposure from DXA scans is minimal. The National Council of Radiation Protection and Measurements (NCRP) has recommended that the annual effective dose limit for infrequent exposure of the general population is 5,000 μSv and that an annual effective dose of 10 μSv be considered a negligible individual dose. The effective dose of a dual-energy X-ray absorptiometry whole body scan on an adult is 2.1 μSv. Studies have shown that quality assurance is an important issue in the use of DXA scans to determine body composition including lean body mass and bone mineral density. DXA instrument manufacturer and model should remain consistent, and their calibration should be monitored throughout treatment. Use of a standardized scan acquisition protocol and appropriate and unchanging scan acquisition and analysis software is essential to achieve consist results.
3. *Dietary intake* must be assessed at baseline and periodical intervals by conducting random weekly, 2 weekdays + 1 weekend day, 24-h dietary recalls (gold standard for collecting dietary data) using a five-step multipass procedure (which has been found to assess mean energy intake within 10% of actual intake) and using the frequently updated University of Minnesota Nutrition Data System for Research (NDS-R) version database for analysis of nutrient composition. Food portion visuals can be provided to patients to estimate portion sizes of foods while monitoring intake.
4. *Symptom log* may be completed daily and collected from patients on a monthly basis. Based on these symptoms, all anticipated and unanticipated, grades of

constitutional, dermatological, gastrointestinal (GI), metabolic, and pain symptoms can be continuously monitored including those symptoms affecting nutritional intake and utilization.

5. *Monthly CMP and CBC* should be monitored to assess electrolytes and organ function. Test for anemia periodically.

6. *Functional markers (Karnofsky performance score)*: Evaluation of patients' functional status and barriers to obtaining adequate nutrients are also necessary. A physical exam combined with personal interview should include the evaluation of functional status such as the ability to chew and swallow, dental or oral problems causing odynophagia or dysphagia, signs of muscle wasting or anasarca, presence of edema, presence of skin or mouth lesion, and ability to perform instrumental activities of daily living (IADLs) such as cooking shopping and feeding self. It is critical to assess activities of daily living, physical activity, exercise, sleep, and ability to work and perform other functional roles. Limitations in the activities of daily living have been identified secondary to and as a cause of weight loss in cancer patients. Cancer and other chronic diseases pose difficulties specifically for the cancer patient receiving treatment and the elderly in carrying out activities of daily living. A loss of postural and locomotive muscle mass has been observed within 7 days of inactivity. The Karnofsky Performance Scale Index allows patients to be classified as to their functional impairment. This has been used to compare effectiveness of different therapies and to assess the prognosis in individual patients and has been validated in cancer patient populations.

7. *Godin Leisure-Time Exercise Questionnaire* weekly to monitor physical activity.

8. *Handgrip strength dynamometry assessment*: A validated tool commonly used to assess handgrip strength is the Jamar dynamometer, which is a fast, reliable, and easy-to-perform device commonly used by our team to measure improvements in functional strength. The Jamar dynamometer has a lower % coefficient of variation and is thus a more precise device than other handgrip dynamometers.

9. *Biochemical markers of protein status (serum albumin and transferrin)*: Assessment of protein status is critical in the identification and treatment of abnormalities in protein metabolism. There is substantial evidence of the correlation between serum hepatic proteins and inflammation making these the most relevant biomarkers in cancer patient populations. Serum transferrin, prealbumin, and albumin have been observed as intermediate endpoint biomarkers and independently associated with clinical outcomes. Measurements of body composition combined with more objective and sensitive measure of protein nutriture is ideal for the biochemical assessment of intravascular and visceral protein stores. We have thus included the three major valid intermediate endpoint biomarkers (IEBs) that represent intravascular and visceral protein pools – transferrin, prealbumin, and albumin – as the biochemical indicators of protein status. Although transferrin levels are affected by iron status, serum transferrin, either singly or as part of a multiparameter index, is the strongest predictor of cancer patient morbidity and mortality.

10. *Immune and inflammatory markers*: A range of metabolic responses triggered by inflammatory and immunological responses in cancer patients. Cytokines can be measured in a panel including IL-1, IL-4, IL-6, IL-8, IL-10, GM-CSF, IFN-κ, TNF-α, and CRP (BioRad-Bioplex). All of these biomarkers have been shown to increase with disease, aging, and cytotoxic agents. Though we realize these intermediate endpoint biomarkers of cytokines cannot be reliably interpreted, as over 70% of the subjects as observed in our studies were on active treatment with cytotoxic agents, these variables are important to determine as they may provide useful information and contribute to the better understanding of the mechanistic process.

11. *Quality of life* should be measured at baseline and monthly using the Rand Short Form (SF)-36 (Medical Outcomes Study SF36) [140]. The SF-36 has been used extensively with general, high-risk, and cancer populations and has available norms for mail and telephone versions and comparisons between group and individual scores. Scores are calculated and transformed to a 0–100 scale, with higher scores indicating increased health status. Reliability of the SF-36 scales was measured by Cronbach α coefficient and the results ranged from 0.78 in general health perceptions to 0.91 in the physical functioning domain.

12. *Analysis of biomarkers (optional)*: A number of biomarkers of oxidative stress and inflammation have been shown to change with age and disease. *Studies have correlated peripheral markers of inflammation, immune function, and oxidative stress in serum/plasma with central inflammation and central nervous system functioning* [135–137].

13. *Examples of Biomarkers of oxidative stress (optional)*: Isoprostanes are a family of eicosanoids formed in vivo from the free radical catalyzed peroxidation of arachidonic acid that is independent of cyclooxygenase activity. They appear to be reliable markers of lipid peroxidation. Levels of 8-isoprostane increase with age in some but not all studies and are reduced by diets high in fruits and vegetables. Ideally measured with GC-mass spectroscopy, isoprostanes can also be measured by ELISA. Other markers of lipid peroxidation include malondiadehyde that can easily be measured, although it may reflect some enzyme-dependent peroxidation, and inflammation is still a valuable measure for comparison with other studies. Markers of protein oxidation and nitration have also been shown to increase with age, and two markers routinely measured are protein carbonyls and 3-nitrotyrosine (3-NT). Furthermore, oxidative DNA damage is another marker measured in aging as it is widely thought that oxidative damage to DNA is a significant contributor to age-related disease as well as cancer. Oxidative DNA damage markers are also decreased in humans following diets high in fruits and vegetables. Markers of inflammation are also useful and also show upregulation with age and disease.

14. *Since fatigue, depression, and anemia* are co-occurring symptoms with NI, patients should be periodically screened for this symptom cluster and treated for the same.

9.5.5   Follow-up

Patients must be seen by the multidisciplinary team on a regularly scheduled basis to monitor progress and to review compliance to intervention including diet intake adequacy, symptom logs, physical activity, change in concomitant medications, and any other symptoms related to treatment. Reassessment/reevaluation for monitoring and evaluation of response to nutritional therapy and CT must include monitoring of clinical, functional, dietary, and behavioral outcomes that were identified by the comprehensive nutritional assessment.

9.6   Future Directions

In spite of the large body of literature demonstrating NI to be a significant and distressing problem for patients with cancer and posttreatment for cancer, currently there are no proven treatments or preventive measures for this symptom of cancer. Although several patients are aware of this symptom, based on hearing about "cancer treatment fog" or "chemo brain" from friends and support groups, in a qualitative study, Munir et al. [138] found less than 33% of the population report having received any information about the possible effects of chemotherapy on cognition or any advice about methods of coping with these problems. There is thus a need for well-validated treatments and interventions targeting specific populations. With our knowledge of the mechanism of treatment-induced NI, several groups, including our research team, are evaluating the safety, effectiveness, and timing of interventions with CT and nutritional agents with botanical and biological nutrient-derived substances used to ameliorate the NI.

> **Summary for the Clinician**
> In spite of the large body of literature demonstrating CI to be a significant and distressing problem for patients with cancer and posttreatment for cancer, currently there are no proven treatments or preventive measures for this side effect.
>
> Although several patients are aware of this side effect, based on advice from friends and support groups, less than one third of the population report having received any information about the possible effects of chemotherapy on cognition or any advice about methods of coping with these problems.
>
> It is clear that tissue injury due to oxidative stress and inflammation has been demonstrated to occur during active treatment. Although it is logical to initiate interventions with antioxidants and anti-inflammatory agents during chemotherapy, in theory, these agents, especially antioxidants, may decrease the efficacy of these cytotoxic agents by quenching free radicals.
>
> There is thus a concern that antioxidants might counteract the effect of cytotoxic agents especially those which mediate their action by generating

free radicals such as alkylating agents and antimetabolites. There are no standard interventions to treat neurocognitive impairment.

Based on these theoretical principles, timing of intervention must begin posttreatment with chemotherapy or radiation therapy.

Current strategies include a multidisciplinary approach lead by the patient's primary oncologist with referrals to neuropsycho-oncologist, nutritionist, physical therapist, and clinical pharmacist.

Recommended treatment approaches must be multimodal, involving a thorough screening, intervention using cognitive training, nutritional intervention, and physical therapy to include cardiorespiratory as well strength training exercises.

There is thus a need for well-validated treatments and interventions targeting specific populations. With our knowledge of the mechanism of treatment-induced NI, several groups, including our research team, are evaluating the safety, effectiveness, and timing of interventions with CT and nutritional agents with botanical and biological nutrient-derived substances to ameliorate the NI.

References

1. Jansen CE, Cooper BA, Dodd MJ, Miaskowski CA (2010) A prospective longitudinal study of chemotherapy-induced cognitive changes in breast cancer patients. Support Care Cancer 19(10):1647–1656 [Epub ahead of print]
2. Ahles TA, Saykin AJ (2007) Candidate mechanisms for chemotherapy-induced cognitive changes. Nat Rev 7:192–201
3. Joshi G, Aluise CD, Cole MP, Sultana R, Pierce WM, Vore M, St Clair DK, Butterfield DA (2010) Alterations in brain antioxidant enzymes and redox proteomic identification of oxidized brain proteins induced by the anti-cancer drug adriamycin: implications for oxidative stress-mediated chemobrain. Neuroscience 166(3):796–807, Epub 2010 Jan 20
4. Fardell JE, Vardy J, Johnston IN, Winocur G (2011) Chemotherapy and cognitive impairment: treatment options. Clin Pharmacol Ther. doi:10.1038/clpt.2011.112 [Epub ahead of print]
5. Falleti MG, Sanfilippo A, Maruff P, Weih L, Phillips KA (2005) The nature and severity of cognitive impairment associated with adjuvant chemotherapy in women with breast cancer: a meta-analysis of the current literature. Brain Cogn 59(1):60–70, Epub 2005 Jun 21. Review
6. Aziz NM (2007) Cancer survivorship research: state of knowledge, challenges and opportunities. Acta Oncol 46(4):417–432, Review. PMID: 17497308
7. Nelson CJ, Nandy N, Roth AJ (2007) Chemotherapy and cognitive deficits: mechanisms, findings, and potential interventions. Palliat Support Care 5(3):273–280, Review. PMID: 17969831
8. Boykoff N, Moieni M, Subramanian SK (2009) Confronting chemobrain: an in-depth look at survivors' reports of impact on work, social networks, and health care response. J Cancer Surviv 3(4):223–232, PMCID: PMC2775115
9. Deprez S, Amant F, Smeets A, Peeters R, Leemans A, Van Hecke W, Verhoeven JS, Christiaens MR, Vandenberghe J, Vandenbulcke M, Sunaert S (2012) Longitudinal assessment of chemotherapy-induced structural changes in cerebral white matter and its correlation with impaired cognitive functioning. J Clin Oncol 30(3):274–281
10. Vearncombe KJ, Rolfe M, Wright M, Pachana NA, Andrew B, Beadle G (2009) Predictors of cognitive decline after chemotherapy in breast cancer patients. J Int Neuropsychol Soc 15(6):951–962

11. Reid-Arndt SA (2009) Breast cancer and "chemobrain": the consequences of cognitive difficulties following chemotherapy and the potential for recovery. Mo Med 106(2): 127–131

12. Phillips KM, Jim HS, Small BJ, Laronga C, Andrykowski MA, Jacobsen PB (2011) Cognitive functioning after cancer treatment: a 3-year longitudinal comparison of breast cancer survivors treated with chemotherapy or radiation and noncancer controls. Cancer. doi: 10.1002/cncr.26432. [Epub ahead of print]

13. Jansen C, Miaskowski C, Dodd M, Dowling G, Kramer J (2005) Potential mechanisms for chemotherapy-induced impairments in cognitive function. Oncol Nurs Forum 32(6): 1151–1163, Review

14. Vardy J, Dhillon H (2010) The fog hasn't lifted on "chemobrain" yet: ongoing uncertainty regarding the effects of chemotherapy and breast cancer on cognition. Breast Cancer Res Treat 123(1):35–37, Epub 2010 Jan 6

15. Kurita K, Meyerowitz BE, Hall P, Gatz M (2011) Long-term cognitive impairment in older adult twins discordant for gynecologic cancer treatment. J Gerontol A Biol Sci Med Sci 66(12):1343–1349, 1758–535X

16. Vardy JL et al (2010) Cognitive function and fatigue in cancer patients after chemotherapy: a longitudinal cohort study in patients with colorectal cancer (CRC), ICCTF, Cognition and Cancer Conference, New York

17. Wefel JS, Vardy J, Ahles T, Schagen SB (2011) International Cognition and Cancer Task Force recommendations to harmonise studies of cognitive function in patients with cancer. Lancet Oncol 12(7):703–708, Epub 2011 Feb 25

18. Nathan PC, Patel SK, Dilley K et al (2007) Guidelines for identification of, advocacy for, and intervention in neurocognitive problems in survivors of childhood cancer: a report from the Children's Oncology Group. Arch Pediatr Adolesc Med 161(8):798–806 [PUBMED Abstract]

19. Robinson KE, Kuttesch JF, Champion JE et al (2010) A quantitative meta-analysis of neurocognitive sequelae in survivors of pediatric brain tumors. Pediatr Blood Cancer 55(3): 525–531 [PUBMED Abstract]

20. Reeves CB, Palmer SL, Reddick WE et al (2006) Attention and memory functioning among pediatric patients with medulloblastoma. J Pediatr Psychol 31(3):272–280 [PUBMED Abstract]

21. Ellenberg L, Liu Q, Gioia G et al (2009) Neurocognitive status in long-term survivors of childhood CNS malignancies: a report from the Childhood Cancer Survivor Study. Neuropsychology 23(6):705–717 [PUBMED Abstract]

22. Whitney KA, Lysaker PH, Steiner AR, Hook JN, Estes DD, Hanna NH (2008) Is "chemobrain" a transient state? A prospective pilot study among persons with non-small cell lung cancer. J Support Oncol 6(7):313–321

23. Il'yasova D, Mixon G, Wang F, Marcom PK, Marks J, Spasojevich I, Craft N, Arredondo F, DiGiulio R (2009) Markers of oxidative status in a clinical model of oxidative assault: a pilot study in human blood following doxorubicin administration. Biomarkers 14(5):321–325, PMICD: PMC2716435

24. Oeffinger KC, Hudson MM, Landier W (2009) Survivorship: childhood cancer survivors. Prim Care 36(4):743–780, Review

25. Oeffinger KC, Nathan PC, Kremer LC (2010) Challenges after curative treatment for childhood cancer and long-term follow up of survivors. Hematol Oncol Clin North Am 24(1):129–149

26. Ries LAG, Melbert D, Krapcho M et al (2007) SEER cancer statistics review, 1975–2004. National Cancer Institute, Bethesda

27. Gurney JG, Severson RK, Davis S, Robison LL (1995) Incidence of cancer in children in the United States. Sex-, race-, and 1-year age-specific rates by histologic type. Cancer 75:2186–2195

28. Greenlee RT, Hill-Harmon MB, Murray T, Thun M (2001) Cancer statistics, 2001. CA Cancer J Clin 51:15–36

29. Hewitt M, Weiner SL, Simone JV (2003) Childhood cancer survivorship: improving care and quality of life. National Academy of Sciences, Washington DC

30. Jemal A, Siegel R, Ward E et al (2006) Cancer statistics, 2006. CA Cancer J Clin 56:106–130

31. Kumar NB, Allen KA, Riccardi D, Bercu B, Cantor A, Minton S, Balducci L, Jacobsen P (2004) Fatigue, weight gain, lethargy and amenorrhea in breast cancer patients on chemotherapy: is subclinical hypothyroidism the culprit? Breast Cancer Res Treat 83:149–159

32. O'Shaughnessy JA, Vukelja SJ, Holmes FA, Savin M, Jones M, Royall D, George M, Von Hoff D (2005) Feasibility of quantifying the effects of epoetin alfa therapy on cognitive function in women with breast cancer undergoing adjuvant or neoadjuvant chemotherapy. Clin Breast Cancer 5(6):439–446

33. Seyb KI, Ansar S, Bean J, Michaelis ML (2006) beta-Amyloid and endoplasmic reticulum stress responses in primary neurons: effects of drugs that interact with the cytoskeleton. J Mol Neurosci 28(2):111–123

34. Small BJ, Rawson KS, Walsh E, Jim HS, Hughes TF, Iser L, Andrykowski MA, Jacobsen PB (2011) Catechol-O-methyltransferase genotype modulates cancer treatment-related cognitive deficits in breast cancer survivors. Cancer 117(7):1369–1376. doi: 10.1002/cncr.25685. Epub 2010 Nov 8

35. Abushamaa AM, Sporn TA, Folz RJ (2002) Oxidative stress and inflammation contribute to lung toxicity after a common breast cancer chemotherapy regimen. Am J Physiol Lung Cell Mol Physiol 283(2):L336–L345

36. Mustafa S, Walker A, Bennett G, Peter M (2008) Wigmore5-Fluorouracil chemotherapy affects spatial working memory and newborn neurons in the adult rat hippocampus. Eur J Neurosci 28:323–330

37. Monje ML, Vogel H, Masek M, Ligon KL, Fisher PG, Palmer TD (2007) Impaired human hippocampal neurogenesis after treatment for central nervous system malignancies. Ann Neurol 62:515–520

38. Joseph JA, Denisova N, Fisher D, Bickford P, Prior R, Cao G (1998) Age-related neurodegeneration and oxidative stress: putative nutritional intervention. Neurol Clin 16(3):747–755

39. Olanow CW (1993) A radical hypothesis for neurodegeneration. Trends Neurosci 16: 439–444

40. Markesbery WR (1997) Oxidative stress hypothesis in Alzheimer's disease. Free Radic Biol Med 23:134–147

41. de Ruiter MB et al (2010) Cerebral hyporesponsiveness and cognitive impairment 10 years after chemotherapy for breast cancer. Hum Brain Mapp 32(8):1206–1219; e-pub ahead of print 28 July 2010

42. Kreukels BP et al (2006) Effects of high-dose and conventional-dose adjuvant chemotherapy on long-term cognitive sequelae in patients with breast cancer: an electrophysiologic study. Clin Breast Cancer 7:67–78

43. Abraham J, Haut MW, Moran MT, Filburn S, Lemiuex S, Kuwabara H (2008) Adjuvant chemotherapy for breast cancer: effects on cerebral white matter seen in diffusion tensor imaging. Clin Breast Cancer 8:88–91

44. Inagaki M et al (2007) Smaller regional volumes of brain gray and white matter demonstrated in breast cancer survivors exposed to adjuvant chemotherapy. Cancer 109:146–156

45. Cohen ME, Duffner PK (1991) Long-term consequences of CNS treatment for childhood cancer, part I: pathologic consequences and potential for oncogenesis. Pediatr Neurol 7(3):157–163 [PUBMED Abstract]

46. Kadan-Lottick NS, Brouwers P, Breiger D et al (2009) Comparison of neurocognitive functioning in children previously randomly assigned to intrathecal methotrexate compared with triple intrathecal therapy for the treatment of childhood acute lymphoblastic leukemia. J Clin Oncol 27:5986–5992

47. Bostrom BC, Sensel MR, Sather HN et al (2003) Dexamethasone versus prednisone and daily oral versus weekly intravenous mercaptopurine for patients with standard-risk acute lymphoblastic leukemia: a report from the Children's Cancer Group. Blood 101:3809–3817

48. Waber DP, Carpentieri SC, Klar N et al (2000) Cognitive sequelae in children treated for acute lymphoblastic leukemia with dexamethasone or prednisone. J Pediatr Hematol Oncol 22:206–213

49. Brown RT, Madan-Swain A, Pais R et al (1992) Chemotherapy for acute lymphocytic leukemia: cognitive and academic sequelae. J Pediatr 121(6):885–889 [PUBMED Abstract]

50. Kadan-Lottick NS, Zeltzer LK, Liu Q et al (2010) Neurocognitive functioning in adult survivors of childhood non-central nervous system cancers. J Natl Cancer Inst 102(12):881–893

51. Kadan-Lottick NS, Brouwers P, Breiger D et al (2009) A comparison of neurocognitive functioning in children previously randomized to dexamethasone or prednisone in the treatment of childhood acute lymphoblastic leukemia. Blood 114:1746–1752

52. Sapolsky RM, Uno H, Rebert CS, Finch CE (1990) Hippocampal damage associated with prolonged glucocorticoid exposure in primates. J Neurosci 10:2897–2902

53. Hajek T, Kopecek M, Preiss M, Alda M, Hoschl C (2006) Prospective study of hippocampal volume and function in human subjects treated with corticosteroids. Eur Psychiatry 21: 123–128

54. Butler RW, Hill JM, Steinherz PG et al (1994) Neuropsychologic effects of cranial irradiation, intrathecal methotrexate, and systemic methotrexate in childhood cancer. J Clin Oncol 12(12):2621–2629, [PUBMED Abstract]

55. Kaleita TA, Reaman GH, MacLean WE et al (1999) Neurodevelopmental outcome of infants with acute lymphoblastic leukemia: a Children's Cancer Group report. Cancer 85(8): 1859–1865 [PUBMED Abstract]

56. Buizer AI, de Sonneville LM, Veerman AJ (2009) Effects of chemotherapy on neurocognitive function in children with acute lymphoblastic leukemia: a critical review of the literature. Pediatr Blood Cancer 52(4):447–454 [PUBMED Abstract]

57. von der Weid N, Mosimann I, Hirt A et al (2003) Intellectual outcome in children and adolescents with acute lymphoblastic leukaemia treated with chemotherapy alone: age- and sex-related differences. Eur J Cancer 39(3):359–365 [PUBMED Abstract]

58. Armstrong GT, Conklin HM, Huang S et al (2011) Survival and long-term health and cognitive outcomes after low-grade glioma. Neuro Oncol 13(2):223–234 [PUBMED Abstract]

59. Seruga B, Zhang H, Bernstein LJ, Tannock IF (2008) Cytokines and their relationship to the symptoms and outcome of cancer. Nat Rev Cancer 8(11):887–899, Epub 2008 Oct 10

60. Myers JS (2010) The possible role of cytokines in chemotherapy-induced cognitive deficits. Adv Exp Med Biol 678:119–123

61. Seigers R, Fardell JE (2011) Neurobiological basis of chemotherapy-induced cognitive impairment: a review of rodent research. Neurosci Biobehav Rev 35(3):729–741, Epub 2010 Oct 1

62. Hudis CA, Vogel CL, Gralow JR, Williams D, Procrit Study Group (2005) Weekly epoetin alfa during adjuvant chemotherapy for breast cancer: effect on hemoglobin levels and quality of life. Clin Breast Cancer 6(2):132–142

63. Sargin D, El-Kordi A, Agarwal A, Müller M, Wojcik SM, Hassouna I, Sperling S, Nave KA, Ehrenreich H (2011) Expression of constitutively active erythropoietin receptor in pyramidal neurons of cortex and hippocampus boosts higher cognitive functions in mice. BMC Biol 9:27

64. Massa E, Madeddu C, Lusso MR, Gramignano G, Mantovani G (2006) Evaluation of the effectiveness of treatment with erythropoietin on anemia, cognitive functioning and functions studied by comprehensive geriatric assessment in elderly cancer patients with anemia related to cancer chemotherapy. Crit Rev Oncol Hematol 57(2):175–182

65. Mancuso A, Migliorino M, De Santis S, Saponiero A, De Marinis F (2006) Correlation between anemia and functional/cognitive capacity in elderly lung cancer patients treated with chemotherapy. Ann Oncol 17(1):146–150

66. Iconomou G, Koutras A, Karaivazoglou K, Kalliolias GD, Assimakopoulos K, Argyriou AA, Ifanti A, Kalofonos HP (2008) Effect of epoetin alpha therapy on cognitive function in anaemic patients with solid tumours undergoing chemotherapy. Eur J Cancer Care (Engl) 17(6):535–541

67. Lower EE, Fleishman S, Cooper A, Zeldis J, Faleck H, Yu Z, Manning D (2009) Efficacy of dexmethylphenidate for the treatment of fatigue after cancer chemotherapy: a randomized clinical trial. J Pain Symptom Manage 38(5):650–662
68. Berger MM (2004) Can oxidative damage be treated nutritionally? Clin Nutr 24:172–183
69. Weis J (2011) Cancer-related fatigue: prevalence, assessment and treatment strategies. Expert Rev Pharmacoecon Outcomes Res 11(4):441–446
70. Mehnert A, Scherwath A, Schirmer L, Schleimer B, Petersen C, Schulz-Kindermann F, Zander AR, Koch U (2007) The association between neuropsychological impairment, self-perceived cognitive deficits, fatigue and health related quality of life in breast cancer survivors following standard adjuvant versus high-dose chemotherapy. Patient Educ Couns 66(1): 108–118
71. Mar Fan HG, Clemons M, Xu W, Chemerynsky I, Breunis H, Braganza S, Tannock IF (2008) A randomized, placebo-controlled, double-blind trial of the effects of d-methylphenidate on fatigue and cognitive dysfunction in women undergoing adjuvant chemotherapy for breast cancer. Support Care Cancer 16(6):577–583, PMID: 17972110
72. Ferguson RJ, Ahles TA, Saykin AJ, McDonald BC, Furstenberg CT, Cole BF, Mott LA (2007) Cognitive-behavioral management of chemotherapy-related cognitive change. Psychooncology 16(8):772–777
73. Cotman CW, Berchtold NC, Christie LA (2007) Exercise builds brain health: key roles of growth factor cascades and inflammation. Trends Neurosci 30:464–472
74. Galantino ML, Cannon N, Hoelker T, Quinn L, Greene L (2008) Effects of Iyengar yoga on measures of cognition, fatigue, quality of life, flexibility, and balance in breast cancer survivors: a case series. Rehab Oncol 26:18–27
75. Fardell JE, Vardy J, Shah JD, Johnston IN (2010) Exercise ameliorates oxaliplatin and 5-fluorouracil induced cognitive deficits in laboratory rodents. Cognition and cancer conference, international cognition and cancer taskforce, New York, 8–9 March 2010
76. Colcombe S, Kramer AF (2003) Fitness effects on the cognitive function of older adults: a meta-analytic study. Psychol Sci 14:125–130
77. Erickson KI et al (2009) Aerobic fitness is associated with hippocampal volume in elderly humans. Hippocampus 19:1030–1039
78. Jacobson SA, Sabbagh MN (2008) Donepezil: potential neuroprotective and disease-modifying effects. Expert Opin Drug Metab Toxicol 4:1363–1369
79. Minzenberg MJ, Carter CS (2008) Modafinil: a review of neurochemical actions and effects on cognition. Neuropsychopharmacology 33:1477–1502
80. Repantis D, Schlattmann P, Laisney O, Heuser I (2010) Modafinil and methylphenidate for neuroenhancement in healthy individuals: a systematic review. Pharmacol Res 62: 187–206
81. Wagner LI, Cella D (2004) Fatigue and cancer: causes, prevalence and treatment approaches. Br J Cancer 91:822–828
82. Rebok GW, Rasmusson DX, Brandt J (1996) Prospects for computerized memory training in normal elderly: effects of practice on explicit and implicit memory tasks. Appl Cogn Psychol 10(3):211–223
83. Rasmusson DX, Rebok GW, Bylsma FW, Brandt J (1999) Effects of three types of memory training in normal elderly. Aging, Neuropsychol, Cognit 6:56–66
84. Labouvie-Veif G, Gonda JN (1976) Cognitive strategy training and intellectual performance in the elderly. J Gerontol 31(3):3327–3332
85. Kramer AF, Larish JL, Stayer DL (1995) Training for attentional control in dual task settings: a comparison of young and older adults. J Exp Psychol Appl 1(1):50–76
86. Schaie KW, Hertzog C, Willis SL, Schulenberg J (1987) Effects of cognitive training on primary mental ability structure. Psychol Aging 2(3):233–242
87. Ball KK, Berch DB, Helmers KF, Jobe JB, Leveck MD, Marsiske M, Morris JN, Rebok GW, Smith DM, Tennstedt SL, Unverzagt FW, Willis SL, Advanced Cognitive Training for Independent and Vital Elderly Study Group (2002) Effect of cognitive training interventions with older adults: a randomized controlled trial. J Am Med Assoc 288:2271–2281

88. Ball KK, Edwards JD, Ross LA (2007) The impact of speed of processing training on cognitive and everyday functions. J Gerontol B Psychol Sci Soc Sci 62B:19–31, PMID: 16019280

89. Edwards JD, Wadley VG, Myers R, Roenker DL, Cissell GM, Ball KK (2002) Transfer of a speed of processing intervention to near and far cognitive functions. Gerontology 48: 329–340

90. Edwards JD, Wadley VG, Vance DE, Roenker DL, Ball KK (2005) The impact of speed of processing training on cognitive and everyday performance. Aging Ment Health 9:262–271

91. Roenker DL, Cissell GM, Ball KK, Wadley VG, Edwards JD (2003) Speed-of-processing and driving simulator training result in improved driving performance. Hum Factors 45(2):218–233

92. Wolinsky FD, Unverzagt FW, Smith DM, Jones R, Stoddard A, Tennstetdt SL (2006) The ACTIVE cognitive training trial and health-related quality of life: protection that lasts for 5 years. J Gerontol A Biol Sci Med Sci 61:1324–1329

93. Wolinsky FD, Unverzagt FW, Smith DM, Jones R, Wright E, Tennstetdt SL (2006) The effects of the ACTIVE cognitive training trial on clinically relevant declines in health-related quality of life. J Gerontol A Biol Sci Med Sci 61B(5):S281–S287

94. Fan HG, Park A, Xu W, Yi QL, Braganza S, Chang J, Couture F, Tannock IF (2009) The influence of erythropoietin on cognitive function in women following chemotherapy for breast cancer. Psychooncology 18(2):156–161

95. Wald DS, Kasturiratne A, Simmonds M (2010) Effect of folic acid, with or without other B vitamins, on cognitive decline: meta-analysis of randomized trials. Am J Med 123(6): 522–527

96. Lawenda BD, Kelly KM, Ladas EJ, Sagar SM, Vickers A, Blumberg JB (2008) Should supplemental antioxidant administration be avoided during chemotherapy and radiation therapy? J Natl Cancer Inst 100(11):773–783

97. Greenlee H, Gammon MD, Abrahamson PE, Gaudet MM, Terry MB, Hershman DL, Desai M, Teitelbaum SL, Neugut AI, Jacobson JS (2009) Prevalence and predictors of antioxidant supplement use during breast cancer treatment: the Long Island Breast Cancer Study Project. Cancer 115(14):3271–3282, PMCID:PMC2763503

98. Roenker DL, Cissell GM, Ball KK, Wadley VG, Edwards JD (2003) Speed-of-processing and driving simulator training result in improved driving performance. Hum Factors 45(2):218–213. Summer

99. Shytle RD, Ehrhart J, Tan J, Vila J, Cole M, Sanberg CD, Sanberg PR, Bickford PC (2007) Oxidative stress of neural, hematopoietic, and stem cells: protection by natural compounds. Rejuvenation Res 10(2):173–178

100. Morris MC, Evans DA, Schneider JA, Tangney CC, Bienias JL, Aggarwal NT (2006) Dietary folate and vitamins B-12 and B-6 not associated with incident Alzheimer's disease. J Alzheimers Dis 9(4):435–443

101. Shaik YB, Castellani ML, Perrella A, Conti F, Salini V, Tete S, Madhappan B, Vecchiet J, De Lutiis MA, Caraffa A, Cerulli G (2006) Role of quercetin (a natural herbal compound) in allergy and inflammation. J Biol Regul Homeost Agents 20:47–52

102. Ortiz D, Shea TB (2004) Apple juice prevents oxidative stress induced by beta-amyloid in culture. J Alzheimers Dis 6:27–30

103. Joseph JA, Shukitt-Hale B, Denisova NA, Prior RL, Cao G, Martin A, Taglialatela G, Bickford PC (1998) Long-term dietary strawberry, spinach, or vitamin E supplementation retards the onset of age-related neuronal signal-transduction and cognitive behavioral deficits. J Neurosci 18:8047–8055

104. Gemma C, Bickford PC (2007) Interleukin-1beta and caspase-1: players in the regulation of age-related cognitive dysfunction. Rev Neurosci 18(2):137–148

105. Cartford MC, Gemma C, Bickford PC (2002) Eighteen-month-old Fischer 344 rats fed a spinach-enriched diet show improved delay classical eyeblink conditioning and reduced expression of tumor necrosis factor alpha (TNFalpha) and TNFbeta in the cerebellum. J Neurosci 22(14):5813–5816

106. Joseph JA, Shukitt-Hale B, Willis LM (2009) Grape juice, berries, and walnuts affect brain aging and behavior. J Nutr 139(9):1813S–1817S

107. Willis LM, Shukitt-Hale B, Joseph JA (2009) Dietary polyunsaturated fatty acids improve cholinergic transmission in the aged brain. Genes Nutr 4(4):309–314, PMCID:PM2775891

108. Kumar NB, Krischer JP, Allen K, Riccardi D, Besterman-Dahan K, Salup R, Kang L, Xu P, Pow-Sang J (2007) A phase II randomized, placebo-controlled clinical trial of purified isoflavones in modulating steroid hormones in men diagnosed with prostate cancer. Nutr Cancer 59(2):163–168, PMCID: PMC2435485

109. Kumar NB, Krischer JP, Allen K, Riccardi D, Besterman-Dahan K, Salup R, Kang L, Xu P, Pow-Sang J (2007) Safety of purified isoflavones in men with early stage prostate cancer. Nutr Cancer 59(2):169–175, PMCID: PMC2442460

110. Kumar NB, Cantor A, Allen K, Riccardi D, Besterman-Dahan K, Seigne J, Helal M, Salup R, Powsang J (2004) The specific role of isoflavones in reducing prostate cancer risk. Prostate 59(2):141–147

111. Kumar NB, Allen KA, Cantor A, Riccardi D, Cox CE (2002) The specific role of isoflavones on estrogen metabolism in pre-menopausal women. Cancer 94(4):1166–1174

112. Kumar NB, Besterman-Dahan K, Kang L, Pow-Sang J, Xu P, Allen K, Riccardi D, Krischer JP (2008) Results of a randomized clinical trial of the action of several doses of lycopene in localized prostate cancer: administration prior to radical prostatectomy. Clin Med Urol 1: 1–14, http://la-press.com/journal.php?journal_id=75. PMCID:PMC2846655

113. Kumar NB, Besterman-Dahan K, Kang L, Pow-Sang J, Xu P, Allen K, Riccardi D, Krischer JP (2010) Results of a randomized clinical trial of the action of several doses of isoflavones in localized prostate cancer: administration prior to radical prostatectomy. J Soc Integr Oncol 8(1):3–13

114. Janle EM, Lila MA, Grannan M, Wood L, Higgins A, Yousef GG, Rogers RB, Kim H, Jackson GS, Ho L, Weaver CM (2010) Pharmacokinetics and tissue distribution of 14C-labeled grape polyphenols in the periphery and the central nervous system following oral administration. J Med Food 13:926–933

115. Milbury PE, Kalt W (2010) Xenobiotic metabolism and berry flavonoid transport across the blood–brain barrier. J Agric Food Chem 58:3950–3956

116. Andres-Lacueva C, Shukitt-Hale B, Galli RL, Jauregui O, Lamuela-Raventos RM, Joseph JA (2005) Anthocyanins in aged blueberry-fed rats are found centrally and may enhance memory. Nutr Neurosci 8:111–120

117. Kalt W, Blumberg JB, McDonald JE, Vinqvist-Tymchuk MR, Fillmore SA, Graf BA, O'Leary JM, Milbury PE (2008) Identification of anthocyanins in the liver, eye, and brain of blueberry-fed pigs. J Agric Food Chem 56:705–712

118. Prasain JK, Peng N, Dai Y, Moore R, Arabshahi A, Wilson L, Barnes S, Michael WJ, Kim H, Watts RL (2009) Liquid chromatography tandem mass spectrometry identification of proanthocyanidins in rat plasma after oral administration of grape seed extract. Phytomedicine 16:233–243

119. Lin LC, Wang MN, Tseng TY, Sung JS, Tsai TH (2007) Pharmacokinetics of (–)-epigallocatechin-3-gallate in conscious and freely moving rats and its brain regional distribution. J Agric Food Chem 55(4):1517–1524

120. Mandel S, Amit T, Reznichenko L, Weinreb O, Youdim MB (2006) Green tea catechins as brain-permeable, natural iron chelators-antioxidants for the treatment of neurodegenerative disorders. Mol Nutr Food Res 50:229–234

121. Willis LM, Shukitt-Hale B, Joseph JA (2009) Recent advances in berry supplementation and age-related cognitive decline. Curr Opin Clin Nutr Metab Care 12(1):91–94

122. Shukitt-Hale B, Cheng V, Joseph JA (2009) Effects of blackberries on motor and cognitive function in aged rats. Nutr Neurosci 12(3):135–140

123. Willis LM, Shukitt-Hale B, Joseph JA (2009) Modulation of cognition and behavior in aged animals: role for antioxidant- and essential fatty acid-rich plant foods. Am J Clin Nutr 89(5):1602S–1606S, Review. PMID: 19339395

124. Joseph JA, Fisher DR, Cheng V, Rimando AM, Shukitt-Hale B (2008) Cellular and behavioral effects of stilbene resveratrol analogues: implications for reducing the deleterious effects of aging. J Agric Food Chem 56(22):10544–10551

125. Kumar NB, Kazi A, Smith T, Crocker T, Yu D, Reich RR, Reddy K, Hastings S, Exterman M, Balducci L, Dalton K, Bepler G (2010) Cancer cachexia: traditional therapies and novel molecular mechanism-based approaches to treatment. Curr Treat Options Oncol 11(3–4): 107–117. Review

126. Mazza M, Pomponi M, Janiri L, Bria P, Mazza S (2007) Omega-3 fatty acids and antioxidants in neurological and psychiatric diseases: an overview. Prog Neuropsychopharmacol Biol Psychiatry 31:12–26

127. Gadoth N (2008) On fish oil and omega-3 supplementation in children: the role of such supplementation on attention and cognitive dysfunction. Brain Dev 30:309–312

128. Acosta S, Jernberg J, Sanberg CD, Sanberg PR, Small BJ, Gemma C, Bickford PC (2010) NT-020, a natural therapeutic approach to optimize spatial memory performance and increase neural progenitor cell proliferation and decrease inflammation in the aged rat. Rejuvenation Res 13(5):581–588, Epub ahead of print. PMID: 20586644

129. Block KI, Koch AC, Mead MN, Tothy PK, Newman RA, Gyllenhaal C (2008) Impact of antioxidant supplementation on chemotherapeutic toxicity: a systematic review of the evidence from randomized controlled trials. Int J Cancer 123(6):1227–1239

130. Willis LM, Shukitt-Hale B, Cheng V, Joseph JA (2008) Dose-dependent effects of walnuts on motor and cognitive function in aged rats. Br J Nutr 9:1–5

131. Calon F, Lim GP, Yang F, Morihara T, Teter B, Ubeda O, Rostaing P, Triller A, Salem N Jr, Ashe KH, Frautschy SA, Cole GM (2004) Docosahexaenoic acid protects from dendritic pathology in an Alzheimer's disease mouse model. Neuron 43(5):633–645

132. Johnson EJ, Schaefer EJ (2006) Potential role of dietary $n - 3$ fatty acids in the prevention of dementia and macular degeneration. Am J Clin Nutr 83(6 Suppl):1494S–1498S

133. Lim WS, Gammack JK, Van Niekerk J, Dangour AD (2006) Omega 3 fatty acid for the prevention of dementia. Cochrane Database Syst Rev 1:CD005379, Review

134. Barton D, Loprinzi C (2002) Novel approaches to preventing chemotherapy-induced cognitive dysfunction in breast cancer: the art of the possible. Clin Breast Cancer Suppl 3:S121–S127, Review

135. Flirski M, Sobow T (2005) Biochemical markers and risk factors of Alzheimer's disease. Curr Alzheimer Res 2:47–64

136. Irizarry MC (2004) Biomarkers of Alzheimer disease in plasma. NeuroRx 1:226–234

137. Ray S, Britschgi M, Herbert C, Takeda-Uchimura Y, Boxer A, Blennow K, Friedman LF, Galasko DR, Jutel M, Karydas A, Kaye JA, Leszek J, Miller BL, Minthon L, Quinn JF, Rabinovici GD, Robinson WH, Sabbagh MN, So YT, Sparks DL, Tabaton M, Tinklenberg J, Yesavage JA, Tibshirani R, Wyss-Coray T (2007) Classification and prediction of clinical Alzheimer's diagnosis based on plasma signaling proteins. Nat Med 13:1359–1362

138. Munir F, Kalawsky K, Lawrence C, Yarker J, Haslam C, Ahmed S (2011) Cognitive intervention for breast cancer patients undergoing adjuvant chemotherapy: a needs analysis. Cancer Nurs 34(5):385–392

139. Balducci L (2010) Anemia, fatigue and aging. Transfus Clin Biol 17(5–6):375–381, Epub 2010 Nov 9. Review

140. Garratt AM, Ruta DA, Abdalla MI, Buckingham JK, Russell IT (1993) The SF36 health survey questionnaire: an outcome measure suitable for routine use within the NHS? BMJ 306(6890):1440–1444

Dysfunction of the Bowel/Constipation

10

Core Messages

Constipation is commonly defined as having a bowel movement fewer than three times per week and characterized by stools that are hard, dry, small in size, and difficult and painful to eliminate. Individuals who are constipated experience straining, bloating, and the sensation of a full bowel.

The physical sequelae of constipation range from hemorrhoids, diverticular disease, fecal impaction, abdominal pain, reflux, nausea and vomiting, insomnia, and fatigue (Bell TJ) to poor quality of life in this patient population and contributing to the burden of the condition and often require treatment.

Anywhere from 15% to 90% of cancer patients report constipation. The variation observed in the prevalence rates reported can be attributed to varying trial designs (prospective and retrospective), population heterogeneity (age, gender), underlying pathology, choice, dose and route of administration of opioid, duration of treatment, and individual variation in perception of the symptom.

The etiology of constipation in cancer patients can be attributed to several factors but broadly classified as related to somatopathic, functional causes or medication-induced constipation.

Constipation is frequently the result of autonomic neuropathy caused by the vinca alkaloids, taxanes, and thalidomide. Other drugs such as opioid analgesics or anticholinergics (antidepressants and antihistamines) may lead to constipation by causing decreased sensitivity to the defecation reflexes and decreased gut motility.

Physiologic factors such as dehydration and metabolic disturbances such as hyperkalemia can contribute to this symptom.

Mechanical causes such as tumor or treatments such as radiation therapy and other symptoms such as cancer anorexia, cachexia, nausea, and vomiting can exacerbate symptoms of constipation in this patient population.

N.B. Kumar, *Nutritional Management of Cancer Treatment Effects*,
DOI 10.1007/978-3-642-27233-2_10, © Springer-Verlag Berlin Heidelberg 2012

In patients who are hospitalized or living in locations other than home to receive serial treatments, unfamiliar environments, use of bedpan, and lack of privacy have also been observed to be contributors in oncology cancer patient populations in clinical settings. Depression due to chronic illness, immobility, anorexia, and use of antidepressants has also been associated to constipation.

10.1　Definition

Constipation is commonly defined as having a bowel movement fewer than three times per week and characterized by stools that are hard, dry, small in size, and difficult and painful to eliminate. Individuals who are constipated experience straining, bloating, and the sensation of a full bowel [1]. In attempting to define constipation using a more comprehensive approach, the Rome diagnostic criteria for constipation not only encompass bowel movement frequency but also capture the discomfort associated with constipation (Table 10.1) [2]. The physical sequelae of constipation range from hemorrhoids, diverticular disease, fecal impaction, abdominal pain, reflux, nausea and vomiting, insomnia, and fatigue [3] to poor quality of life in this patient population and contributing to the burden of the condition and often require

Table 10.1　Rome II and III criteria for chronic constipation [2]

Diagnostic criteria	Symptoms
Rome II in at least 12 weeks, which need not be consecutive, in the preceding 12 months, ≥2 symptoms must be present	Straining in >25% of bowel movements
	Hard or lumpy stools in >25% of bowel movements
	Sensation of incomplete evacuation in >25% of bowel movements
	Sensation of anorectal obstruction/blockade in >25% of bowel movements
	Manual maneuvers to facilitate >25% of bowel movements (digital disimpaction)
	<3 bowel movements per week
	Loose stool is not present, and criteria for irritable bowel syndrome are not fulfilled
Rome III presence of ≥2 symptoms	Straining during ≥25% of defecations
	Lumpy or hard stools in ≥25% of defecations
	Sensation of incomplete evacuation for ≥25% of defecations
	Sensation of anorectal obstruction/blockage for ≥25% of defecations
	Manual maneuvers to facilitate ≥25% of defecations (digital manipulations, pelvic floor support)
	<3 evacuations per week
	Loose stools are rarely present without the use of laxatives
	Insufficient criteria for irritable bowel syndrome
	Criteria fulfilled for the last 3 months, and symptom onset ≥6 months prior to diagnosis

treatment [4]. In patients with cancer diagnosis, constipation is the most common and often most debilitating adverse effect associated with opioid therapy for the management of chronic pain [5–7]. Even after aggressive therapies to improve bowel function have been implemented, many patients continue to experience symptoms of opioid-induced bowel disorders such as constipation (OIC). Uncontrolled OIC necessitates the need for rectal invasive procedures (enema, manual evacuation) that lead not only to increased health-care costs, but most importantly, cause severe patient suffering [8]. To avoid these unwanted effects, some even choose to decrease or discontinue therapy with opioid analgesics, and experience inadequate pain control [9]. Chronic constipation is classified as functional (primary) or secondary. Functional constipation can be divided into normal transit, slow transit, or outlet constipation. Possible causes of secondary chronic constipation include medication use, as well as medical conditions, such as hypothyroidism [58] or irritable bowel syndrome. Frail older patients may present with nonspecific symptoms of constipation, such as delirium, anorexia, and functional decline. Risk factors for constipation include female gender, older age, inactivity, low caloric intake, low-fiber diet, low income, low educational level, and taking a large number of medications [10, 11].

10.2 Prevalence

Since constipation is a multifactorial syndrome, it is challenging to obtain accurate estimates of the prevalence of constipation in cancer patients. Estimates of the frequency of constipation vary from 15% to 90% in patients receiving opioids [12–14]. In a multinational, internet-based survey that was designed to assess the prevalence, frequency, severity, and impact of opioid-induced bowel dysfunction (OBD) in patients receiving opioid therapy for chronic pain and taking laxatives, Bell et al. [15] surveyed 322 patients, of whom 81% reported constipation and 58% reported straining to pass a bowel movement (58%) with a third of patients had missed, decreased, or stopped using opioids in order to make it easier to have a bowel movement. In another study to examine the prevalence of opioid-induced bowel disorders (OBD), including constipation, 593 cancer patients receiving treatment were assessed according to WHO guidelines [15]. Constipation was one of the most frequent side effects of opioid treatment, observed in 23% of patients. In yet another series of studies conducted in a large US hospice found that 40–63% of patients with cancer had opioid-induced constipation [16]. In a study of over 2,000 patients on treatment with opioids, nonsteroidal anti-inflammatory drugs (NSAIDs) or other therapies for chronic pain demonstrated that 63.5% of patients were experiencing constipation despite 89.5% of patients receiving laxatives. Similar rates were reported in cancer patients treated with opioids and prophylactic laxatives resulting in 37.8–50.0% incidence of constipation [17]. The variation observed in the prevalence rates reported can be attributed to varying trial designs (prospective and retrospective), population heterogeneity (age, gender and underlying pathology, choice, dose and route of administration of opioid, duration of treatment, and individual variation in perception of the symptom [18]. Overall bowel disorders such as constipation are common symptoms that are distressing cancer patients.

10.3 Etiology

Heterogenic group of diseases and drugs can contribute to constipation. The etiology of constipation in cancer patients can be attributed to several factors but broadly classified as related to somatopathic, functional causes or medication-induced constipation [19]. A significant number of therapies used to treat cancer patients can also be classified as medication-induced constipation, i.e., opioid-induced constipation is caused by linkage of the opioid to opioid receptors in the bowel and the central nervous system [19]. Constipation is frequently the result of autonomic neuropathy caused by the vinca alkaloids, taxanes, and thalidomide. Other drugs such as opioid analgesics and anticholinergics (antidepressants and antihistamines) may lead to constipation by causing decreased sensitivity to the defecation reflexes and decreased gut motility. Physiologic factors such as dehydration and metabolic disturbances such as hyperkalemia can contribute to this symptom. Mechanical causes such as tumor or treatments such as radiation therapy and other symptoms such as cancer anorexia, cachexia, nausea, and vomiting can exacerbate symptoms of constipation in this patient population. Psychological factors such as depression, distress and change in environment, decreased functional capacity, and loss of privacy have also been associated to constipation (Fig. 10.1).

10.3.1 Medications for Cancer Treatment

Although constipation is a well-recognized symptom of cancer treatment, very few studies have characterized this symptom as it relates specifically to chemotherapy regimens. Chemotherapy-induced constipation is recognized as being a combination of reduced frequency of bowel motility and increased stool consistency [20]. Several cytotoxic agents that can cause autonomic nervous system changes such as vinca alkaloids, oxaliplatins, taxanes, and thalidomide have been observed clinically to contribute to constipation. Contributing factors associated with cytotoxic therapies have been hypothesized to occur secondary to alteration in the balance of the normal gut function. Decreased oral intake due to cancer anorexia, dehydration, decreased motility, neuropathy, increased resorption, blockage, overtreated diarrhea, and antiemetics may all contribute to constipation in this population. Increased transit time due to alteration in gut motility can result in bowel content being in communication with the bowel wall for a longer period of time, leading to increased fluid absorption resulting in constipation [20]. In a study to compare the effects on QOL of weekly versus thrice-weekly sequential neoadjuvant docetaxel, weekly docetaxel is well tolerated and has less distressing side effects such as constipation, without compromising therapeutic responses [21].

Several research studies over the past two decades have documented symptoms of constipation in cancer patient population administered with opioids to treat cancer pain or sedatives. The highest prevalence of constipation was reported in cancer patients whose pain is managed with opioids, especially those patients treated with morphine, whereas the lowest was observed in patients on oxycodone CR and

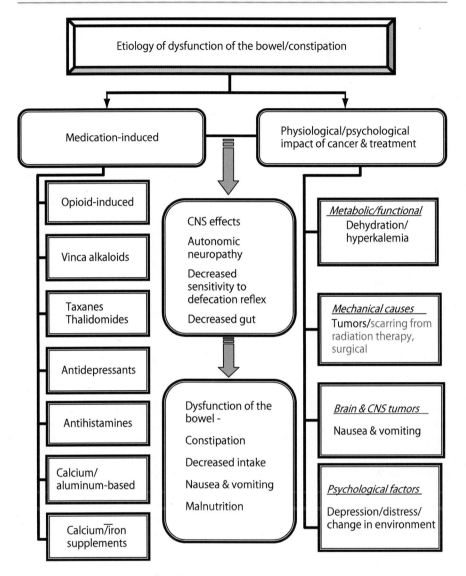

Fig. 10.1 Etiology of dysfunction of the bowel/constipation

buprenorphine TTS [11]. Existing disease-related constipation has also been reported to be exacerbated by opioid therapy [5, 21, 22]. Heterogeneous diseases including cancer and drugs such as opioids, immunomodulators, and taxanes/vinca alkaloids increase the risk of acute large bowel ischemia consistent with multifactorial pathogenesis [23].

Opioid analgesics are a cornerstone of pain therapy in the hospice and palliative care cancer patient population [7, 9, 18]. Despite proven analgesic efficacy, opioid use is associated with frequently dose-limiting bowel dysfunction that seriously impacts patients' quality of life (QOL). Opioids produce varying degrees of constipation, suggesting a dose-related phenomenon [22]. Kandemir et al. [24] reported 30.4% constipation in patients who received OND plus DEX, compared with 9.3% -treated with MCL plus DEX ($p < 0.01$). Constipation was observed in 8.6% patients receiving OND, 3.6% GRA, and 6.2% TRO [25]. In a trial that evaluated the effect of long-term treatment with oral sustained-release hydromorphone, transdermal fentanyl, and transdermal buprenorphine on nausea, emesis, and constipation, gastrointestinal symptoms of cancer pain patients undergoing an opioid therapy were found to be related to multifactorial causes. Transdermal opioids showed no benefit over oral controlled-release hydromorphone with regard to gastrointestinal symptoms. The conversion ratios for transdermal fentanyl, transdermal buprenorphine, and oral hydromorphone did not accord to the literature, because of differing occurrences of opioid tolerance after long-term therapy [26]. In a prospective, multicentric study to assess the prevalence of OBD in patients on analgesic therapy for the treatment of pain from any cause and identify the factors associated with the onset of this side effect, Rosti et al. reported that female gender and age >70 years also appeared as risk factors. The logistic analysis indicated that cancer-related pain, increased age, and the use of fentanyl are positive predictors of the presence of this bowel disorder, whereas the administration of oxycodone CR was associated with a decreased incidence of these symptoms [11]. The etiology of opioid-induced bowel disorder is based on the physiology of the GI tract, and the role of the endogenous opioid system in the alimentary canal is critical for the management of opioid-induced bowel disorders, including identification of targeted therapies. In a comprehensive review of the pathophysiology, Panchal et al. [18] summarize the current data on our understanding of the etiology of bowel disorders in cancer patients treated with opioids. The GI tract is amply innervated by the enteric nervous system, which is composed of the myenteric plexus, located between circular and longitudinal smooth muscle layers of the bowel, and the submucosal plexus, located in the submucosa [27, 28, 56]. Enteric neurons also synthesize endogenous opioid peptides and their transmitters such as met-enkephalin, leu-enkephalin, β-endorphin, and dynorphin, all of which have been localized to both neurons and endocrine cells of the mucosa in the GI tract [27]. Laboratory as well as clinical trials have demonstrated that these endogenous opioids inhibit enteric nerve activity and inhibit both propulsive motor and secretory activities [27–29], thus playing a critical role in coordinating the contractile process under normal conditions and suppressing intestinal motility when required (such as during inflammation, stress, and trauma) [27, 30]. Immunocytochemistry and mRNA quantification techniques have also identified receptors that mediate the effects of both endogenous and exogenous opioids on bowel function [27, 28, 56]. Three major and distinct classes of opioid receptors have been identified in the enteric nervous system: delta, kappa, and mu [31, 32], of which the enteric mu-opioid receptor appears to be the principal mediator of opioid agonist effects on the GI tract [31, 33, 57]. When opioid agonists bind to these receptors, an inhibition of the release of excitatory and inhibitory neurotransmitters is observed, interrupting the coordinated rhythmic contractions required for intestinal motility and reducing mucosal secretions [28, 34].

Administration of exogenous opioids can cause OBD by decreasing peristalsis [29], which in combination with reduced secretions into the gut and increased reabsorption of fluid from the gut (as the stool remains in the intestinal lumen for extended periods) leads to the formation of dry, hard stools that are difficult to pass. The understanding of the pathophysiology of the effects of opioid therapy in the GI tract has provided the opportunity for newer targeted therapies addressing the underlying opioid receptor–mediated cause of bowel dysfunction for the management of opioid-induced bowel disorders, specifically constipation that does not respond nor is relieved by laxative therapy. Newer agents such as utilizing mu-opioid receptor antagonists have evolved to manage opioid-induced constipation. The combination of the strong opioid oxycodone and the opioid antagonist naloxone has been shown to have the potential to prevent opioid-induced bowel dysfunction (OIBD) while maintaining analgesic efficacy [18, 35].

Anticholinergic preparations (e.g., gastrointestinal antispasmodics and antidepressants), phenothiazines, calcium- and aluminum-based antacids, diuretics, vitamin supplements (e.g., iron and calcium), tranquilizers and sleeping medications, and pudendal blocks are agents administered to cancer patients demonstrated to contribute to symptoms of constipation. Additionally fatigue, cancer anorexia, inadequate fluid intake, prolonged immobility, and inadequate exercise can exacerbate symptoms of constipation [5, 36].

10.3.2 Tumor or Tumor-Radiation-Induced Constipation

Narrowing of colon lumen related to scarring from radiation therapy, surgical anastomosis, or compression from growth of extrinsic tumors, neurological lesions (cerebral tumors) and spinal cord injury or compression have been observed to contribute to constipation. Inability to increase intra-abdominal pressure secondary to emphysema, any neuromuscular impairment of the diaphragm or abdominal muscles, or massive abdominal hernias can also contribute to symptoms of constipation. Atony of muscles has been associated with malnutrition, cachexia, anemia, and carcinoma. In addition, senility has also been associated with atony of muscles contributing to constipation. Metabolic disorders such as hypothyroidism, dehydration, hypercalcemia, hypokalemia, and hyponatremia have also been observed in clinical settings to contribute to constipation.

10.3.3 Psychological Factors

In patients who are hospitalized or living in locations other than home to receive serial treatments, unfamiliar environments, use of bedpan, and lack of privacy have also been observed to be contributors in oncology cancer patient populations in clinical settings. Depression due to chronic illness, immobility, anorexia, and use of antidepressants have also been associated to constipation [10, 11, 37].

10.4   Current Treatment for Cancer or Treatment-Induced Constipation

Current management of cancer constipation includes a comprehensive assessment of the symptom and treatment based on the etiology of constipation. The primary approach to treat constipation includes bulk producers that are natural or semisynthetic polysaccharide and cellulose, laxatives (saline, stimulant, and lubricant), fecal softeners, lactulose (Cholac, Cephulac), polyethylene glycol and electrolytes (Golytely, Colyte), and opioid antagonists (naloxone, methylnaltrexone). The treatment consists of basic measures and the application of laxatives using a laxative ladder for stepwise selection of choice of laxatives based on the etiology [19]. It has also been suggested that clinicians should not base laxative prescribing on the opioid dose, but rather should titrate the laxative according to bowel function. Lower doses of opioids or weaker opioids, such as codeine, are just as likely to cause constipation [22]. For these reasons, it is important that palliative care practitioners have an adequate understanding of normal GI function and the underlying mechanisms responsible for OBD, the burden of OBD in the context of appropriate and effective pain management, and the benefits provided by effective pharmacotherapy. Several real-world cases are discussed to illustrate the application of optimal symptom management and the use of strategies that minimize the effects of OBD and improve patient QOL [9].

10.4.1 Assessment

The evaluation of constipation is a multidisciplinary endeavor. Assessment includes a comprehensive history and physical examination including major symptoms related and resulting from constipation such as evidence of bleeding, unintended weight loss, iron deficiency anemia, acute onset constipation in older patients, colonic ischemia, and rectal prolapse [10]. Several tools have been used by institutions treating this patient population to assess and to characterize the extent and severity of the condition with supportive standards to be used as a reference for diagnostic criteria. The Patient Assessment of Constipation Quality of Life (PAC-QOL) was developed to address the need for a standardized, patient-reported outcome measure to evaluate the burden of constipation on patients' everyday functioning and well-being over time. The Patient Assessment of Constipation Symptoms (PAC-SYM) questionnaire is used to assess the symptoms and severity of constipation. Both the PAC-QOL and PAC-SYM instruments have been shown to be reliable, valid, and responsive measures of constipation and opioid-induced constipation, respectively [38, 39]. In addition, these brief instruments have been easy to administer and provide health professionals an opportunity to initiate activity and implement treatment. Rome criteria II-III is a more comprehensive definition that should ideally form the basis of any tool used to assess constipation associated with OBD [2].

The Bowel Function Index (BFI) numerical analogue scale (0–100), calculated as the mean of three variables (ease of defecation, feeling of incomplete bowel evacuation, and personal judgment of constipation), was developed to evaluate bowel function in opioid-treated patients with pain. This clinician-administered tool allows easy measurement of OIC from the patient's perspective [40]. In a study to evaluate the psychometric characteristics of the BFI using data from clinical studies of oral prolonged-release (PR) oxycodone/naloxone, BFI was observed to be a valid and reliable instrument for the assessment of opioid-induced constipation in chronic pain patients. Psychometric analyses from clinical trials support the BFI's psycho-metric properties. A change of less than five points in BFI was indicative of high reproducibility. Correlations between BFI item and total scores to stool frequency were statistically significant and in the low-to-moderate range (OXN2401 −0.23 to −0.29, $p < 0.001$; OXN3401 range −0.26 to −0.40, $p < 0.001$; OXN3001 −0.14 to −0.15, $p < 0.05$). Data indicate that a BFI score change of ≥ 12 points represents a clinically meaningful change in symptoms of constipation. Although validated only by using three clinical trials, these instruments appear promising not only to develop assessment tools but also to monitor response to treatment regimens [41].

A new tool, the Victoria Bowel Performance Scale (BPS), was designed as an ordinal nine-point scale from −4 (severe constipation) to +4 (severe diarrhea) and includes three parameters: visual stool characteristics, bowel pattern, and ability to control defecation. This study tested the reliability of BPS using case scenarios in a test-retest format [42, 43]. Results of early validation of this tool demonstrated that the raters were consistent in their scoring over time, with an average Cohen's kappa of 0.70 over all of the raters. The average Pearson correlation coefficient between time periods 1 and 2 scores was 0.92. Further prospective testing in day-to-day clinical care is needed to further confirm the reliability and clinical utility of the BPS. A BPS management guideline has been developed to assist with decision mak-ing for each BPS score, which also requires validation [42]. The Victoria BPS was also found to be an acceptable and a useful bowel function assessment tool, uniquely incorporating the patient's usual bowel function. Modifications to the scale have been made to improve clarity and allow for the expected drop in bowel activity seen in end-of-life care. Considerable educational effort and appropriate organization of the charts are required for optimal implementation. The proportion of revised BPS scores ranging from −1 to +1 is proposed as an indicator of satisfactory bowel man-agement for clinical, audit, and research purposes [43]. With the early validation studies appearing promising, further prospective testing in day-to-day clinical care is needed to further confirm the reliability and clinical utility of this scale. A BPS management guideline has been developed to assist with decision making for each BPS score, which also requires further validation.

10.4.2 Pharmacological Interventions

10.4.2.1 Bulk Producers

Bulk producers are natural or semisynthetic polysaccharide and cellulose. They work with the body's natural processes to hold water in the intestinal tract, soften the stool, and increase the frequency of the passage of stool. Bulk producers are not recommended for use in a regimen to counteract the bowel effects of opioids. Methylcellulose (Cologel), polycarbophil calcium (FiberCon®), barley malt extract

(Maltsupex), or psyllium products such as psyllium hydrophilic mucilloid (Metamucil®) are commonly recommended. Bulk-forming laxatives are not recommended for use in palliative care patients, for such patients are normally not able to take in the required amount of fluids [19].

10.4.2.2 Laxatives

Saline or osmotic laxatives consist of high osmolarity compounds combined with saline to attract water into the lumen of the intestines. The fluid accumulation alters the stool consistency, distends the bowel, and induces peristaltic movement. Side effects of saline laxatives include cramps; repeated use can alter fluid and electrolyte balance and mostly contraindicated in renal function as well those patients with edema, congestive heart failure, megacolon, or hypertension. Osmotic laxatives are divided into (magnesium) salts, saccharine, alcohols, and macrogols. Lactulose is a synthetic disaccharide that passes to the colon undigested. When it is broken down in the colon, it produces lactic acid, formic acid, acetic acid, and carbon dioxide. These products increase the osmotic pressure, thus increasing the amount of water held in the stool, which softens the stool and increases the frequency of passage. Although lactulose was one of the most frequently used saccharine laxative, associated side effects such as flatulence, bloating, and abdominal cramping have restricted use [19]. On the other hand, orally administered macrogol is not metabolized, and pH value and bowel flora remain unchanged. It has been shown to hydrate hardened stools, increase stool volume, decrease the duration of colon passage, and dilate the bowel wall that then triggers the defecation reflex. Because of its high effectiveness and tolerance, even when administered over time, macrogol has become the laxative of first choice in palliative care patients, especially when normal fluid intake levels can be maintained [19]. In a systematic review and meta-analysis to assess efficacy of polyethylene glycol (PEG) in adults with nonorganic constipation versus placebo, PEG was found to be a more effective laxative than lactulose in adult patients with constipation [44]. Similarly, laxative management in ambulatory cancer patients on opioid therapy was examined in a prospective, open-label investigation of polyethylene glycol, sodium picosulfate (SPS), and lactulose. In spite of opioid therapy, the incidence of constipation was low in these ambulatory cancer pain patients at an early disease stage. For prevention of constipation, PEG or SPS is recommended instead of lactulose [26]. Lee-Robichaud [45] completed a meta-analysis of all relevant data from randomized clinical trials in order to determine whether lactulose or polyethylene glycol is more effective at treating chronic constipation and fecal impaction and confirmed that polyethylene glycol is better than lactulose in outcomes of stool frequency per week, form of stool, relief of abdominal pain, and the need for additional products. On subgroup analysis, this was seen in both adults and children, except for relief of abdominal pain. In another trial, Movicol, a polyethylene glycol (PEG)+electrolyte solution (PEG+E), was evaluated as treatment for severe constipation and fecal impaction. Chen et al. [46] observed that PEG+E, administered orally at a dose equivalent to eight 13.8 g sachets (1 L) per day over 3 days, was a highly effective and well-tolerated therapy for the treatment of severe constipation and fecal impaction. Both lactulose and polyethylene glycol are more effective in promoting defecation than placebo. Patients receiving polyethylene glycol had a slightly lower incidence of acute intestinal pseudoobstruction, whereas length of stay was shorter in lactulose-treated patients. Morphine administration was associated with delayed defecation except in the polyethylene glycol–treated group. Irrespective of study medication, early defecation was associated with a shorter length of stay [47]. Stimulant laxatives on the other hand increase motor activity of the bowels by direct action on the intestines. However, prolonged use of these drugs causes laxative dependency and loss of normal bowel function and may also cause cramping. Specifically, long-term use of danthron discolors rectal mucosa and discolors alkaline urine red. Lubricant laxatives such as mineral oil lubricate intestinal mucosa and soften stool and mostly used in combination with laxatives prophylactically to prevent straining in patients for whom straining would be dangerous and still considered important in palliative care patients. Despite the wealth of management approaches available to treat constipation, an estimated 54% of patients treated for OBD do not achieve the "desired result" with medication even half the time [5].

10.4.2.3 Opioid Agonists

Methylnaltrexone is a selective mu-opioid receptor antagonist that has restricted ability to cross the blood–brain barrier, thus enabling reversal of opioid-induced peripheral effects, such as constipation, without affecting the central effects, such as pain relief [9]. Subcutaneous methylnaltrexone, 0.15 mg/kg of body weight, can be administered daily or every other day to treat opioid-induced constipation. In a study of palliative care patients, including those with cancer and noncancer etiologies, approximately one-half of patients defecated within 4 h of receiving the injection, with 30% of patients having a bowel movement within the first 30 min. Studies in palliative care patients' patient populations observed no evidence of withdrawal or other central effects of the opioid, and pain scores remained unchanged [48, 49].

A study of prolonged-release naloxone in an oxycodone:naloxone ratio of 2:1 (average results of 40:20 mg, 60:30 mg, and 80:40 mg oxycodone:naloxone combination relative to placebo) demonstrated improved bowel function without reversal of analgesia [50]. Other studies [7, 51] have shown that treatment with subcutaneous methylnaltrexone relative to placebo significantly increased the rescue-free laxation response rate within 4 h of the first dose (primary endpoint) in adult patients with opioid-induced constipation and advanced illness in two randomized, double-blind, placebo-controlled, multicentre, and phase III studies: one was a single-dose study ($n = 154$) and the other a multiple-dose study ($n = 133$). In the multiple-dose study, rescue-free laxation response rates within 4 h after at least two of the first four doses (coprimary endpoint) were also significantly higher in methylnaltrexone recipients than in placebo recipients. Moreover, median time to laxation after the first dose was significantly shorter in methylnaltrexone recipients than in placebo recipients in both studies. Methylnaltrexone was not associated with any significant changes in pain scores or central opioid withdrawal in these studies. Methylnaltrexone was generally well tolerated in clinical trials; most adverse events were of mild to moderate severity. Similar findings were reported in patients with advanced illness [7] where subcutaneous methylnaltrexone rapidly induced laxation in patients with advanced illness and opioid-induced constipation. Treatment did not appear to affect central analgesia or precipitate opioid withdrawal. Response rates among methylnaltrexone-treated patients who had responded to all previous doses were 57–100% for doses two to seven. Among methylnaltrexone-treated patients who did not respond to the first or to the first two consecutive doses, 35% and 26% responded to the second and third dose, respectively. Higher percentages of patients and clinicians rated bowel status as improved in the methylnaltrexone than the placebo group. Fewer methylnaltrexone than placebo patients reported use of common laxative types, particularly enemas, during the study. Subcutaneous methylnaltrexone promptly and predictably induced laxation, improved constipation distress, and was associated with less laxative use in patients with advanced illness and OIC [52]. In a recently reported review, Candy et al. [53] included seven studies involving 616 participants; all underreported methodological features. In four studies, the laxatives lactulose, senna, co-danthramer, misrakasneham, and magnesium hydroxide with liquid paraffin were evaluated. In three methylnaltrexone. In studies comparing the different laxatives, evidence was inconclusive. Evidence on subcutaneous methylnaltrexone was clearer; in combined analysis (287 participants), methylnaltrexone, in comparison with a placebo, significantly induced laxation at 4 h (odds ratio 6.95; 95% confidence interval 3.83–12.61). In combined analyses, there was no difference in the proportion experiencing side effects, although participants on methylnaltrexone suffered more flatulence and dizziness. No evidence of opioid withdrawal was found. In one study, severe adverse events, commonly abdominal pain, were reported that were possibly related to methylnaltrexone. A serious adverse event considered to be related to the methylnaltrexone also occurred; this involved a participant having severe diarrhea, subsequent dehydration, and cardiovascular collapse. The authors concluded that their 2010 update found that evidence on laxatives for management of constipation remains limited due to insufficient RCTs. However, the conclusions found that subcutaneous methylnaltrexone is effective in inducing laxation in palliative care patients with opioid-induced constipation and where conventional laxatives have failed [53]. However, the safety of this product is not fully evaluated, and large, rigorous, and independent trials are needed.

10.4.2.4 Antiemetics

Since nausea, vomiting, and gastroesophageal reflux are also symptoms associated with opioid use, studies have examined the effect of antiemetics in relieving symptoms of constipation, although their utility in an OBD population has yet to be validated. Aprepitant (Emend) is the first commercially available drug from a new class of agents, the neurokinin NK(1) receptor antagonists. Oral aprepitant, in combination with other agents, is indicated for the prevention of acute and delayed chemotherapy-induced nausea and vomiting (CINV) associated with highly emetogenic chemotherapy in adults [54] (Dando TM). In a meta-analysis including 10 studies involving 4,376 oncology patients, the incidence of constipation was lower ($p = 0.002$) in patients treated with aprepitant for chemotherapy-induced nausea and vomiting, demonstrating some benefits of antiemetics in treating symptom clusters including constipation [55].

10.4.3 Nonpharmacological Approaches

Nonpharmacological approaches which involve nutritional strategies including increased nutritional intake, fluids, and fiber; increasing physical activity and exercises if appropriate; and improving the environment of the patient to provide privacy, support, and encouragement have all been observed to improve symptoms clinically as well as the quality of life of the cancer patient.

10.5 Guidelines

The evaluation of constipation is a multidisciplinary endeavor. Multiple, systematic assessment and approaches are currently followed in various institutions around the world. The following guidelines are considered best practice standards. Improved management of constipation may require a *multimodal approach by multidisciplinary teams*. These include specific and comprehensive assessment, nutritional guidelines, pharmacotherapy, and physical activity, in addition to monitoring and closely assessing patients for change in status. Nonpharmacological strategies for constipation in cancer patients include interventions such as increased dietary fiber, fluid intake, encouraging mobility and ambulation, and encouraging daily bowel movements at the same time every day [13, 45]. However, pharmacological approaches with bulking agents, laxatives, antiemetics, stool softeners, and opioid receptor agonists are often necessary. The basic goal in the management of this symptoms is to establish the patient's normal bowel pattern and habits (time of day for normal bowel movement, consistency, color, and amount); explore the patient's level of understanding and compliance relating to exercise level, mobility, and diet (fluid, fruit, and fiber intake); determine normal or usual use of laxatives, stimulants, or enemas; determine laboratory values, specifically looking at platelet count; and conduct a physical assessment of the rectum (or stoma) to rule out impaction. All assessment and reassessment should be conducted continuously taking into consideration change in medications and medical status of the cancer patient.

10.5.1 Comprehensive Assessment

A comprehensive assessment by a multidisciplinary team including an MD, RD, PharmD, RNs, PT, and psychosocial workers must include physical assessment of subjective information of normal bowel pattern (nature and frequency of bowel movements daily, in addition to straining, pain, and bleeding symptoms that may accompany defecation), dietary assessment (changes in nutritional, fiber, and fluid intake), current medications (opioids, chemotherapy, or radiation therapy and change in medications) and other symptoms such as distention, flatus, cramping, absence of bowel sounds, and rectal fullness. A digital rectal examination should always be done to rule out fecal impaction at the level of the rectum. A test for occult blood to determine presence of a possible intraluminal lesion and a thorough examination of the gastrointestinal tract is necessary if cancer is suspected.

Physical assessment will determine the presence or absence of bowel sounds, flatus, or abdominal distention. Patients with colostomies should also be assessed for constipation including monitoring of irrigation of the colostomy for proper technique. The initial physical exam may systematically assess stool impaction (constipation with diarrhea with overflow around impaction) and obstruction (physical exam and X-ray). Patients may also be assessed for hypercalcemia, hypokalemia, hypothyroidism, and diabetes as these conditions may exacerbate constipation.

The following questions may provide a useful assessment guide:

1. What is normal for the patient (frequency, amount, and timing)?
2. When was the last bowel movement? What was the amount, consistency, and color? Was blood passed with it?
3. Has the patient been having any abdominal discomfort, cramping, nausea or vomiting, pain, excessive gas, or rectal fullness?
4. Does the patient regularly use laxatives or enemas? What does the patient usually do to relieve constipation? Does it usually work?
5. What type of diet does the patient follow? How much and what type of fluids are taken on a regular basis?
6. What medication (dose and frequency) is the patient taking? Is the patient taking any opioids?
7. Is this symptom a recent change?
8. How many times a day is flatus passed?
9. Does the patient strain more than normal to defecate?
10. Is there pain accompanying passing of stool?
11. Has the environment of patient changed?
12. Does patient have a sense of control over stools?
13. Does the patient use a private bathroom, bedside commode, or bedpan?
14. Does patient have a colostomy?

Patients should be assessed by a multidisciplinary team at admission and periodically as treatments including medications and nutritional and fluid intake may change. Establish the patient's normal bowel pattern and habits (time of day for normal bowel movement, consistency, color, and amount). If a patient is on opioids or admitted with a symptom of constipation, bowel movements must be recorded daily.

10.5.2 Pharmacotherapy

Based on the assessment, etiology of constipation must be identified and pharmacological approaches targeted to the etiology of this symptom. Preventive interventions with laxatives and stool softeners are provided to patients who are anticipated to begin treatments that can produce changes in bowel function with a goal of at least 1 nonforced bowel once in 1–2 days. Several institutions have developed and adapted a practice consensus algorithm for the prevention and management of opioid-induced constipation. A series of combinations of laxatives, stool softeners, and bulking agents are introduced proactively and modified based on individual response to intervention. The following is a current list of agent used:

- *Cathartics and laxatives*:
  - Bisacodyl (Dulcolax®)
  - Magnesium citrate (Citrate of Magnesia®)
  - Magnesium hydroxide (MOM, Milk of Magnesia®)
  - Senna (Senokot®)
  - Sodium phosphate (Fleet Phospho Soda®, Fleet Enema®)
  - Sorbitol
  - Lactulose (causes less problems with melanosis coli and has been shown to contribute to future colonic inertia. It works as an osmotic laxative. It should only be used in patients without significant bowel obstruction).
  - Miralax (Can be used on an intermittent and/or long-term basis. It causes less dependence post long-term use).
- *Bulk-producing agents*:
  - Polycarbophil calcium (FiberCon®)
  - Psyllium hydrophilic mucilloid (Metamucil®)
  - Methylcellulose (Cologel)
  - Barley malt extract (Maltsupex)
- *Lubricants*:
  - Glycerin (rectal suppository)
  - Mineral oil
- *Surfactant/stool softener*:
  - Docusate sodium (Colace®)
- *Opioid agonists*:
  - Methylnaltrexone
  - Naloxone

10.5.3 Nonpharmacological Interventions

Nonpharmacological approaches such as nutritional intake, physical activity, fluid intake, and changes in the environment have been found to be clinically effective in managing constipation.

10.5.3.1 Nutrition Guidelines

- Screen patient within 24 h of admission. This order for screening has been a standard order for all cancer patient admissions to avoid delay in timing of screening.
- Assess all symptoms: gastrointestinal tract: taste alterations, smell alterations, dysphagia, dyspnea, other pain, early satiety, dry mouth, too much saliva production, anorexia, diarrhea, constipation, nausea, vomiting, dehydration, fatigue, height, weight, recent weight loss, anthropometrics, and others (mid-arm muscle circumference, body composition [DEXA], grip strength); psychosocial: family/caregiver support, depression, and ADL.

- Screen, assess current nutritional status, and estimate caloric, protein, and multivitamin/mineral needs (refer to Chap. 2).
- Provide adequate nutrition by including "calorie" and "protein" booster education material and nutritional supplements to ensure intake of proteins (recommended 0.8 g–1.0 g/kg/day). Provide dense caloric supplements up to 400 cal/day containing 1.5 kcal/mL. If intake is insufficient in proteins intake, supplement with modular protein supplements, adding this to favorite beverage (http://www.nestle-nutrition.com/Products/Default.aspx; http://abbottnutrition.com/). The choice of nutritional supplements can be based in the personal choice of the patient, patient needs, tolerance to product, as well as other comorbidities.
- If more calories or protein are needed to meet nutritional needs, introduce nutritional supplements with fiber, i.e., Ensure® with fiber.
- Include a standard multivitamin/mineral supplementation to prevent any further deficits and meet increased needs.
- Assess adequacy of intake and provide an appetite stimulant (megestrol acetate 20 mg–800 mg/day or alternate) if patient has cancer anorexia to ensure adequate intake and prevent further weight loss.
- Provide each patient with nutritional guidelines to ensure adequate intake of calories and proteins and a list of suggested high-calorie and high-protein nutritional supplements to choose from, taking into consideration taste alterations, early satiety, nausea, and vomiting that are common symptoms observed in this patient population.
- Proactive measures to provide alternate mode of nutritional support must be planned during acute phase of treatment when it would be a greater risk to feed patient via the oral route. Selection of route of feeding may be informed based on general guidelines and criteria provided in Table 2.6.
- Other strategies to improve nutritional intake.
- Meals must be eaten at regular times each day.

Soluble and insoluble fiber intake
- Ingestion of a normal diet rich in both soluble and insoluble fiber-containing foods is recommended.
- Encourage adequate fiber intake. Experts recommend that healthy adults consume 20–35 g of fiber per day (average consumption is 11 g).
- While there are no specific fiber recommendations for cancer patients, they should also be encouraged to eat more high-fiber foods such as fruits (e.g., raisins, prunes, peaches, and apples), vegetables (e.g., squash, broccoli, carrots, and celery), and 100% whole-grain cereals, breads, and bran. Increased fiber intake must be accompanied by increased fluid intake, or constipation may result.
- Additional fiber may not be recommended with certain chemotherapeutic drugs or narcotics The meal plan should be made with consideration for when patient will ingest the fiber and include the gradual increase of the fiber.
- Fiber intake may be planned after determining etiology of constipation. High-fiber intake is contraindicated in patients at increased risk for bowel obstruction, such as those with a history of bowel obstruction or status postcolostomy. Recommend eating a minimum of 5 g/serving of fiber from bran cereals or

cereals like shredded wheat. Also include foods made with whole grains such as bulgur or wheat berries, beans such as kidney beans, chickpeas, lentils, fresh fruit and vegetables, and dried fruit.

- Soaking beans first in water and discarding the water may help to reduce flatulence from this food group.
- Use a bulking agent, such as fiber supplements or a laxative/stool softener. Research indicates that a high-fiber diet with laxatives and lubricants such as mineral oil do not adversely affect nutritional status over a 6-month period [8].
- If mineral oil is used, supplements of fat-soluble vitamins (A, D, and E) may be indicated.

Fluids

- As fiber intake help hydrate stools, a high-fiber intake requires increased fluid volumes in the diet.
- Recommended fluid consumption is 8–10 cups of noncaffeinated beverages each day, e.g., water, prune juice, warm juices, and tea.
- Provide a warm or hot drink, preferably water with flavor, approximately one-half hour before time of patient's usual defecation.

10.5.3.2 Physical Activity

- Encourage regular exercise, including abdominal exercises in bed or moving from bed to chair if the patient is not ambulatory.

10.5.3.3 Environmental Changes

Private area and time

- Provide privacy and quiet time at the patient's usual or planned time for defecation.
- Provide toilet or bedside commode and appropriate assistive devices; avoid bedpan use whenever possible.

10.5.4 Markers and Instruments for Patient Monitoring and Assessment of Response to Treatment by the Interdisciplinary Medical Team

1. *Anthropometric measurements* such as participant's height, weight, and body mass index can be performed at admission and at regular intervals established by the medical team.
2. *Body composition by DXA scan*: DXA should be used to assess both total lean body mass (LBM), fat mass (FM), and total bone mineral density (BMD).Total bone mineral density (BMD) is a valid indirect measure of skeletal muscle and patient activity. Total LBM is sometimes called total fat-free mass (FFM) depending upon specific DXA manufacturer. DXA instruments use an X-ray source that generates or is split into two energies to measure bone mineral mass and soft tissue from which fat and fat-free mass are estimated. The exam is quick (1–2 min), precise (0.5–1%), and noninvasive. DXA scanners have the precision required to

detect changes in muscle mass as small as 5%. Radiation exposure from DXA scans is minimal. The National Council on Radiation Protection and Measurements (NCRP) has recommended the annual effective dose limit for infrequent exposure of the general population is 5,000 μSv and that an annual effective dose of 10 μSv be considered a negligible individual dose. The effective dose of a dual-energy X-ray absorptiometry whole body scan on an adult is 2.1 μSv. Studies have shown that quality assurance is an important issue in the use of DXA scans to determine body composition including lean body mass and bone mineral density. DXA instrument manufacturer and model should remain consistent, and their calibration should be monitored throughout treatment. Use of a standardized scan acquisition protocol and appropriate and unchanging scan acquisition and analysis software is essential to achieve consist results.

3. *Dietary intake* must be assessed at baseline and periodical intervals by conducting random weekly, 2 weekdays + 1 weekend day, 24-h dietary recalls (gold standard for collecting dietary data) using a 5-step multipass procedure (which has been found to assess mean energy intake within 10% of actual intake) and using the frequently updated University of Minnesota Nutrition Data System-Research version (NDS-R) database for analysis of nutrient composition. Food portion visuals can be provided to patients to estimate portion sizes of foods while monitoring intake.

4. *Symptom log* may be completed daily and collected from patients on a monthly basis. Based on these symptoms, all anticipated and unanticipated, grades of constitutional, dermatological, gastrointestinal (GI), metabolic, and pain symptoms can be continuously monitored including those symptoms affecting nutritional intake and utilization.

5. *Monthly* CMP and CBC should be monitored to assess electrolytes and organ function.

6. *Functional markers* (*Karnofsky performance score*): Evaluation of patients' functional status and barriers to obtaining adequate nutrients is also necessary. A physical exam combined with personal interview should include the evaluation of functional status such as the ability to chew and swallow, dental or oral problems causing odynophagia or dysphagia, signs of muscle wasting or anasarca, presence of edema, presence of skin or mouth lesion, and ability to perform instrumental activities of daily living (IADLs) such as cooking, shopping, and self-feeding. It is critical to assess activities of daily living, physical activity, exercise, sleep, and ability to work and perform other functional roles. Limitations in the activities of daily living have been identified secondary to and as a cause of weight loss in cancer patients. Cancer and other chronic diseases pose difficulties specifically for the cancer patient receiving treatment and the elderly in carrying out activities of daily living. A loss of postural and locomotive muscle mass has been observed within 7 days of inactivity. The Karnofsky Performance Scale Index allows patients to be classified as to their functional impairment. This has been used to compare effectiveness of different therapies and to assess the prognosis in individual patients and has been validated in cancer patient populations. This has been used to compare effectiveness of different therapies and to assess the prognosis in individual patients and has been validated in cancer patient populations.

7. *Godin Leisure-Time Exercise Questionnaire* weekly to monitor physical activity.

8. *Handgrip Strength Dynamometry Assessment*: A validated tool commonly used to assess handgrip strength is the Jamar dynamometer, which is a fast, reliable, and easy-to-perform device commonly used by our team to measure improvements in functional strength. The Jamar dynamometer has a lower percent coefficient of variation and is thus a more precise device than other handgrip dynamometers.

9. *Biochemical markers of protein status (serum albumin and transferrin)*: Assessment of protein status is critical in the identification and treatment of abnormalities in protein metabolism. There is substantial evidence of the correlation between serum hepatic proteins and inflammation, making these the most relevant biomarkers in cancer patient populations. Serum transferrin, prealbumin, and albumin have been observed as intermediate endpoint biomarkers and independently associated with clinical outcomes. Measurements of body composition combined with more objective and sensitive measure of protein nutriture are ideal for the biochemical assessment of intravascular and visceral protein stores. We have thus included the three major valid intermediate endpoint biomarkers (IEBs) that represent intravascular and visceral protein pools – transferrin, prealbumin, and albumin – as the biochemical indicators of protein status. Although transferrin levels are affected by iron status, serum transferrin, either singly or as part of a multiparameter index, is the strongest predictor of cancer patient morbidity and mortality.

10. *Immune and inflammatory markers*: A range of metabolic responses triggered by inflammatory and immunological responses in cancer patients. Cytokines can be measured in a panel including IL-1, IL-4, IL-6, IL-8, IL-10, GM-CSF, IFN-κ, TNFα, and CRP (BioRad-Bioplex). All of these biomarkers have been shown to increase with disease, aging, and cytotoxic agents. Though we realize these intermediate endpoint biomarkers of cytokines cannot be reliably interpreted, as over 70% of the subjects as observed in our studies were on active treatment with cytotoxic agents, these variables are important to determine, as they may provide useful information and contribute to the better understanding of the mechanistic process.

11. *Quality of life*: should be measured at baseline and monthly using the Rand Short Form (SF)-36 (Medical Outcomes Study SF-36) [59]. The SF-36 has been used extensively with both general, high-risk, and cancer populations and has available norms for mail and telephone versions and comparisons between group and individual scores. Scores are calculated and transformed to a 0–100 scale, with higher scores indicating increased health status. Reliability of the SF-36 scales was measured by Cronbach α coefficient, and the results ranged from 0.78 in general health perceptions to 0.91 in the physical functioning domain.

12. *Assessment of stool frequency*: A comprehensive assessment by a multidisciplinary team including of normal bowel pattern, including nature and frequency of bowel movements daily, in addition to straining, pain, and bleeding symptoms that may accompany defecation; dietary assessment, including changes in

nutritional, fiber, and fluid intake; current medications, including opioids, chemotherapy or radiation therapy, and change in medications; other symptoms such as distention, flatus, cramping, absence of bowel sounds, and rectal fullness; and a digital rectal examination that should always be done to rule out fecal impaction at the level of the rectum.

13. *Occult blood*: A test for occult blood to determine presence of a possible intraluminal lesion and a thorough examination of the gastrointestinal tract is necessary.

14. *GI function – stool impaction/obstruction*: Physical assessment will determine the presence or absence of bowel sounds, flatus, or abdominal distention. Patients with colostomies should also be assessed for constipation including monitoring of irrigation of the colostomy for proper technique. The follow-up physical exam may monitor for stool impaction (constipation with diarrhea with overflow around impaction) and obstruction (physical exam and X-ray).

10.5.5 Follow-up

Patients must be seen by the multidisciplinary team on a regularly scheduled basis to monitor progress and to review compliance to intervention including diet intake adequacy, symptom logs, change in concomitant medications, and any other issues related to treatment. Improved management of malnutrition with nutritional therapy may require a multimodal intervention by multidisciplinary teams using a comprehensive and integrated approach. If constipation is resolved, continue therapy. If constipation persists, reassess patient for etiology and severity of constipation and recheck for impaction and obstruction. Reassessment/reevaluation for monitoring and evaluation of nutritional therapy must include monitoring of clinical, functional, dietary, and behavioral outcomes that were identified by the comprehensive nutritional assessment

10.6   Future Directions

In spite of a large number of bulking, softening, and laxatives used to relieve constipation, a significant number of cancer patients still suffer from this side effect, some even reportedly reducing or abandoning their pain medications potentially sacrificing their anagogic to get relief of this symptom. The understanding of the pathophysiology of the effects of opioid therapy in the GI tract has provided the opportunity for newer targeted therapies addressing the underlying opioid receptor–mediated cause of bowel dysfunction for the management of opioid-induced bowel disorders, specifically constipation that does not respond nor is relieved by laxative therapy. Newer agents such as utilizing mu-opioid receptor antagonists have evolved to manage opioid-induced constipation. As treatment regimens continue to evolve, the adverse symptoms continue to become recognized. Future research should continue to evaluate these targeted therapies to alleviate these symptoms and improve quality of survival of this patient population.

Summary for the Clinician

Current management of cancer constipation includes a comprehensive assessment of the symptom and treatment based on the etiology of constipation. Assessment should record nature and frequency of bowel movements daily, in addition to straining, pain, and bleeding symptoms that may accompany defecation.

The primary approach to treat constipation includes bulk producers that are natural or semisynthetic polysaccharide and cellulose, laxatives (saline, stimulant, and lubricant), fecal softeners, lactulose (Cholac, Cephulac), polyethylene glycol and electrolytes (Golytely, Colyte), and opioid antagonists (naloxone, methylnaltrexone).

Since nausea, vomiting, and gastroesophageal reflux are also symptoms associated with opioid use, studies have examined the effect of antiemetics in relieving symptoms of constipation, although their utility in an OBD population has yet to be validated.

The treatment consists of basic measures and the application of laxatives using a laxative ladder for stepwise selection of choice of laxatives based on the etiology. It has also been suggested that clinicians should not base laxative prescribing on the opioid dose, but rather should titrate the laxative according to bowel function since lower doses of opioids or weaker opioids, such as codeine, are just as likely to cause constipation.

Although several nonpharmacological approaches are in use, pharmacological approaches with bulking agents, laxatives, antiemetics, stool softeners, and opioid receptor agonists are often necessary.

Nonpharmacological strategies for constipation in cancer patients include interventions such as increased dietary fiber, fluid intake, encouraging mobility and ambulation, and encouraging daily bowel movements at the same time every day.

The basic goal in the management of this symptoms is to establish the patient's normal bowel pattern and habits (time of day for normal bowel movement, consistency, color, and amount); explore the patient's level of understanding and compliance relating to exercise level, mobility, and diet (fluid, fruit, and fiber intake); determine normal or usual use of laxatives, stimulants, or enemas; determine laboratory values, specifically looking at platelet count; and conduct a physical assessment of the rectum (or stoma) to rule out impaction.

All assessment and reassessment should be conducted continuously taking into consideration change in medications and medical status of the cancer patient.

In spite of a large number of bulking, softening agents, and laxatives used to relieve constipation, a significant number of cancer patients still suffer from this side effect, some even reportedly reducing or abandoning their pain medications potentially sacrificing their anagogic to get relief of this symptom.

References

1. Mahan KL, Escott-Stump S (2000) Krause's food nutrition and diet therapy, 10th edn. W.B. Saunders Company, Philadelphia, pp 649–665
2. Longstreth GF (2006) Functional bowel disorders. Gastroenterology 130:1480–1491
3. Bell TJ, Panchal SJ, Miaskowski C, Bolge SC, Milanova T, Williamson R (2009) The prevalence, severity, and impact of opioid-induced bowel dysfunction: results of a US and European patient survey (PROBE 1). Pain Med 10(1):35–42, Epub 2008 Aug 18
4. Basson M (2007) Constipation. http://www.emedicine.com/med/topic2833.htm. Accessed March 2007
5. Pappagallo M (2001) Incidence, prevalence, and management of opioid bowel dysfunction. Am J Surg 182:11S–18S
6. Walsh TD (1990) Prevention of opioid side effects. J Pain Symptom Manage 5:362–367
7. Tuteja AK, Biskupiak J, Stoddard GJ, Lipman AG (2010) Opioid-induced bowel disorders and narcotic bowel syndrome in patients with chronic non-cancer pain. Neurogastroenterol Motil 22(4):424–430, e96. Epub 2010 Jan 21
8. Leppert W (2010) The role of opioid receptor antagonists in the treatment of opioid-induced constipation: a review. Adv Ther 27(10):714–730, Epub 2010 Aug 26
9. Thomas JR, Cooney GA, Slatkin NE (2008) Palliative care and pain: new strategies for managing opioid bowel dysfunction. J Palliat Med 11(1):S1–S19, quiz S21–2
10. Jamshed N, Lee ZE, Olden KW (2011) Diagnostic approach to chronic constipation in adults. Am Fam Physician 84(3):299–306
11. Rosti G, Gatti A, Costantini A, Sabato AF, Zucco F (2010) Opioid-related bowel dysfunction: prevalence and identification of predictive factors in a large sample of Italian patients on chronic treatment. Eur Rev Med Pharmacol Sci 14(12):1045–1050
12. Moore RA (2005) Prevalence of opioid adverse events in chronic non-malignant pain: systematic review of randomised trials of oral opioids. Arthritis Res Ther 7:R1046–R1051
13. Kalso E (2004) Opioids in chronic non-cancer pain: systematic review of efficacy and safety. Pain 112:372–380
14. Allan L et al (2001) Randomised crossover trial of transdermal fentanyl and sustained release oral morphine for treating chronic non-cancer pain. BMJ 322:1154–1158
15. Meuser T (2001) Symptoms during cancer pain treatment following WHO-guidelines: a longitudinal follow-up study of symptom prevalence, severity and etiology. J Pain 93:247–257
16. McMillan SC (2004) Assessing and managing opiate-induced constipation in adults with cancer. Cancer Control 11:3–9
17. Myotoku M, Nakanishi A, Kanematsu M, Sakaguchi N, Hashimoto N, Koyama F, Yamaguchi S, Ikeda K, Konishi H, Hirotani Y (2010) Reduction of opioid side effects by prophylactic measures of palliative care team may result in improved quality of life. J Palliat Med 13(4):401–406
18. Panchal SJ, Müller-Schwefe P, Wurzelmann JI (2007) Opioid-induced bowel dysfunction: prevalence, pathophysiology and burden. Int J Clin Pract 61(7):1181–1187
19. Klaschik E, Nauck F, Ostgathe C (2003) Constipation – modern laxative therapy. Support Care Cancer 11(11):679–685, Epub 2003 Sep 20
20. Gibson RJ, Keefe DM (2006) Cancer chemotherapy-induced diarrhoea and constipation: mechanisms of damage and prevention strategies. Support Care Cancer 14(9):890–900, Epub 2006 Apr 8
21. Walker LG, Eremin JM, Aloysius MM, Vassanasiri W, Walker MB, El-Sheemy M, Cowley G, Beer J, Samphao S, Wiseman J, Jibril JA, Valerio D, Clarke DJ, Kamal M, Thorpe GW, Baria K, Eremin O (2011) Effects on quality of life, anti-cancer responses, breast conserving surgery and survival with neoadjuvant docetaxel: a randomised study of sequential weekly versus three-weekly docetaxel following neoadjuvant doxorubicin and cyclophosphamide in women with primary breast cancer. BMC Cancer 11:179
22. Bennett M, Cresswell H (2003) Factors influencing constipation in advanced cancer patients: a prospective study of opioid dose, danthron dose and physical functioning. Palliat Med 17(5):418–422

23. Longstreth GF, Yao JF (2010) Diseases and drugs that increase risk of acute large bowel isch-emia. Clin Gastroenterol Hepatol 8(1):49–54, Epub 2009 Sep 16

24. Herndon CM (2002) Management of opioid-induced gastrointestinal effects in patients receiv-ing palliative care. Pharmacotherapy 22(2):240–250

25. Raynov J, Danon S, Valerianova Z (2002) Control of acute emesis in repeated courses of mod-erately emetogenic chemotherapy. J BUON 7(1):57–60

26. Wirz S, Wittmann M, Schenk M, Schroeck A, Schaefer N, Mueller M, Standop J, Kloecker N, Nadstawek J (2009) Gastrointestinal symptoms under opioid therapy: a prospective compari-son of oral sustained-release hydromorphone, transdermal fentanyl, and transdermal buprenor-phine. Eur J Pain 13(7):737–743, Epub 2008 Oct 31

27. Holzer P (2007) Treatment of opioid-induced gut dysfunction. Expert Opin Investig Drugs 16: 181–194

28. Sternini C (2004) The opioid system in the gastrointestinal tract. Neurogastroenterol Motil 16(Suppl 2):3–16

29. Mehendale SR (2006) Opioid-induced gastrointestinal dysfunction. Dig Dis 24:105–112

30. Sanger GJ (2004) The role of endogenous opioids in the control of gastrointestinal motility: predictions from in vitro modelling. Neurogastroenterol Motil 16(Suppl 2):38–45

31. De Schepper HU (2004) Opioids and the gut: pharmacology and current clinical experience. Neurogastroenterol Motil 16:383–394

32. Holzer P (2004) Opioids and opioid receptors in the enteric nervous system: from a problem in opioid analgesia to a possible new prokinetic therapy in humans. Neurosci Lett 361:192–195

33. Shook JE (1987) Peptide opioid antagonist separates peripheral and central opioid antitransit effects. J Pharmacol Exp Ther 243:492–500

34. De Luca A (1996) Insights into opioid action in the intestinal tract. Pharmacol Ther 69:103–115

35. Clemens KE, Mikus G (2010) Combined oral prolonged-release oxycodone and naloxone in opioid-induced bowel dysfunction: review of efficacy and safety data in the treatment of patients experiencing chronic pain. Expert Opin Pharmacother 11(2):297–310

36. Pettit M (2005) Treatment of gastroesophageal reflux disease. Pharm World Sci 27:432–435

37. Klepstad P (2000) Effects on cancer patients' health-related quality of life after the start of morphine therapy. J Pain Symptom Manage 20:19–26

38. Slappendel R (2006) Validation of the PAC-SYM questionnaire for opioid-induced constipa-tion in patients with chronic low back pain. Eur J Pain 10:209–217

39. Marquis P (2005) Development and validation of the patient assessment of constipation qual-ity of life questionnaire. Scand J Gastroenterol 40:540–551

40. Ueberall MA, Müller-Lissner S, Buschmann-Kramm C, Bosse B (2011) The bowel function index for evaluating constipation in pain patients: definition of a reference range for a non-constipated population of pain patients. J Int Med Res 39(1):41–50

41. Rentz AM, Yu R, Müller-Lissner S, Leyendecker P (2009) Validation of the bowel function index to detect clinically meaningful changes in opioid-induced constipation. J Med Econ 12(4):371–383

42. Downing GM, Kuziemsky C, Lesperance M, Lau F, Syme A (2007) Development and reli-ability testing of the Victoria bowel performance scale (BPS). J Pain Symptom Manage 34(5): 513–522, Epub 2007 Jul 30

43. Hawley P, Barwich D, Kirk L (2011) Implementation of the Victoria bowel performance scale. J Pain Symptom Manage 42(6):946–953

44. Belsey JD, Geraint M, Dixon TA (2010) Systematic review and meta analysis: polyethylene glycol in adults with non-organic constipation. Int J Clin Pract 64(7):944–955

45. Lee-Robichaud H, Thomas K, Morgan J, Nelson RL (2010) Lactulose versus polyethylene glycol for chronic constipation. Cochrane Database Syst Rev (7):CD007570

46. Chen CC, Su MY, Tung SY, Chang FY, Wong JM, Geraint M (2005) Evaluation of polyethyl-ene glycol plus electrolytes in the treatment of severe constipation and faecal impaction in adults. Curr Med Res Opin 21(10):1595–1602

47. van der Spoel JI, Oudemans-van Straaten HM, Kuiper MA, van Roon EN, Zandstra DF, van der Voort PH (2007) Laxation of critically ill patients with lactulose or polyethylene glycol: a two-center randomized, double-blind, placebo-controlled trial. Crit Care Med 35(12):2726–2731

48. Thomas J, Karver S, Cooney GA et al (2008) Methylnaltrexone for opioid-induced constipation in advanced illness. N Engl J Med 358(22):2332–2343
49. Portenoy RK, Thomas J, Moehl Boatwright ML et al (2008) Subcutaneous methylnaltrexone for the treatment of opioid-induced constipation in patients with advanced illness: a double-blind, randomized, parallel group, dose-ranging study. J Pain Symptom Manage 35(5):458–468
50. Meissner W, Leyendecker P, Mueller-Lissner S et al (2009) A randomised controlled trial with prolonged-release oral oxycodone and naloxone to prevent and reverse opioid-induced constipation. Eur J Pain 13(1):56–64
51. Garnock-Jones KP, McKeage K (2010) Methylnaltrexone. Drugs 70(7):919–928. doi:10.2165/11204520-000000000-00000
52. Chamberlain BH, Cross K, Winston JL, Thomas J, Wang W, Su C, Israel RJ (2009) Methylnaltrexone treatment of opioid-induced constipation in patients with advanced illness. J Pain Symptom Manage 38(5):683–690, Epub 2009 Aug 26
53. Candy B, Jones L, Goodman ML, Drake R, Tookman A (2011) Laxatives or methylnaltrexone for the management of constipation in palliative care patients. Cochrane Database Syst Rev (1):CD003448
54. Dando TM, Perry CM (2004) Aprepitant: a review of its use in the prevention of chemotherapy-induced nausea and vomiting. Drugs 64(7):777–794
55. Fang ZW, Zhai SD (2010) A meta-analysis of aprepitant for prevention of chemotherapy-induced nausea and vomiting. Beijing Da Xue Xue Bao 42(6):756–763
56. Wood JD (2004) Function of opioids in the enteric nervous system. Neurogastroenterol Motil 16(Suppl 2):17–28
57. Camilleri M (2005) Alvimopan, a selective peripherally acting mu-opioid antagonist. Neurogastroenterol Motil 17(2):157–165
58. Ebert EC (2010) The thyroid and the gut. J Clin Gastroenterol 44(6):402–406
59. Garratt AM, Ruta DA, Abdalla MI, Buckingham JK, Russell IT (1993) The SF36 health survey questionnaire: an outcome measure suitable for routine use within the NHS? BMJ 306(6890):1440–1444

Dysphagia

Core Messages

Dysphagia, derived from the Greek word "phagein," meaning "to eat," characterized by the multidimensional symptom complex including impairment of the swallowing mechanism, is a common symptom of several cancers, in addition to consequences of neuromuscular disorders.

In cancer patient populations, dysphagia is one of the most frequently occurring syndromes in oral, esopharyngeal, head and neck, and brain tumors or as a sequela of chemoradiation or surgery for these malignancies or generalized weakness due to nonuse or reduced use of muscles in the region.

Based on the origin of dysphagia, it is classified as oropharyngeal or esophageal. Oropharyngeal dysphagia is difficulty emptying material from the oropharynx into the esophagus; it results from abnormal function proximal to the esophagus. Patients complain of difficulty initiating swallowing, nasal regurgitation, and tracheal aspiration followed by coughing. Esophageal dysphagia is characterized by difficulty passing food down the esophagus. It results from either a motility disorder or a mechanical obstruction.

Dysphagia may be attributed to tumor location and size and the extent of penetration to adjoining tissue. On the other hand, the magnitude of treatment-related effects is dependent on the extent of insult and the capacity of the patient to compensate.

Prolonged dysphagia often leads to inadequate and compromised nutritional intake and can lead to malnutrition, weight loss, and exacerbating medical condition and treatment outcomes. Swallowing difficulties negatively impact quality of life functioning.

Dysphagia, when unidentified and not treated, can lead to tracheal aspiration of ingested material, oral secretions, or both. Aspiration can cause acute pneumonia; recurrent aspiration may eventually lead to chronic lung disease.

Once etiology of dysphagia is identified and if dysphagia is due to location and size of tumor, initial treatment strategies include surgical and mechanical interventions to restore the esophageal lumen, antineoplastic treatments

N.B. Kumar, *Nutritional Management of Cancer Treatment Effects*,
DOI 10.1007/978-3-642-27233-2_11, © Springer-Verlag Berlin Heidelberg 2012

including preoperative chemotherapy for organ preservation, and intensity-modulated radiotherapy aimed at reducing organ damage.

Current strategies for management of symptoms of dysphagia also include the introduction of compensatory strategies and direct therapy techniques. Compensatory strategies include postural changes, sensory enhancements, changing feeding strategies, and diet changes. Therapy procedures include exercise programs and swallowing maneuvers that have been implemented to facilitate the physiology of swallowing.

11.1   Definition/Description

Dysphagia, derived from the Greek word "phagein," meaning "to eat," characterized by the multidimensional symptom complex including impairment of the swallowing mechanism, is a common symptom of several cancers, in addition to consequences of neuromuscular disorders. The intricate mechanism of swallowing can be divided into three phases and involves over 50 muscles and nerves: (a) oral phase (voluntary) where food is chewed, masticated, moistened by saliva, and pushed to the pharynx; (b) pharyngeal phase (beginning of swallowing reflex); and (c) esophageal phase. Dysphagia is a disruption in the swallowing process, which includes difficulty in transporting (or a lack of transporting) a food or liquid bolus from the mouth through the pharynx and esophagus into the stomach [1–5]. Dysphagia is a condition resulting in a disturbance in the normal transfer of food from the oral cavity to the stomach. Symptoms include difficulty in swallowing resulting from the abnormalities in any one of the normal phases of swallowing. Dysphagia should not be confused with globus sensation, a feeling of having a lump in the throat, which is unrelated to swallowing and occurs without impaired transport [6]. Dysphagia, when unidentified and treated, can lead to tracheal aspiration of ingested material, oral secretions, or both. Aspiration can cause acute pneumonia; recurrent aspiration may eventually lead to chronic lung disease. Since depressed cough reflex is one of the features of dysphagia, clinical manifestations of aspiration may be unreliable and insidious [7, 8]. Prolonged dysphagia often leads to inadequate and compromised nutritional intake and can lead to malnutrition, weight loss, and exacerbating medical condition and treatment outcomes [1–5, 7, 8].

Based on the origin of dysphagia, it is classified as oropharyngeal or esophageal (Fig. 11.1). The oropharyngeal swallow involves a rapid, highly coordinated set of neuromuscular actions beginning with lip closure and terminating with opening of the upper esophageal sphincter [9]. Oropharyngeal dysphagia is difficulty emptying material from the oropharynx into the esophagus; it results from abnormal function proximal to the esophagus. Patients complain of difficulty initiating swallowing, nasal regurgitation, and tracheal aspiration followed by coughing. Esophageal dysphagia is characterized by difficulty passing food down the esophagus. It results from either a motility disorder or a mechanical obstruction [1, 6, 10]. Swallowing

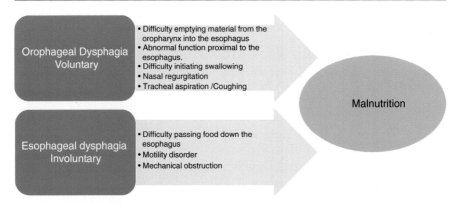

Fig. 11.1 Classification of dysphagia

difficulties negatively impact quality of life functioning [11]. Impaired swallowing can cause significant morbidity and mortality [12].

11.2 Prevalence

The exact prevalence of dysphagia is unknown, especially in cancer patient populations where it is predominantly underdiagnosed. Dysphagia may be attributed to tumor location and size and the extent of penetration to adjoining tissue [13]. On the other hand, the magnitude of treatment-related effects is dependent on the extent of insult and the capacity of the patient to compensate [1]. In cancer patient populations, dysphagia is one of the most frequently occurring syndrome in oral, esopharyngeal, head and neck, and brain tumors [13–15] or as a consequence of chemoradiation or surgery for these malignancies [16–19] or generalized weakness due to nonuse or reduced use of muscles in the region [20, 21]. Impairment of swallowing function is a common multidimensional symptom complex seen in 50–75% of head and neck cancer (HNC) survivors [22]. The prevalence of dysphagia markedly increases with age and presents particular problems in this older cancer patient population [23–26] potentially compromising nutritional status, increasing the risk of aspiration pneumonia, and undermining the quality of life. Oropharyngeal dysphagia was present in 50.6% of patients, mostly to solid foods (72.4%). Silent aspiration of thin fluids is common in patients with nasopharyngeal cancers post radiation therapy [27]. Patients with total glossectomy and chemoradiotherapy had the highest rate of dysphagia [25]. Other tumors that affect swallowing are usually located in the skull base or brainstem such as brainstem glioma, brainstem metastasis, ependymoma, choroid plexus, papilloma, large pineal region tumors, and neoplasms of the cerebellopontine angle [28]. Depending on their location, benign or malignant tumors may cause oral or pharyngeal dysphagia [13]. In other cases, there may be only temporary discomfort due to pain and swelling. Dysphagia is also a common, debilitating, and potentially life-threatening sequela of concurrent chemoradiation for head and neck malignancy. Approximately ten million Americans are evaluated each year with swallowing difficulties [6] for cancer and other etiologies.

11.3   Etiology

In cancer patient populations, dysphagia commonly occurs in oral, esopharyngeal, head and neck, brain, and in some lung malignancies, when the esophagus is involved (Table 11.1).

11.3.1 Tumor Location–Related Effects

The neuroanatomical etiology of dysphagia in patients with brain tumors is probably attributable to reduced awareness of oral sensory feedback cues due to mastication, contralateral weakness of the face and tongue, and oral apraxia with impaired motor programming ability for oral lingual feeding [28]. Direct tumor compression causes impairment of the brainstem circuitry that underlies swallowing. Newton et al. [13] observed that many brain tumor patients lose the neurological feedback needed to cough or to swallow properly. They may have lost sensation in the mouth or throat, or they may have a reduced level of consciousness, or they may have lost the coordination to chew and swallow properly. Although these patients may not be identified by self or by clinical observations to be dysphagic, they may be at highest risk for aspiration. On the other hand, patients who developed swallowing difficulties following surgery may experience transient dysphagia related to swelling of the brain postsurgery and experience only mild problems, and showed significant improvement with time. These patients tended to have tumors that occurred external to the brain [13, 28].

Tumors of the oral cavity, on the other hand, include those of the anterior tongue, buccal mucosa, alveolar ridge, and anterior palate, and treatment of oral carcinomas can often restore structure and function and may not have a significant long-term impact on dysphagia, since this portion that encompasses the first stage of swallow is primarily voluntary and is associated mostly with bolus manipulation and mastication. In addition, with the advent of laser surgical techniques, with the exception of reduced tongue range of motion, it is estimated that [29] 92% of patients were able to return to normal diets after transoral laser excision of tongue base tumors. Surgical resection can have devastating effects on swallowing for those patients requiring total glossectomy and if resection extends beyond the tongue to laryngeal or pharyngeal structures or replacement with placement of a flap, where tissues are adynamic and at least initially insensate [1].

Oropharynx, on the other hand, which includes the tongue base, tonsillar fossas, and posterior pharyngeal wall is involuntary, and dysphagia attributed to deficits in the oropharyngeal swallow is much more complex, as sensory and motor deficits lead to significant limitations in bolus pressure and propulsion. In head and neck cancer patients, dysphagia may be caused by surgical ablation of muscular [30], bony, cartilaginous, or nervous structures where tumor may be located and is attributed to the combination of disrupted normal anatomy secondary to mass effect, nerve involvement, soft tissue tethering, or tumor-induced pain. The majority of head and neck malignancies are mucosally based and are squamous cell carcino-

Table 11.1 Etiology of dysphagia

Tumor-related	Treatment-related factors contributing to dysphagia	Lifestyle
Brain tumors/skull or brain stem	*Surgery*	History of heavy alcohol consumption
Brainstem glioma	Loss or part removal of organ	
Brainstem metastasis	Total glossectomy	
Ependymoma	Edema of the brain following surgery	
Choroid plexus	Base of tongue surgery	
Papilloma	Permanent placement of flap-adynamic tissue/insensate	
Large pineal region tumors	Odynophagia (pain) during mastication and swallowing	
Neoplasms of the cerebellopontine angle	Bleeding	
	Dry mouth	
Oral cavity	*Chemotherapy and other drugs*	
Anterior tongue	Antimetabolites	
Buccal mucosa	Radiosensitive chemotherapy regimens	
Alveolar ridge	Antineoplastic agents	
Anterior palette	Agents to treat insomnia	
	Agents to treat epilepsy	
	Steroid therapies	
Oropharynx	*Radiation therapy/chemoradiation therapies*	
Tongue base	Significant soft-tissue fibrosis	
Tonsillar fossas	Mucosal scarring	
Posterior pharyngeal wall	Xerostomia	
Pharyngeal esophageal	Edema	
	Reduced muscle size	
	Reduced salivary flow	
	Longer oral transit times	
	Increased pharyngeal residue	
	Reduced circopharyngeal opening times	
	Reduced glottic closure	
	Pharyngoesophageal spasms	
	Impaired taste	
	Impaired smell	
	Trismus	
	Tooth decay	
	Tissue stiffness	
	Tissue damage from radiation	
	Epiglottic dysmotility	
	Vallecular residue	
	Laryngeal penetration or aspiration	

(continued)

Table 11.1 (continued)

Tumor-related	Treatment-related factors contributing to dysphagia	Lifestyle
Head and neck	*General weakness and pain*	
Muscular	Odonophagia	
Bone	Contralateral weakness of face and tongue	
Cartiliginous	Reduced or nonuse	
Neural structures	Reduced awareness	
Penetration to lymph nodes	Impaired motor programming	
Others	*Infection/inflammation*	
Elderly cancer patient population	Candidiasis	
	Graft-versus-host disease	

mas. These lesions can be exophytic or infiltrative in nature and often metastasize to cervical lymph nodes requiring treatment of not only the primary location but also draining lymphatics [30].

11.3.2 Chemotherapy-Related Effects

The severity and persistence of swallowing deficits after treatment are related to the size and location of tumor, magnitude of surgical intervention or soft tissue, tumor response to nonsurgical therapies such as radiation and chemotherapy [1], and the nature of reconstruction. Chemotherapy-related side effects such as mucositis resulting in odynophagia (pain) during mastication and swallowing and bleeding, dry mouth, skin damage from radiation, infections, and graft-versus-host disease may all contribute to dysphagia. The cytotoxic agents most commonly associated with oral, pharyngeal, and esophageal symptoms of dysphagia are the antimetabolites such as methotrexate and fluorouracil. The radiosensitizer chemotherapies, designed to heighten the effects of radiation therapy, also heighten the side effects of the radiation mucositis [31, 32]. Additionally, similar to the effect of neuromuscular disorder, generalized weakness due to nonuse or reduced use of muscles in the region [20, 21] has received attention in patients with dysphagia. Dysphagia can also be triggered by antiepileptic agents as well those used to treat insomnia. Dysphagia can also be attributed to inflammatory causes such as candidiasis of the oral mucosa, caused by inflammation and irritants such as radiation therapy or chemotherapy, or steroid therapy.

11.3.3 Radiation and Chemoradiation Therapy–Related Effects

Dysphagia can be more protracted and severe as a sequel of nonsurgical therapies such as chemoradiation for these malignancies [17–19]. External-beam radiation has both early and late side effects producing significant soft tissue fibrosis, mucosal scaring, and xerostomia that can impact swallowing function. The effects of postoperative radiation have been observed to significantly reduce oral and pharyngeal functions including longer oral transit times, increased pharyngeal residue, and reduced cricopharyngeal opening times. Impaired function has also been attributed to radiation effects such as edema and reduced salivary flow. Swallowing function continues to deteriorate over time, even many years after radiation therapy in patients with nasopharyngeal carcinoma. The late effect of reduced blood supply to the muscle can result in fibrosis and reduced muscle size and dramatically affect swallowing years after treatment with a fixation of the hyolaryngeal complex, reduced glottic closure, and cricopharyngeal relaxation, resulting in potential for aspiration [30]. Dysphagia disorders in patients with cancer of the oropharynx are significantly affected by the radiation therapy dose to the superior and middle constrictor muscle [33]. A steep dose-effect relationship, with an increase of the probability of dysphagia of 19% with every additional 10 Gy, was observed [33]. The severity of swallowing problems may vary depending on the type of surgery and whether one has undergone radiation or chemotherapy treatments. In subjects undergoing high-dose chemoradiotherapy for head and neck cancers reported more severe dysphagia than those who received radiation treatment alone, with lasting effects of dysphagia reported well into 1 year posttreatment [19]. Similarly, the degree of dysphagia postlaryngectomy and post-radiation therapy decreased over 3 years in 50% of the patients, with the remaining patients continuing to experience pharyngoesophageal spasms [34]. Swallowing function was of high priority in this patient population [19]. Although combined treatments improved tumor control [34–37], the long-term sequelae of radiotherapy can include loss of energy, pain, xerostomia, impaired taste, impaired smell, trismus, tooth decay, tissue stiffness, edema, and impairments in speech, voice, and swallowing with poor response to convention treatments for dysphagia [37, 38]. Evaluated patients were treated with radiation therapy for nasopharyngeal cancer, and over 90% were found to have a definable abnormality on endoscopic swallowing examination. Several fluoroscopy studies showed *all* movements comprising the swallow were impaired [39] with the location of the tumor having very little effect on the severity of dysphagia. Pharyngeal transport dysfunction and anterior segment abnormalities manifested by epiglottic dysmotility, vallecular residue, laryngeal penetration, or aspiration were all common after aggressive concomitant chemotherapy and radiation therapy in head and neck cancer patients [40]. In examining impact of demographics, tumor characteristics, and treatment factors on swallowing disorder in patients treated with radiation therapy or chemoradiation therapy for head and neck cancers, Frowen et al. [41] observed that swallowing was best at baseline, significantly worse at 3 months, and improving at 6 months posttreatment. They observed that worse dysphagia was associated with living in rural areas, history of heavy alcohol consumption, bilateral radiation to the oropharnx, hypopharyngeal tumor site, large particularly T4 tumors, nonconformal radiotherapy, bilateral radiation to the pharynx, and longer radiotherapy fields. More recently, strategies to include preoperative chemotherapy for organ preservation [42, 43] and intensity-modulated radiotherapy aimed at reducing organ damage [43, 44] have demonstrated relatively better improvement in the symptoms of dysphagia in esophageal and head and neck cancer patient populations. A disadvantage of preoperative chemotherapy is in the delay to potentially control disease treatment outcome using chemoradiation therapy).

11.4   Current Treatment Strategies for Dysphagia

Since dysphagia can result from tumor, psychosocial, and treatment-related factors or can be attributed to a multifactorial etiology, multimodal management of dysphagia by multidisciplinary teams is ideal, targeting the specific etiology of dysphagia. The basic approach to managing patients with dysphagia is to prevent dehydration and malnutrition and to avoid aspiration and related complications such as pneumonia. Most recommendations for diagnosis and management of swallowing dysfunction requires timely and careful screening using detailed history and clinical examination by integrated, multidisciplinary teams consisting of treating oncologists (surgeons, radiation oncologists, medical oncologists), dentists, speech pathologist, clinical pharmacist, psychosocial worker, physical therapist, radiologist, and dietitian for comprehensive symptom assessment, established nutritional guidelines, pharmacotherapy, psychosocial intervention, and physical activity, in addition to monitoring and closely assessing patients for change in status. Treatment strategies can include surgical interventions, chemotherapy, radiation therapy, chemoradiation therapies as well as introduction of compensatory strategies and direct therapy techniques. Compensatory strategies include postural changes, sensory enhancements, changing feeding strategies, and diet changes. Therapy procedures include exercise programs and swallowing maneuvers that have been implemented to facilitate the physiology of swallowing.

11.4.1 Screening and Initial Assessment

Several validated screening tools have been used to evaluate the nature and extent of dysphagia thoroughly, with much of the validation studies coming from the stroke literature. (Swallowing Disturbance Questionnaire (SDQ) [45] and The Acute Stroke Dysphagia Screen) [46]. In essence, elements of a thorough clinical swallow assessment include a detailed history of subjective complaints and medical status, pertinent clinical observations, and a physical examination by the medical team. Although several clinical bedside swallowing assessments have been suggested, videofluoroscopic swallowing studies are the gold standard for characterizing the specific swallowing abnormalities. This is performed in the radiology department by a radiologist and speech pathologist. This technique not only allows estimation of risks of aspiration and respiratory complications but also helps in determining dietary and compensatory strategies and valuable in identifying the clinical or instrumental assessment of swallowing function and makes recommendations for therapeutic intervention, including ascertaining the need for nonoral nutrition [47].

Although several protocols for performing videofluoroscopic swallowing studies exist in various institutions, the principles are focused on oropharyngeal swallow physiology assessment with an ultimate goal to identify possible management of pathophysiologies. Swallowing trials are initiated with a range of food textures, with the order of bolus presentation or modifications to the procedures based on individual patient performance, aspiration risks, abnormalities identified, and patient tolerance [30, 47]. Benefits include the ability to view the complex interaction of the phases of swallowing, describe the anatomy changes and dynamics of the swallow, identify the etiology of aspiration, and assess the benefit of treatment strategies during the study. Evaluation of the oropharyngeal swallow usually involves the use of a modified barium swallow radiographic study with the goals of (a) defining the patient's swallow anatomy and physiology causing the dysphagia and (b) evaluating the immediate effectiveness of treatment procedures including compensatory strategies and direct therapy techniques.

More recently, fiberoptic endoscopic evaluation of swallowing (FEES) has been used as the state-of-the-art nonradioactive alternative to modified barium swallow studies. Flexible laryngoscopy reveals some unique aspects of swallowing and complements the fluoroscopy procedure. This exam allows for direct assessment of the motor and sensory aspects of the swallow in order to precisely guide the dietary and behavioral management of patients with swallowing problems to decrease the risk of aspiration pneumonia. Velopharyngeal closure, anatomy of the base of the tongue and hypopharynx, abduction and adduction of the vocal folds, pharyngeal musculature, and the patient's ability to manage his/her own secretions are assessed. Laryngopharyngeal reflux (LPR) can also be visualized. It consists of passing a thin, flexible endoscope into the pharynx and observing the act of swallowing. It provides excellent visualization of postsurgical or aching maneuvers that may facilitate swallowing and prevent aspiration in a patient. It can also be used as biofeedback to retrain swallowing function. FEES is a safe, valid, and reliable procedure that can be used in patient populations, including cancer patient populations [20]. Scintigraphy, manofluorography, and ultrasound have all been used as methods of assessment. However, they are generally used as an adjunct to modified barium swallow or FEES rather than alternative associated treatments [47, 48]. Future studies should examine whether routine posttherapy videofluoroscopy or FEES and/or training aspirating patients in safe swallowing strategies can better diagnose and allow for interventions targeting the etiology of dysphagia, avoiding compromise of nutrition status and hydration, and preventing aspiration-related complications.

Once etiology of dysphagia is identified and if dysphagia is due to location and size of tumor, initial treatment strategies include surgical and mechanical interventions to restore the esophageal lumen [44, 49], antineoplastic treatments including preoperative chemotherapy for organ preservation [42, 43], and intensity-modulated radiotherapy aimed at reducing organ damage [43, 44]. These strategies have demonstrated relatively better improvement in the symptoms of dysphagia in esophageal and head and neck cancer patient populations. A disadvantage of preoperative chemotherapy is in the delay to potentially control disease treatment outcome using chemoradiation therapy. In patients with early squamous cell carcinoma of the esophagus, growing evidence suggests that esophageal stricture often develops after endoscopic submucosal dissection requiring multiple dilations and risk for perforation [50]. Medications and surgery have a very limited role in the treatment of oropharyngeal dysphagia [9].

In esophageal cancer patients, self-expanding metal stent insertion has been observed to be safe, effective, and quicker in palliating dysphagia compared to other modalities [49, 51]. This modality was observed to be effective specifically in the palliation of dysphagia in selected patients with malignant esophageal strictures [49, 51]. However, high-dose intraluminal brachytherapy may be a suitable alternative and might provide additional survival benefit with a better quality of life [18, 51]. Self-expanding metal stent insertion and brachytherapy provide comparable palliation to endoscopic ablative therapy but are preferable due to the reduced requirement for reinterventions [10, 49, 51]. Rigid plastic tube insertion, dilatation alone or in combination with other modalities, chemotherapy alone, combination chemoradiotherapy, laser, photodynamic therapy, and bypass surgery are not recommended for palliation of dysphagia due to a high incidence of delayed complications and recurrent dysphagia [10, 49, 51]. In patients with inoperable esophageal cancer, palliative combination treatment of dysphagia with argon plasma coagulation (APC) and high-dose-rate brachytherapy was more efficient and well tolerated than APC alone resulting in fewer complications and better quality of life [18]. Based on these limitations and in addition to these management modalities, several behavioral management of swallowing disorders including the introduction of compensatory strategies and direct therapy techniques have been evaluated. Compensatory strategies include postural changes, sensory enhancements, changing feeding strategies, and diet changes. Therapy procedures include exercise programs and swallowing maneuvers that have been implemented to facilitate the physiology of swallowing.

11.4.2 Nutritional Interventions

Adjunct to surgical intervention, direct nutritional therapy to prevent and treat malnutrition, aspiration and consequences of aspiration, and introduction of compensatory strategies such as sensory enhancement, postural changes, and changing feeding strategies form the basis of nutritional interventions to facilitate the physiology of swallowing. In patients with dysphagia, (a) where oral intake is contraindicated and for many patients where (b) oral intake will only continue to present a challenge to provide adequate nutrition during treatment with radiotherapy or chemoradiation due to toxicity of treatment or (c) obstruction caused by tumor or treatment and (d) when it is anticipated that oral intake will only deteriorate in the next 7 days and not improve, alternate routes of feeding has been a rational approach to meet nutritional needs. In a recent review [52] of research using the Cochrane database, Nugent et al. [52] compared the effectiveness of different enteral feeding methods (nasogastric vs. percutaneous endoscopic gastrostomy) used in the treatment of patients with head and neck cancers receiving radiotherapy and chemoradiation using clinical outcomes, nutritional status, quality of life, and rates of complications. They observed that there was no sufficient evidence to determine the optimal method of enteral feeding for this patient population, and more studies are needed with larger sample sizes. Similarly, Logemann et al. observed that there is little evidence regarding specific criteria or guidelines that clinicians can use to determine route of feeding of patients with dysphagia, such as oral or nonoral in patients with oropharyngeal dysphagia [53]. In a study of a group of experienced clinicians treating oropharyngeal cancers on an average of 14 years, criteria that were considered critical to determine route of nutritional intervention were (a) amount of aspiration, (b) acuity of medical condition, (c) history of pneumonia, (d) alertness, (e) cough ability, (f) frequency of aspiration, (g) respiratory status, (g) patient wishes, (h)secretion management, (i) silent aspiration, (j) recovery prognosis, (k) ability to complete postures/maneuvers, and (l) diagnosis [53]. Given this criteria, clinicians used aspiration and medical diagnosis as the most important criteria for selecting feeding route. However, there was still no consensus among this group in determining if they would recommend oral, partial, or no oral feeing for the patient, establishing a need for systematic research, education, and training of clinicians. Langmore et al. [20] observed that dependence on PEG may lead to adverse swallowing ability in postirradiated head and neck cancer patients, potentially due to decreased use of swallowing musculature. Oral chemesthesis is the detection of chemicals that activate temperature and pain receptors in the oral mucosa and influence greater neuromotor activity during the oral phase of swallowing. Thus, presentation of orally chemesthetic liquids has been observed to stimulate a faster, stronger swallow compared to water. Patients with pharyngeal delay have demonstrated some tolerance to carbonated beverages like ginger ale and club soda, supporting the hypothesis that oropharyngeal swallowing can be modulated in response to sensory stimuli [54, 55].

11.4.3 Physical Therapy

The tongue is critical in the swallowing mechanism, playing the role in bolus propulsion through the oral cavity. Thus, any lingual impairment after surgery, chemotherapy, or radiation for head and neck cancers can impair overall oropharyngeal swallow with significant reduction in lingual strength. Lazarus et al. [56] observed that mean maximum tongue strength dropped a nonsignificant amount immediately after treatment, and then increased significantly at 6 and 12 months post treatment completion. Studies have also reported that contralateral weakness of face and tongue, reduced or nonuse of these muscles due to odynophagia, reduced awareness, and impaired motor programming in patients with head and neck and oropharyngeal cancers may also contribute to dysphagia or exacerbation of these symptoms [20, 21]. Adjunct to nutritional interventions, based on the stage of swallowing affected, rehabilitative techniques such as swallow maneuvers (supraglottic swallow; effortful swallow), exercises (to increase strength of muscle groups), and sensory stimulation techniques (thermal-tactile stimulation; low-level electrical stimulation) have been found effective [20, 53] in improving dysphagia. A wide range of postures and maneuvers were recommended as critical by a group of experienced clinicians in a pilot study [53] including effortful swallow, head turn, chin tuck, super supraglottic swallow, supraglottic swallow, and repeat swallow for managing oropharyngeal dysphagia [53]. Preoperative education and training, using swallowing exercises [21, 30], have been found to improve quality of life as well as symptoms related to dysphagia [53]. If weakness of muscles due to treatment is anticipated, exercises to strengthen the jaw and tongue such as jaw range of motion, tongue base range of motion exercises, and effortful swallow exercises, tongue holding maneuver, Mendelsohn maneuver, and super supraglottic swallow [21, 30] have been helpful to patients. Postural behavior modification, instructing patients to always sit up straight while eating and drinking, not to lie down after a meal nor recline, not to go to bed only after 3 h after a meal, and to stand up if food gets stuck and stretch the upper body and walk around have also been found to reduce symptoms of dysphagia. Exercise programs may be helpful, but their immediate effects cannot be examined during the initial evaluation and may have to be evaluated periodically [9, 30, 53] and modified in oropharyngeal cancer patients.

11.4.4 Pharmacotherapies

Palliative chemoradiotherapy has been observed to be effective in stage IVB esophageal cancer postesophagectomy, reporting an improvement in dysphagia in over 72% of patients, with acceptable toxicity and favorable survival [57, 58]. Antineoplastic treatments including preoperative chemotherapy for organ preservation have been observed to prevent or reduce dysphagia [42, 43]. Dysphagia can also be triggered by antiepileptic agents as well those used to treat insomnia. Dysphagia can also be attributed to inflammatory causes such as candidiasis of the oral mucosa, caused by inflammation and irritants such as radiation therapy or chemotherapy or for those patients on steroid therapy. However, there is insufficient evidence to claim or refute a benefit for any antifungal agent in treating candidiasis [59]. Further well-designed, placebo-controlled trials assessing the effectiveness of old and new interventions for treating oral candidiasis are needed to inform clinical practice targeting patients receiving treatment for cancer. Since oral pain (odynophagia) is a classic symptom accompanying dysphagia, systemic analgesics like opiates must be considered via the transdermal route. Since dehydration is also common in this patient population, IV or subcutaneous fluid replacements are critical to maintain hydration, especially in the absence of poor tolerance to liquids.

11.5   Guidelines

The following guidelines are considered best practice standards based on available review of the current research literature. Due to the multifactorial etiology of dysphagia, there is no single standard of therapy established to treat the symptoms of dysphagia in cancer patients. Diagnosis and management of swallowing dysfunction requires timely and careful screening using detailed history and clinical examination by integrated, multidisciplinary teams consisting of treating oncologists (surgeons, radiation oncologists, medical oncologists), dentists, speech pathologist, clinical pharmacist, psychosocial worker, physical therapist, radiologist, and dietitian for comprehensive symptom assessment, established nutritional guidelines, pharmacotherapy, psychosocial intervention and physical activity, in addition to monitoring and closely assessing patients for change in status. In addition to mechanical interventions to restore the esophageal lumen [44, 49] and antineoplastic treatments if applicable, several supportive and behavioral interventions have been implemented to facilitate the physiology of swallowing. Some of the basic principles to managing patients with dysphagia are to prevent dehydration and malnutrition and to avoid aspiration and related complications such as pneumonia. Treatment plan must be targeted to the specific etiology of dysphagia. In addition, the intervention must be proactive and based on ongoing evaluations to monitor patient's change in status based on disease stage, response to treatment, and treatment outcomes as well as use of concomitant medications.

11.5.1 Nutrition Guidelines

Nutritional screening must be performed within 24 h of admission of the patient by a registered dietitian/nutritionist:

1. Screen patient within 24 h of admission. This order for screening has been a standard order for all cancer patient admissions to avoid delay in timing of screening.
2. Assess all symptoms. Gastrointestinal tract: taste alterations, smell alterations, dysphagia, dyspnea, other pain, early satiety, dry mouth, too much saliva production, anorexia, diarrhea, constipation, nausea, vomiting, dehydration, fatigue, height, weight, recent weight loss, anthropometrics, and others (mid-arm muscle circumference, body composition [DEXA], grip strength); psychosocial: family/caregiver support, depression, and ADL.
3. Assess current nutritional status and estimate caloric, protein, and multivitamin/mineral needs.
4. If dysphagia is identified or suspected based on bedside observation or as reported by family, patient, or other members of the medical team, refer patient to speech pathologist for more thorough evaluation prior to starting to feed patient.
5. It is critical to obtain a baseline evaluation of any swallowing abnormality in the patient prior to the start of any treatment for cancer using a validated tool to obtain this information (Swallowing Disturbance Questionnaire (SDQ) [45] and The Acute Stroke Dysphagia Screen) [46]. In essence, a thorough clinical swallow assessment includes a detailed history of subjective complaints and medical status, pertinent clinical observations, and a physical examination by the medical team. Once dysphagia is identified, all oral nutrition interventions must be held until swallowing studies have been completed and the recommendations are obtained from the speech pathologist/radiologist team.

11.5.2 Speech Pathologist/Radiologist

Although several clinical bedside swallowing assessments have been suggested, videofluoroscopic swallowing study is the gold standard for characterizing the specific swallowing abnormalities. This is performed in the radiology department by a radiologist and speech pathologist. This technique not only allows estimation of risks of aspiration and respiratory complications but also helps in determining dietary and compensatory strategies and valuable in identifying the clinical or instrumental assessment of swallowing function and makes recommendations for therapeutic intervention, including ascertaining the need for nonoral nutrition [47]. Fiberoptic endoscopic evaluation of swallowing (FEES) has been used as the state-of-the-art nonradioactive alternative to modified barium swallow studies. Flexible laryngoscopy reveals some unique aspects of swallowing and complements the fluoroscopy procedure. This exam allows for direct assessment of the motor and sensory aspects of the swallow in order to precisely guide the dietary and behavioral management of patients with swallowing problems to decrease the risk of aspiration pneumonia. Velopharyngeal closure, anatomy of the base of the tongue and hypopharynx, abduction and adduction of the vocal folds, pharyngeal musculature, and the patient's ability to manage his/her own secretions are assessed. Laryngopharyngeal reflux (LPR) can also be visualized. It consists of passing a thin, flexible endoscope into the pharynx and observing the act of swallowing. It provides excellent visualization of postsurgical or aching maneuvers that may facilitate swallowing and prevent aspiration in a patient. It can also be used as biofeedback to retrain swallowing function. FEES is a safe, valid, and reliable procedure that can be used in patient populations, including cancer patient populations [20]. Scintigraphy, manofluorography, and ultrasound have all been used as methods of assessment. However, they are generally used as an adjunct to modified barium swallow or FEES rather than alternative associated treatments [47, 48]. These evaluations allow the speech pathologist and radiologist to diagnose and allow for interventions targeting the etiology of dysphagia, avoiding compromise of nutrition status and hydration, and preventing aspiration-related complications.

11.5.3 Nutrition Intervention

Based on the results of the swallowing assessment and recommendations, nutritional intervention must be planned accordingly. It is important to schedule a series of evaluation of swallowing and specifically the stage of swallowing that may be impaired posttreatment.

Based on the stage of swallowing affected, nutritional guidelines can be adopted to guide intervention by using compensatory techniques such as by modifying bolus volume, consistency, and viscosity; changing method of food/liquid delivery; modifying sequence of delivery, changing rate of food/liquid delivery; and altering patient behaviors such as dry/clearing swallows and postural changes.

Proactive measures to provide alternate mode of nutritional support must be planned during the acute phase of treatment when it would be a greater risk to feed patient via the oral route. Selection of route of feeding may be informed based on general guidelines and criteria provided in Table 2.6.

11.5.3.1 General Principles for Nutritional Intake Adequacy

1. Screen and assess current nutritional status and estimate caloric, protein, and multivitamin/mineral needs (refer to Chap. 2).
2. Provide adequate nutrition by including "calorie" and "protein" boosters education material and nutritional supplements to ensure intake of proteins (recommended 0.8 g–1.0 g/kg/day). Provide dense caloric supplements up to 400 cal/day containing 1.5 kcal/mL; if intake is insufficient in proteins, supplement with modular protein supplements, adding this to favorite beverage (http://www.nestlenutrition.com/Products/Default.aspx; http://abbottnutrition.com/). The choice of nutritional supplements can be based on the personal choice of the patient, patient needs, tolerance to product, as well as other comorbidities.
3. Include a standard multivitamin/mineral supplementation to prevent any further deficits and meet increased needs.
4. Assess adequacy of intake and provide an appetite stimulant (megestrol acetate 20 mg–800 mg/day or alternate) if patient has cancer anorexia to ensure adequate intake and prevent further weight loss.
5. Provide each patient with nutritional guidelines to ensure adequate intake of calories and proteins and a list of suggested high-caloric and high-protein nutritional supplements to choose from, taking into consideration taste alterations, early satiety, nausea, and vomiting that are common symptoms observed in this patient population.
6. If chemoradiation is considered as treatment plan and if symptoms of dysphagia are anticipated to be protracted, feedings via percutaneous gastrostomy or TPN may be planned during the acute treatment phase and thereafter until symptoms of dysphagia no longer limits oral feedings.
7. However, in patients not receiving curative antineoplastic therapy, with end-stage disease, nutritional intervention must be based on informed decision made by the patient and family. Patients may view nutritional support as a palliative measure, as hydration support, or as a means of delivering necessary medications. Patients and family must be educated about anticipated consequences of not receiving hydration or nutrition as well as risks involved in administering support.
8. If patients decide to not go through PEG or other tube or IV nutrition, they must be allowed to eat for enjoyment, as tolerated.
9. Introduce compensatory strategies such as postural changes, sensory enhancements, changing feeding strategies, and diet changes.

11.5.3.2 Specific Recommendations Based on Capacity to Swallow

If the condition is a slow/weak uncoordinated swallow:
- Include highly seasoned, flavorful, aromatic foods; add sugar and spices to maximize stimulus for swallow.

- Serve food at cold temperatures.
- Include highly textured foods, such as diced, cooked vegetables and fruits.
- Maintain a semisolid consistency that forms a cohesive bolus, such as egg or tuna salad, soufflés, quiches, soft cheeses, and vegetables in sauces.
- Avoid foods that fall apart in the pharynx, such as crackers, plain raw vegetables and fruits, crumbly breads, and dry scrambled eggs.
- Avoid sticky or bulky foods to reduce airway obstruction.
- Exercise caution with thin liquids, such as water, juices, carbonated beverages, as they are unpredictable, difficult to control, and may spill into the pharynx prior to the swallow reflex.
- Small frequent meals may minimize fatigue.
- Patient should sit as upright as possible.

Weakened or poor oral-muscular control:
- Maintain a semisolid consistency that forms cohesive bolus as these require less oral manipulation; purees are difficult to control.
- Avoid slippery, sticky foods, such as peanut butter, fresh white bread, or refried beans.
- Avoid thin liquids as above.
- Small frequent meals will minimize fatigue and maximize nutrient intake.
- Refer to physical therapy for exercises to strengthen the oral and facial muscles.

Reduced oral sensation:
- Position food in the most sensitive area of the mouth to maximize sensation.
- Do not mix textures, such as vegetable soups, to minimize risk of aspiration and to simplify swallowing.
- Use cold temperature foods to maximize sensation.
- Use highly seasoned, flavorful foods.

Cricopharyngeal dysfunction:
- Maintain liquid-pureed diet if no other contraindication is present as these pass through the esophagus more easily.
- Patients with pharyngeal delay have demonstrated some tolerance to carbonated beverages like ginger ale and club soda, supporting the hypothesis that oropharyngeal swallowing can be modulated in response to sensory stimuli. Oral chemesthesis is the detection of chemicals that activate temperature and pain receptors in the oral mucosa and influence greater neuromotor activity during the oral phase of swallowing. Thus, presentation of orally chemesthetic liquids has been observed to stimulate a faster, stronger swallow compared to water.

Decreased laryngeal elevation:
- Limit diet to medium-spoon thick liquids, such as yogurt, sherbet, ice cream, and soft solids, as thin liquids easily penetrate the larynx.
- Avoid sticky or bulky foods or foods that will fall apart to reduce risk of airway obstruction.

Decreased vocal cord closure:
- Avoid thin liquids and avoid foods that will fall apart to reduce risk of small pieces entering the larynx after the swallow.

11.5.4 Dentist

Referral to a dentist must include details regarding current diagnosis, plan of treatment, start date of treatment, limitations of use of medications including antibiotics and other specific information that will assist the dentist to implement dental care safely. If teeth are ill fitting, patients should be referred to the dentist to ensure proper fitting.

Additionally, assure that if dentures or other prosthesis for teeth are used such as partials, patients have these always available and use them.

Fastidious mouth care must be followed to prevent any infections or decay.

11.5.5 Pharmacotherapy

Assessment must be performed within 24 h of admission of the patient by a clinical pharmacist closely working with the registered dietitian.

A thorough medication history must be obtained.

If patient is on antiepileptic or medications for insomnia, this use of medications can trigger dysphagia.

Patients should be screened and treated for candidiasis, especially when patients are on chemotherapy and on steroid therapy.

Recommendations specific for patients with candidiasis:

- Recommend use of a soft toothbrush and rinse your mouth with a diluted 3% hydrogen peroxide solution several times a day.
- Good control of blood sugar levels in persons with diabetes may be needed to clear these infections.
- Prescribe an antifungal mouthwash or lozenges.
- Orabase® or Oral Balance® with or without Kenalog® (covers mouth sores while they are healing).
- Viscous Xylocaine (Lidocaine® 2%) swishes prior to eating may help relieve pain while eating. However, care must be taken and patient instructed that too much of this may also make them too numb and that they may bite their tongue or other parts of their oral cavity.
- Cryotherapy (ice chips) has consistently shown some benefit in reducing pain.

In patients with dysphagia, alternate mode of providing medications, including vitamins and minerals as liquids, gels, suppositories, IV, subcutaneous, IM, or via J-tube or G-tube may be considered.

Since oral pain (odynophagia) is a classic symptom accompanying dysphagia, systemic analgesics like opiates must be considered via the transdermal route.

Since dehydration is also common in this patient population, IV or subcutaneous fluid replacements are critical to maintain hydration, especially in the absence of poor tolerance to liquids.

If patient is able to swallow and has poor appetite, appetite stimulants must be considered.

Current therapies used to improve appetite and to reduce breakdown of muscle proteins (proteolysis):

- *Corticosteroids*
  - Dexamethasone (Decadron®)
  - Methylprednisolone (Solu-Medrol®)
  - Prednisone (Deltasone®)
- *Orexigenic agents*
  - Megestrol acetate (Megace®)
- *Anabolic steroids*
  - Medroxyprogesterone acetate (Provera®, Depo-Provera®)
- *Antiemetics*

11.5.6 Physical Activity

Patients should be proactively receiving a comprehensive assessment of physical status by a licensed physical therapist and therapy initiated within 24 h of assessment.

1. Based on the stage of swallowing affected, rehabilitative techniques such as swallow maneuvers (supraglottic swallow; effortful swallow), exercises (to increase strength of muscle groups), and sensory stimulation techniques (thermal-tactile stimulation; low-level electrical stimulation) can be recommended [20].
2. Refer patients to physical therapy for pretreatment, preoperative education, and training using swallowing exercises [21, 30] which have been found to improve quality of life as well as symptoms related to dysphagia.
3. If weakness of muscles due to treatment is anticipated, recommend and educate exercises to strengthen the jaw and tongue such as jaw range of motion, tongue base range of motion exercises, and effortful swallow exercises, tongue holding maneuver, Mendelsohn maneuver, and super supraglottic swallow [21, 30].
4. Patients should be encouraged to practice these exercises daily during and after treatment since effects of chemoradiation can occur long after treatment completion.
5. Postural recommendations can be made during meal times as indicated. Patients should be instructed to always sit up straight while eating and drinking. They should be instructed not to lie down after a meal nor recline. Patients should be instructed not to go to bed only after 3 h after a meal. Patients should be instructed to stand up if food gets stuck and stretch the upper body and walk around.

11.5.7 Markers and Instruments for Patient Monitoring and Assessment of Response to Treatment by the Interdisciplinary Medical Team

1. *Anthropometric measurements* such as participant's height, weight, and body mass index can be performed at admission and at regular intervals established by the medical team.

2. *Body composition by DXA scan*: DXA should be used to assess both total lean body mass (LBM) and fat mass (FM) and total bone mineral density (BMD). Total bone mineral density (BMD) is a valid indirect measure of skeletal muscle and patient activity. Total LBM is sometimes called total fat-free mass (FFM) depending upon specific DXA manufacturer. DXA instruments use an X-ray source that generates or is split into two energies to measure bone mineral mass and soft tissue from which fat and fat-free mass are estimated. The exam is quick (1–2 min), precise (0.5–1%), and noninvasive. DXA scanners have the precision required to detect changes in muscle mass as small as 5%. Radiation exposure from DXA scans is minimal. The National Council of Radiation Protection and Measurements (NCRP) has recommended that the annual effective dose limit for infrequent exposure of the general population is 5,000 μSv and that an annual effective dose of 10 μSv be considered a negligible individual dose. The effective dose of a dual-energy X-ray absorptiometry whole body scan on an adult is 2.1 μSv. Studies have shown that quality assurance is an important issue in the use of DXA scans to determine body composition including lean body mass and bone mineral density. DXA instrument manufacturer and model should remain consistent, and their calibration should be monitored throughout treatment. Use of a standardized scan acquisition protocol and appropriate and unchanging scan acquisition and analysis software is essential to achieve consist results.

3. *Dietary intake* must be assessed at baseline and periodical intervals by conducting random weekly, 2 weekdays + 1 weekend day, 24-h dietary recalls (gold standard for collecting dietary data) using a 5-step multipass procedure (which has been found to assess mean energy intake within 10% of actual intake) and using the frequently updated University of Minnesota Nutrition Data System for Research (NDS-R) version database for analysis of nutrient composition. Food portion visuals can be provided to patients to estimate portion sizes of foods while monitoring intake.

1. *Symptom log* may be completed daily and collected from patients on a monthly basis. Based on these symptoms, all anticipated and unanticipated, grades of constitutional, dermatological, gastrointestinal (GI), metabolic, and pain symptoms can be continuously monitored including those symptoms affecting nutritional intake and utilization.

2. *Monthly* CMP and CBC should be monitored to assess electrolytes and organ function.

3. *Functional markers (Karnofsky performance score)*: Evaluation of patients' functional status and barriers to obtaining adequate nutrients is also necessary. A physical exam combined with personal interview should include the evaluation of functional status such as the ability to chew and swallow, dental or oral problems causing odynophagia or dysphagia, signs of muscle wasting or anasarca, presence of edema, presence of skin or mouth lesion, and ability to perform instrumental activities of daily living (IADLs) such as cooking, shopping, and self-feeding. It is critical to assess activities of daily living, physical activity, exercise, sleep, and ability to work and perform other functional roles. Limitations in the activities of daily living have been identified secondary to and as a cause of weight loss in cancer patients. Cancer and other chronic diseases pose difficulties

specifically for the cancer patient receiving treatment and the elderly in carrying out activities of daily living. A loss of postural and locomotive muscle mass has been observed within 7 days of inactivity. The Karnofsky Performance Scale Index allows patients to be classified as to their functional impairment. This has been used to compare effectiveness of different therapies and to assess the prognosis in individual patients and has been validated in cancer patient populations. Karnofsky Performance Scale Index allows patients to be classified as to their functional impairment. This has been used to compare effectiveness of different therapies and to assess the prognosis in individual patients and has been validated in cancer patient populations.

4. *Godin Leisure-Time Exercise Questionnaire* weekly to monitor physical activity.

5. *Handgrip strength dynamometry assessment*: A validated tool commonly used to assess handgrip strength is the Jamar dynamometer, which is a fast, reliable, and easy-to-perform device commonly used by our team to measure improvements in functional strength. The Jamar dynamometer has a lower % coefficient of variation and is thus a more precise device than other handgrip dynamometers.

6. *Biochemical markers of protein status (serum albumin and transferrin)*: Assessment of protein status is critical in the identification and treatment of abnormalities in protein metabolism. There is substantial evidence of the correlation between serum hepatic proteins and inflammation, making these the most relevant biomarkers in cancer patient populations. Serum transferrin, prealbumin, and albumin have been observed as intermediate endpoint biomarkers and independently associated with clinical outcomes. Measurements of body composition combined with more objective and sensitive measure of protein nutriture are ideal for the biochemical assessment of intravascular and visceral protein stores. We have thus included the three major valid intermediate endpoint biomarkers (IEBs) that represent intravascular and visceral protein pools – transferrin, prealbumin, and albumin – as the biochemical indicators of protein status. Although transferrin levels are affected by iron status, serum transferrin, either singly or as part of a multiparameter index, is the strongest predictor of cancer patient morbidity and mortality.

7. *Immune and inflammatory markers*: A range of metabolic responses triggered by inflammatory and immunological responses in cancer patients. Cytokines can be measured in a panel including IL-1, IL-4, IL-6, IL-8, IL-10, GM-CSF, IFN-κ, TNF-α, and CRP (BioRad-Bioplex). All of these biomarkers have been shown to increase with disease, aging, and cytotoxic agents. Though we realize these intermediate endpoint biomarkers of cytokines cannot be reliably interpreted, as over 70% of the subjects as observed in our studies were on active treatment with cytotoxic agents, these variables are important to determine, as they may provide useful information and contribute to the better understanding of the mechanistic process.

8. *Quality of life* should be measured at baseline and monthly using the Rand Short Form (SF)-36 (Medical Outcomes Study SF36) [60]. The SF-36 has been used extensively with both general, high-risk, and cancer populations and has available norms for mail and telephone versions and comparisons between group and individual scores. Scores are calculated and transformed to a 0–100 scale, with higher scores indicating increased health status. Reliability of the SF-36 scales was measured by Cronbach α coefficient, and the results ranged from 0.78 in general health perceptions to 0.91 in the physical functioning domain.

11.5.8 Follow-up

Patients must be seen by the multidisciplinary team on a regularly scheduled basis to monitor progress and to review compliance to intervention including diet intake adequacy, symptom logs, change in concomitant medications, and any other issues related to treatment. Improved management of malnutrition with nutritional therapy may require a multimodal intervention by multidisciplinary teams using a comprehensive and integrated approach. Initial screening and knowledge of treatment trajectory of the cancer patient should guide a plan for reassessment of the cancer patient at regularly planned intervals. Subjective and objective data on progress and response to nutritional therapy may be assessed using the indicators used in the comprehensive nutritional assessment. Newly developed symptoms resulting from treatment or progression of disease may require additional monitoring or revision of nutritional therapy. Reassessment/reevaluation for monitoring and evaluation of nutritional therapy must include monitoring of clinical, functional, dietary, and behavioral outcomes that were identified by the comprehensive nutritional assessment.

11.6   Future Directions

With our awareness of the etiology of dysphagia and its consequences, it is important to continue to examine, establish, and continuously evaluate multimodality interventions toward establishing guidelines for the early identification and treatment of dysphagia, in addition to developing treatment strategies to prevent or reduce these symptoms. Future studies should examine whether routine posttherapy videofluoroscopy or FEES and/or training aspirating patients in safe swallowing strategies can better diagnose and allow for interventions targeting the etiology of dysphagia, avoiding compromise of nutrition status and hydration, and preventing aspiration-related complications. These research studies may have a significant impact on mortality, morbidity, and quality of life in this patient population.

Summary for the Clinician

Due to the multifactorial etiology of dysphagia, there is no single standard of therapy established to treat the symptoms of dysphagia in cancer patients.

Diagnosis and management of swallowing dysfunction requires timely and careful screening using detailed history and clinical examination by integrated, multidisciplinary teams consisting of treating oncologists (surgeons, radiation oncologists, medical oncologists), dentists, speech pathologist, clinical pharmacist, psychosocial worker, physical therapist, radiologist, and dietitian.

Some of the basic principles to managing patients with dysphagia are to prevent dehydration and malnutrition and to avoid aspiration and related complications such as pneumonia.

Treatment plan must be targeted to the specific etiology of dysphagia.

Using a comprehensive symptom assessment, it is important to establish compensatory strategies and therapy targeted at the etiology of dysphagia.

In addition to standard medical approaches, nutritional approaches including adequate nutritional support, sensory enhancement, and changing feeding strategies in addition to postural changes must be recommended.

Anticipating treatment-related changes in swallowing ability, therapy procedures including exercise programs and swallowing maneuvers must be implemented to facilitate the physiology of swallowing prior to and posttreatment with chemoradiation therapies.

Patients must be screened and treated for dysphagia-related symptom cluster such as candidiasis, odynophagia, dehydration, and anorexia.

Intervention must be proactive and based on ongoing evaluations to monitor patient's change in status based on disease stage, response to treatment, and treatment outcomes as well as use of concomitant medications.

With our awareness of the etiology of dysphagia and its consequences, it is important to continue to examine, establish, and continuously evaluate multimodality interventions toward establishing guidelines for the early identification and treatment of dysphagia, in addition to developing treatment strategies to prevent or reduce these symptoms.

Future studies should examine whether routine posttherapy videofluoroscopy or FEES and/or training aspirating patients in safe swallowing strategies can better diagnose and allow for interventions targeting the etiology of dysphagia, avoiding compromise of nutrition status and hydration, and preventing aspiration-related complications. These research studies may have a significant impact on mortality, morbidity, and quality of life in this patient population.

References

1. McCulloch TM, Van Daele D, Ciucci MR (2011) Otolaryngology head and neck surgery: an integrative view of the larynx. Head Neck 33(Suppl 1):S46–S53. doi: 10.1002/hed.21901. Epub 2011 Sep 9
2. Lazarus CL (1993) Effects of radiation therapy and voluntary maneuvers on swallow functioning in head and neck cancer patients. Clin Comm Disord 3:11–20
3. Kumar S (2010) Swallowing and dysphagia in neurological disorders. Rev Neurol Dis 7(1): 19–27, Review
4. Patti F, Emmi N, Restivo DA, Liberto A, Pappalardo A, Torre LM, Reggio A (2002) Neurogenic dysphagia: physiology, physiopathology and rehabilitative treatment. Clin Ter 153(6): 403–419, Review
5. Olszewski J (2006) Causes, diagnosis and treatment of neurogenic dysphagia as an interdisciplinary clinical problem. Otolaryngol Pol 60(4):491–500, Review
6. Domench E, Kelly J (1999) Swallowing disorders. Med Clin N Am 83(1):97–113
7. Nguyen NP, Frank C, Moltz CC, Karlsson U, Nguyen PD, Ward HW, Vos P, Smith HJ, Huang S, Nguyen LM, Lemanski C, Ludin A, Sallah S (2009) Analysis of factors influencing dysphagia severity following treatment of head and neck cancer. Anticancer Res 29(8): 3299–3304
8. Nguyen NP, Frank C, Moltz CC, Vos P, Smith HJ, Nguyen PD, Martinez T, Karlsson U, Dutta S, Lemanski C, Nguyen LM, Sallah S (2009) Analysis of factors influencing aspiration risk following chemoradiation for oropharyngeal cancer. Br J Radiol 82(980):675–680, Epub 2009 Mar 30
9. Logemann JA, Larsen K (2011) Oropharyngeal dysphagia: pathophysiology and diagnosis for the anniversary issue of diseases of the esophagus. Dis Esophagus. doi: 10.1111/j.1442-2050.2011.01210.x
10. Eroglu A, Turkyilmaz A, Subasi M, Karaoglanoglu N (2010) The use of self-expandable metallic stents for palliative treatment of inoperable esophageal cancer. Dis Esophagus 23(1):64–70, Epub 2009 May 15
11. Lovell SJ, Wong HB, Loh KS et al (2005) Impact of dysphagia on quality of life in nasopharyngeal carcinoma. Head Neck 27(10):864–872
12. Palmer JB, Drennan JC, Baba M (2000) Evaluation and treatment of swallowing impairments. Am Fam Physician 61:2453–2462
13. Newton HB, Newton C, Pearl D, Davidson T (1994) Swallowing assessment in primary brain tumor patients with dysphagia. Neurology 44(10):1927–1932
14. Sink J, Kademani D (2011) Maxillofacial oncology at the University of Minnesota: treating the epidemic of oral cancer. Northwest Dent 90(3):13–16, 38
15. Arias F, Manterola A, Domínguez MA, Martínez E, Villafranca E, Romero P, Vera R (2004) Acute dysphagia of oncological origin. Therapeutic management. An Sist Sanit Navar 27 (Suppl 3):109–115
16. Platteaux N, Dirix P, Dejaeger E, Nuyts S (2010) Dysphagia in head and neck cancer patients treated with chemoradiotherapy. Dysphagia 25(2):139–152, Epub 2009 Aug 27
17. Chone CT, Spina AL, Barcellos IH, Servin HH, Crespo AN (2011) A prospective study of long-term dysphagia following total laryngectomy. B-ENT 7(2):103–109
18. Rupinski M, Zagorowicz E, Regula J, Fijuth J, Kraszewska E, Polkowski M, Wronska E, Butruk E (2011) Randomized comparison of three palliative regimens including brachytherapy, photodynamic therapy, and APC in patients with malignant dysphagia (CONSORT 1a) (revised II). Am J Gastroenterol 106(9):1612–1620. doi:10.1038/ajg.2011.178, Epub 2011 Jun 14
19. Wilson JA, Carding PN, Patterson JM (2011) Dysphagia after nonsurgical head and neck cancer treatment: patients' perspectives. Otolaryngol Head Neck Surg 145(5):767–771, Epub 2011 Jul 11
20. Langmore S, Krisciunas GP, Miloro KV, Evans SR, Cheng DM (2011) Does PEG use cause dysphagia in head and neck cancer patients? Dysphagia

21. Kulbersh BD, Rosenthal EL, McGrew BM, Duncan RD, McColloch NL, Carroll WR, Magnuson JS (2006) Pretreatment, preoperative swallowing exercises may improve dysphagia quality of life. Laryngoscope 116(6):883–886

22. Dwivedi RC, St Rose S, Roe JW, Khan AS, Pepper C, Nutting CM, Clarke PM, Kerawala CJ, Rhys-Evans PH, Harrington KJ, Kazi R (2010) Validation of the Sydney Swallow Questionnaire (SSQ) in a cohort of head and neck cancer patients. Oral Oncol 46(4):e10–e14, Epub 2010 Mar 9

23. Manikantan K, Khode S, Sayed SI, Roe J, Nutting CM, Rhys-Evans P, Harrington KJ, Kazi R (2009) Dysphagia in head and neck cancer. Cancer Treat Rev 35(8):724–732, Epub 2009 Sep 13

24. Howden CW (2004) Management of acid-related disorders in patients with dysphagia. Am J Med 117(Suppl 5A):44S–48S, Review

25. García-Peris P, Parón L, Velasco C, de la Cuerda C, Camblor M, Bretón I, Herencia H, Verdaguer J, Navarro C, Clave P (2007) Long-term prevalence of oropharyngeal dysphagia in head and neck cancer patients: impact on quality of life. Clin Nutr 26(6):710–717, Epub 2007 Oct 22

26. Morris H (2006) Dysphagia in the elderly – a management challenge for nurses. Br J Nurs 15(10):558–562, Review

27. Ng LK, Lee KY, Chiu SN, Ku PK, van Hasselt CA, Tong MC (2011) Silent aspiration and swallowing physiology after radiotherapy in patients with nasopharyngeal carcinoma. Head Neck 33(9):1335–1339. doi:10.1002/hed.21627. Epub 2010 Nov 10

28. Mehta MP, Paleologos NA, Mikkelsen T, Robinson PD, Ammirati M, Andrews DW, Asher AL, Burri SH, Cobbs CS, Gaspar LE, Kondziolka D, Linskey ME, Loeffler JS, McDermott M, Olson JJ, Patchell RA, Ryken TC, Kalkanis SN (2010) The role of chemotherapy in the management of newly diagnosed brain metastases: a systematic review and evidence-based clinical practice guideline. J Neurooncol 96(1):71–83, Epub 2009 Dec 4. Review

29. Steiner W, Fierek O, Ambrosch P, Hommerich CP, Kron M (2003) Transoral laser microsurgery for squamous cell carcinoma of the base of the tongue. Arch Otolaryngol Head Neck Surg 129(1):36–43

30. Gaziano JE (2002) Evaluation and management of oropharyngeal dysphagia in head and neck cancer. Cancer Control 9(5):400–409, Review

31. Koiwai K, Shikama N, Sasaki S, Shinoda A, Kadoya M (2009) Risk factors for severe dysphagia after concurrent chemoradiotherapy for head and neck cancers. Jpn J Clin Oncol 39(7):413–417, Epub 2009 Apr 20

32. Nonoshita T, Shioyama Y, Nakamura K, Nakashima T, Ohga S, Yoshitake T, Ohnishi K, Terashima K, Asai K, Honda H (2010) Concurrent chemoradiotherapy with S-1 for T2N0 glottic squamous cell carcinoma. J Radiat Res (Tokyo) 51(4):481–484, Epub 2010 Jun 30

33. Wang X, Hu C, Eisbruch A (2011) Organ-sparing radiation therapy for head and neck cancer. Nat Rev Clin Oncol 8(11):639–648. doi:10.1038/nrclinonc.2011.106 [Epub ahead of print]

34. Eisbruch A et al (2002) Objective assessment of swallowing dysfunction and aspiration after radiation concurrent with chemotherapy for head-and-neck cancer. Int J Radiat Oncol Biol Phys 53(1):23–28

35. Mittal BB et al (2003) Swallowing dysfunction – preventative and rehabilitation strategies in patients with head and neck cancers treated with surgery, radiotherapy, and chemotherapy: a critical review. Int J Radiat Oncol Biol Phys 57:1219–1230, | Article | PubMed |

36. Grobbelaar EJ et al (2004) Nutritional challenges in head and neck cancer. Clin Otolaryngol Allied Sci 29(4):307–313

37. Chang YC, Chen SY, Ting LL, Peng SS, Wang TC, Wang TG (2011) A 2-year follow-up of swallowing function after radiation therapy in patients with nasopharyngeal carcinoma. Arch Phys Med Rehabil 92(11):1814–1819, Epub 2011 Aug 15

38. Ku PK, Vlantis AC, Leung SF, Lee KY, Cheung DM, Abdullah VJ, van Hasselt A, Tong MC (2010) Laryngopharyngeal sensory deficits and impaired pharyngeal motor function predict aspiration in patients irradiated for nasopharyngeal carcinoma. Laryngoscope 120(2):223–228

39. Lazarus CL et al (2000) Swallowing and tongue function following treatment for oral and oropharyngeal cancer. J Speech Lang Hear Res 43:1011–1023

40. Smith RV, Goldman SY, Beitler JJ, Wadler SS (2004) Decreased short- and long-term swallowing problems with altered radiotherapy dosing used in an organ-sparing protocol for advanced pharyngeal carcinoma. Arch Otolaryngol Head Neck Surg 130(7):831–836

41. Frowen J, Cotton S, Corry J, Perry A (2010) Impact of demographics, tumor characteristics, and treatment factors on swallowing after (chemo)radiotherapy for head and neck cancer. Head Neck 32(4):513–528

42. Murry T, Madasu R, Martin A, Robbins KT (1998) Acute and chronic changes in swallowing and quality of life following intraarterial chemoradiation for organ preservation in patients with advanced head and neck cancer. Head Neck 20(1):31–37

43. Robbins KT, Kumar P, Wong FS, Hartsell WF, Flick P, Palmer R, Weir AB 3rd, Neill HB, Murry T, Ferguson R, Hanchett C, Vieira F, Bush A, Howell SB (2000) Targeted chemoradiation for advanced head and neck cancer: analysis of 213 patients. Head Neck 22(7): 687–693

44. Feng FY, Kim HM, Lyden TH, Haxer MJ, Worden FP, Feng M, Moyer JS, Prince ME, Carey TE, Wolf GT, Bradford CR, Chepeha DB, Eisbruch A (2010) Intensity-modulated chemoradiotherapy aiming to reduce dysphagia in patients with oropharyngeal cancer: clinical and functional results. J Clin Oncol 28(16):2732–2738, Epub 2010 Apr 26

45. Cohen JT, Manor Y (2011) Swallowing disturbance questionnaire for detecting dysphagia. Laryngoscope 121(7):1383–1387

46. Schrock JW, Bernstein J, Glasenapp M, Drogell K, Hanna J (2011) A novel emergency department dysphagia screen for patients presenting with acute stroke. Acad Emerg Med 18(6): 584–589

47. Gary D, Gramigna GD (2006) How to perform video-fluoroscopic swallowing studies. PART 1 Oral cavity, pharynx and esophagus. GI Motil Online nature.com. Published 16 May 2006

48. Omari TI, Papathanasopoulos A, Dejaeger E, Wauters L, Scarpellini E, Vos R, Slootmaekers S, Seghers V, Cornelissen L, Goeleven A, Tack J, Rommel N (2011) Reproducibility and agreement of pharyngeal automated impedance manometry with videofluoroscopy. Clin Gastroenterol Hepatol 9(10):862–867, Epub 2011 Jun 6

49. Dobrucali A, Caglar E (2010) Palliation of malignant esophageal obstruction and fistulas with self expandable metallic stents. World J Gastroenterol 16(45):5739–5745

50. Takahashi H, Arimura Y, Okahara S, Uchida S, Ishigaki S, Tsukagoshi H, Shinomura Y, Hosokawa M (2011) Risk of perforation during dilation for esophageal strictures after endoscopic resection in patients with early squamous cell carcinoma. Endoscopy 43(3):184–189, Epub 2011 Jan 13

51. Sreedharan A, Harris K, Crellin A, Forman D, Everett SM (2009) Interventions for dysphagia in oesophageal cancer. Cochrane Database Syst Rev(4):CD005048

52. Nugent B, Parker MJ, McIntyre IA (2010) Nasogastric tube feeding and percutaneous endoscopic gastrostomy tube feeding in patients with head and neck cancer. J Hum Nutr Diet 23(3):277–284, Epub 2010 Mar 10

53. Logemann JA, Rademaker A, Pauloski BR, Antinoja J, Bacon M, Bernstein M, Gaziano J, Grande B, Kelchner L, Kelly A, Klaben B, Lundy D, Newman L, Santa D, Stachowiak L, Stangl-McBreen C, Atkinson C, Bassani H, Czapla M, Farquharson J, Larsen K, Lewis V, Logan H, Nitschke T, Veis S (2008) What information do clinicians use in recommending oral versus nonoral feeding in oropharyngeal dysphagic patients? Dysphagia 23(4):378–384, Epub 2008 Aug 1

54. Sdravou K, Walshe M, Dagdilelis L (2011) Effects of carbonated liquids on oropharyngeal swallowing measures in people with neurogenic dysphagia. Dysphagia

55. Krival K, Bates C (2011) Effects of club soda and ginger brew on linguapalatal pressures in healthy swallowing. Dysphagia. [Epub ahead of print]

56. Lazarus C, Logemann JA, Pauloski BR, Rademaker AW, Helenowski IB, Vonesh EF, Maccracken E, Mittal BB, Vokes EE, Haraf DJ (2007) Effects of radiotherapy with or without chemotherapy on tongue strength and swallowing in patients with oral cancer. Head Neck 29(7):632–637

57. Ikeda E, Kojima T, Kaneko K, Minashi K, Onozawa M, Nihei K, Fuse N, Yano T, Yoshino T, Tahara M, Doi T, Ohtsu A (2011) Efficacy of concurrent chemoradiotherapy as a palliative treatment in stage IVB esophageal cancer patients with dysphagia. Jpn J Clin Oncol 41(8):964–972, Epub 2011 Jul 7

58. Knox JJ, Wong R, Visbal AL, Horgan AM, Guindi M, Hornby J, Xu W, Ringash J, Keshavjee S, Chen E, Haider M, Darling G (2010) Phase 2 trial of preoperative irinotecan plus cisplatin and conformal radiotherapy, followed by surgery for esophageal cancer. Cancer 116(17): 4023–4032

59. Worthington HV, Clarkson JE, Khalid T, Meyer S, McCabe M (2010) Interventions for treating oral candidiasis for patients with cancer receiving treatment. Cochrane Database Syst Rev (7):CD001972

60. Garratt AM, Ruta DA, Abdalla MI, Buckingham JK, Russell IT (1993) The SF36 health survey questionnaire: an outcome measure suitable for routine use within the NHS? BMJ 306(6890):1440–1444

Alterations in Taste and Smell

Core Messages

The epicurean pleasure of taste and smell has been consistently demonstrated to be the primary motivating factor for nutritional intake for sustenance in humans as much as the senses are critical for protecting the human body by detecting and identifying food-borne as well as environmental toxins.

Alterations in taste can be attributed to ageusia (absence of taste perception), hypogeusia (decreased sensitivity to taste perception), dysgeusia (distortion of taste perception), or phantogeusia (perception of taste, often described as metallic or salty, without an external stimulus).

Alterations in odor or smell can be attributed to anosmia (absence of odor perception), hyposmia (decreased sensitivity to odor perception), dysosmia (distorted ability to identify odors), parosmia (altered odor perception in the presence of another odor), agnosia (inability to discriminate perceived odors), and phantosmia (odor perception without the presence of any odor).

Taste alterations are characterized by change in the five tastes: sweet, sour, bitter, salty, and umami.

Cancer patients receiving chemotherapy, radiation therapy, and combination therapies report both taste and smell alterations of varying intensities, time to occurrence, and duration.

Alterations in taste and smell have been reported by 56.3% of patients only receiving chemotherapy, 66.5% receiving radiation therapy, and 76% receiving combination therapy.

Inability to taste (dysgeusia) or decreased taste acuity (hypogeusia) is common a side effect of cancer and cancer treatment and reportedly occurs in 56–76% cancer patients, depending on the type of cancer treatment.

In general, taste and smell abnormalities can be attributed to multiple etiologies including a number of physiological alterations such as normal aging, injuries to the oral/pharyngeal anatomy, neural injury, medications, nutritional and immune disorders, and disease states.

N.B. Kumar, *Nutritional Management of Cancer Treatment Effects*,
DOI 10.1007/978-3-642-27233-2_12, © Springer-Verlag Berlin Heidelberg 2012

Surgery to remove tumors of the oral or nasal cavity or tumors obstructing airflow, cytotoxic and radiation therapy to the head and neck region, infections of the nasopharyngeal and oral cavity, and depression are some of contributors of taste and smell alterations.

Dysfunction of the olfactory sense could also lead to taste changes, and diagnoses such as sinusitis and nasal polyps should be considered. Medications such as antidepressants, antihypertensives, and antiemetics may be responsible for taste changes.

Most cancer patients have increased nutritional intake due to hypermetabolism and multiple nutritional deficits in addition to several symptom clusters that compromise nutritional intake leading to malnutrition.

The loss or marked changes in taste and smell seriously compromise nutritional intake and can lead to increased compromise of nutritional status, leading to disruption in serial treatments, tolerance to treatments, and recovery from therapeutic intervention, as well as quality of life.

12.1   Definition

Taste is the sensory system devoted primarily to a safety and quality check of food to be ingested. The epicurean pleasures of taste and smell have been consistently demonstrated to be the primary motivating factor for nutritional intake for sustenance in humans as much as the senses are critical for protecting the human body by detecting and identifying food-borne as well as environmental toxins [1]. Although aided by smell and visual inspection, the final recognition and selection relies on chemoreceptive events in the mouth [2]. Alterations in taste can be attributed to ageusia (absence of taste perception), hypogeusia (decreased sensitivity to taste perception), dysgeusia (distortion of taste perception), or phantogeusia (perception of taste, often described as metallic or salty, without an external stimulus). Alterations in odor or smell can be attributed to anosmia (absence of odor perception), hyposmia (decreased sensitivity to odor perception), dysosmia (distorted ability to identify odors), parosmia (altered odor perception in the presence of another odor), agnosia (inability to discriminate perceived odors), and phantosmia (odor perception without the presence of any odor) [3, 4]. Taste alterations are characterized by change in the five tastes: sweet, sour, bitter, salty, and umami (savoriness). Alterations in taste and smell including decreased taste sensations and metallic tastes [5] are consistently reported by cancer patients during and posttreatment for cancer. Most commonly, the bitter taste threshold is lowered, while the sweet threshold is increased [6]. Steinbach et al. [7] reported salty taste to be altered most often. However, the patterns and intensity of these alterations vary considerably between patients. Some patients prefer sweet foods, while others are able to tolerate more salty foods. Steinbach et al. [7] found that most food aversion was to meat, followed by chocolate, fruit, and coffee. Taste sensations have also been reported to be varied, with some subjects reporting chemosensory changes as peppery, greasy, soapy, powdery, and chemical taste [8]. Others have reported "saw dust," "toilet paper," and "metal" taste [5]. These alterations in smell and taste in cancer patient are manifested by food aversions and decreased caloric and nutrient intake [5, 9, 10]. Most cancer patients have increased nutritional intake due to hypermetabolism and multiple nutritional deficits in addition to several symptom clusters that compromise nutritional intake, leading to malnutrition. The loss or marked changes in taste and smell seriously compromise nutritional intake and can lead to increased compromise of nutritional status, leading to disruption in serial treatments, tolerance to treatments, and recovery from therapeutic intervention, as well as quality of life [63]. In a recent study to characterize chemosensory alterations and their relationship with dietary intake and quality of life (QOL), Brisbois et al. [11] reported that patients reporting chemosensory alteration consumed 20–25% fewer calories per day, experienced greater weight loss, and had poorer QOL scores compared with patients with no alterations, but results did not vary by chemosensory phenotype. Chemosensory alterations were not related to tumor type, gender, or nausea. Dysgeusia is viewed as extremely frustrating, and patients rank taste change second only to alopecia as a bothersome side effect of chemotherapy [5]. Although alterations in taste and smell are of significant concerns to cancer patients and families, these symptoms are rarely addressed by the healthcare providers, and only 17% of patients received information about dysgeusia before initiating treatments [12].

12.2 Prevalence

Cancer patients receiving chemotherapy, radiation therapy, and combination therapies report both taste and smell alterations of varying intensities, time to occurrence, and duration. Of patients who report alterations in taste and smell, 56.3% are only receiving chemotherapy; 66.5%, radiation therapy; and 76%, combination therapy. Inability to taste (dysgeusia) or decreased taste acuity (hypogeusia) [13–16] is a common side effect of cancer and cancer treatment and reportedly occurs in 56–76% cancer patients, depending on the type of cancer treatment [5, 17]. It is reported that two out of three cancer patients (68%) receiving chemotherapy report altered sensory perception such as decreased or lost taste acuity or metallic taste [18, 19]. It is also estimated that over 50% of patients develop a food aversion after chemotherapy and decreased oral intake leads to involuntary weight loss and ultimately malnutrition [20, 21], leading to prolonged morbidity and chemotherapy-induced side effects, decreased response to therapy, and cancer treatment delays that can result from nutritional compromise [8, 22]. While most taste alterations are transient, lasting less than 3 months after completion of treatment, dysgeusia may persist after drug clearance due to damage to the taste buds [23]. Among cancer patients treated with radiotherapy (RT) in head and neck area, the vast majority report an altered taste sense during and after treatments. In a study of patients with head and neck irradiation, Dirix et al. [24] reported that 63% reported taste loss. The minimal amount of irradiation to produce this taste and smell alterations ranges from 15 to

30 Gy, depending on the treatment condition and disease stage of the individual patient. Taste impairment starts a few weeks after the beginning of irradiation, and almost 90–100% of patients experienced loss of taste acuity at a dose of 60 Gy [25, 26]. Following radiation therapy, taste thresholds peak after 3–5 weeks; however, these thresholds decrease significantly after that period, and sensory recovery returns to baseline sensitivity within 6 months–1 year [27–30, 64]. On the other hand, patients receiving radiation therapy for oropharyngeal cancers were not significantly impacted in their ability to recognize odors, although 7% of patients reported a decrease in smell acuity [28, 31]. Over 80% of breast cancer patients on chemotherapy also report change in food odors and increased sensitivity to odors after chemotherapy [32]. Dysosmia is commonly reported in both radiation and chemotherapy patients, especially in the clinical setting, lasting up to 6–9 months posttreatment, when recovery from this symptom accompanied by increase in smell acuity is reported [32–34].

12.3   Etiology/Common Causes

In general, taste and smell abnormalities can be attributed to several etiologies including a number of physiological alterations such as normal aging, injuries to the oral/pharyngeal anatomy, neural injury, medications, nutritional and immune disorders, and disease states [2, 13–16]. Other causes specific to cancer patient populations include cancers of the oral cavity; surgery of the tongue, palate, and oropharynx; elimination of the olfactory component of taste after laryngectomy; radiotherapy for head and neck cancers, abdomen, or pelvis; presence of oral lesions such as stomatitis, ulcer, necrosis, candidiasis, and/or severe xerostomia; damage to the nervous system following surgery or cerebral lesions; metabolic alterations/disorders; nutritional and immune deficiency; endocrine or neurological diseases influencing taste and/or smell sensitivity; chemotherapy or other drugs affecting taste; local disease in the nose or ears; dental pathology; tobacco use; and plasma and salivary levels of zinc [2, 27, 35–37]. Whatever the type of cancers, duration of treatments differs significantly among patients. In addition, the underlying mechanism of each of these disorders is not clearly understood since the etiological basis of these symptoms is multifactorial [38].

Several investigators have consistently shown the relationship between associated symptoms of cancer, emphasizing the need to evaluate symptom clusters and inventions targeting these clusters to fully resolve symptoms observed in cancer patients.

In researching chemosensory interaction and the impact of acquired olfactory impairment, Landis et al. [39, 40] observed an association between decreased taste function and olfaction, taste and trigeminal function. Trigeminal function is the sensory function of the trigeminal nerve that provides the tactile, proprioceptive, and nociceptive afference of the face and mouth. The motor function activates the muscles of mastication, the tensor tympani, tensor veli palatini, mylohyoid, and anterior belly of the digastric. However, in daily life, they are often activated concomitantly. In health and disease, such as cancer, it has been shown that in two of these senses, the trigeminal and olfactory senses, modification of one sense leads to changes in the other sense, and vice versa. In a study to investigate whether and (if so) how the third modality, taste, is influenced by olfactory impairment, Landis et al. tested 210 subjects with normal ($n = 107$) or impaired ($n = 103$) olfactory function for their taste identification capacities. Validated tests were used for olfactory and gustatory testing (Sniffin' Sticks, taste strips). In an additional experiment, healthy volunteers underwent reversible olfactory cleft obstruction to investigate short-time changes of gustatory function after olfactory alteration. Mean gustatory identification (taste-strip score) for the subjects with impaired olfaction was 19.4 ± 0.6 points and 22.9 ± 0.5 points for those with normal olfactory function ($t = 4.6$, $p < 0.001$). The frequencies of both smell and taste impairments interacted significantly (Chi(2), $F = 16.4$, $p < 0.001$) and olfactory and gustatory function correlated (r (210) $= 0.30$, $p < 0.001$). Neither age nor olfactory impairment cause effects interfered with this olfactory-gustatory interaction. In contrast, after short-lasting induced olfactory decrease, gustatory function remained unchanged. The present study suggests that long-standing impaired olfactory function is associated with decreased gustatory function, confirming the mutual chemosensory interactions between smell and taste senses and implying that, in general, these senses decrease mutually after acquired damage [40] (Fig. 12.1).

12.3.1 Chemotherapy Induced

Chemotherapeutic agents such as cyclophosphamide, dacarbazine, doxorubicin, 5-FU, methotrexate, nitrogen mustard, cisplatin, and vincristine have frequently been associated with taste alterations [5, 6] and heightened sensitivity to one or several odors. While patients on these chemotherapies report dysgeusia, all patients on chemotherapy are at risk for taste alterations due to complications of treatment. Dysgeusia can be a prominent symptom in patients who are receiving chemotherapy or head/neck radiation [41, 42]. The type of chemotherapy is another risk factor for the development of dysgeusia. Steinbach et al. [7] found taxane-based chemotherapies to cause the most severe taste alterations, while Wickham et al. [18] reported cisplatin and doxorubicin to be the agents most likely to cause dysgeusia. Etiology is likely associated with several factors, including direct neurotoxicity to taste buds, xerostomia, infection, and psychological conditioning. Neurotoxicity from systemic chemotherapy probably contributes to dysgeusia. Cranial nerves VII (facial), IX (glossopharyngeal), and X (vagus) control integral sensory functions in the tongue, and damage to them has been implicated in taste alterations [43]. Direct insult to the taste cell receptors is one suggested theory. Some chemotherapy agents are secreted in saliva and gain direct contact with taste receptors. Patients may experience a metallic or "chemical" taste when chemotherapy is delivered, and this is consistent with drug secretion in saliva [43]. Hong et al. [1] suggest that cell damage occurs in three ways: (1) a decrease in the number of normal cell receptors, (2) alteration of

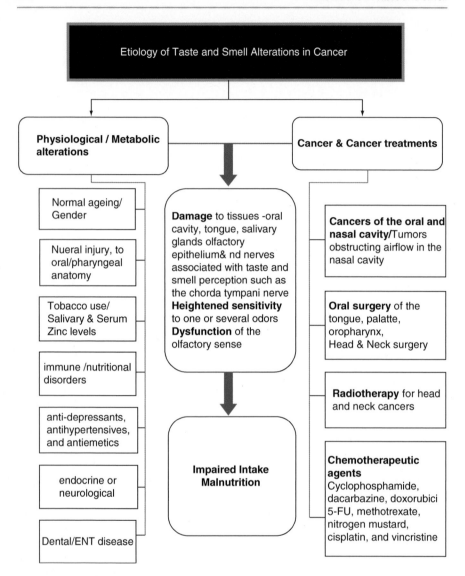

Fig. 12.1 Etiology of taste and smell alterations in cancer

cell structure or receptor surface changes, and (3) interruption of neural coding. The turnover rate of normal human taste bud cells is 10 days, and chemotherapy kills cells with high turnover rates, resulting in taste alteration. Xerostomia or dry mouth has also been implicated in the development of dysgeusia [44]. Decreased saliva secretion alters the amount of chemicals released by the foods, thereby changing the taste. A metallic and or bitter taste is associated with chemotherapy with cyclophosphamide, doxorubicin, 5-fluorouracil, methotrexate, and cisplatin [9, 32]. Over 75% of patients treated with cisplatin alone or in combination with other chemotherapeutic agents reported metallic taste perception [45]. Anywhere from 16% to 55% of cancer patients also complain about odor and unpleasant taste of high-protein foods, especially red meats, and avoid consumption during treatment, implicating a possible relationship between metallic taste and abundant levels of iron compounds such as hemoglobin present in red meats [1, 46, 47]. On the other hand, these patients tolerate proteins from white meats such as chicken, fish, and eggs [1, 46–48]. Chemotherapies such as cyclophosphamide, epirubicin/methotrexate, and 5-fluorouracil when used in the adjuvant setting have been implicated in causing xerostomia, and a 49.9% prevalence rate of xerostomia has been observed in patients undergoing chemotherapy [42]. In addition, taste dysfunction can be associated with damage caused by graft-versus-host disease to the taste perception units [13]. In data derived from a qualitative interview study and a cross-sectional survey of 518 patients, with all patients receiving outpatient cancer chemotherapy in Sweden, 100% of participants reported heightened sensitivity to one or several odors which could not fully be explained by the potential explanatory models of anticipatory nausea and vomiting, pseudohallucination, or increased chemical sensitivity [5]. Although these data do not provide any confirmatory evidence of time to onset and intensity of symptoms enough to compromise nutritional intake, it is clear that most patient populations experience some degree of taste alterations as well as heightened sensitivity to odors during active treatment with cytotoxic therapies.

12.3.2 Radiation Therapy Induced

Similar to chemotherapy, radiation-induced alterations in taste and smell are reported in specific segments of cancer patient populations. Patients receiving radiation therapy for head and neck cancers are potentially at highest risk for alterations of both taste and smell senses with potential or damage to tissues in the oral cavity, tongue, salivary glands and olfactory epithelium, and nerves associated with taste and smell perception such as the chorda tympani [27]. Some studies investigated the four basic taste intensities (sweet, salty, sour, and bitter) and the umami taste, and several of these reports identified diminished threshold sensitivity for at least one taste quality. In a prospective study, Mirza et al. [49] determined whether radiation alters taste function and structure, testing prior to starting radiation and 2 weeks, 2 months, and 6 months after completing radiation. Relative to controls, patients had lower taste identification test scores for bitter, salty, and sour tastes. Sour taste also showed a significant group-by-time interaction ($p=0.03$). Taste pores were decreased in the irradiated group, with a significant group-by-time interaction ($p=0.03$). Head and neck cancer patients have decreased taste function, and radiation adversely affected sour taste and taste pores. Similarly, taste dysfunction in patients receiving radiotherapy was evaluated by Yamashita et al. [50] in a prospective study involving 51 patients undergoing radical head and neck irradiation Taste ability was measured by the taste threshold for the four basic tastes (sweet, sour, salt, and bitter qualities) plus "umami" quality using a filter-paper disk method in patients before, during, and after radiotherapy (RT). All tastes declined on the fifth week after the start of

RT and improved on the 11th week. Anatomic pathologic analyses in rats revealed that taste buds diminished completely on the sixth day after irradiation of 15 Gy in a single fraction, and the appearance of taste buds returned almost to the preirradiation state on the 28th day. The main cause of taste disorder resulting from RT was believed to be a disappearance of taste buds and not damage to the taste nerves. Radiation therapy can damage salivary glands, causing salivary hypofunction and xerostomia. A total fractionated radiation dose higher than 3,000 Gy reduces acuity of sweet, sour, bitter, and salt tastes. Damage to the microvilli and outer surface of the taste cells has been proposed as the principal mechanism for loss of the sense of taste. In many cases, taste acuity returns in 2–3 months after cessation of radiation. However, many other patients develop permanent hypogeusia. Damage to the major salivary glands during head and neck RT leads to disturbance in taste acuity.

The relationship between the time course and the degree of taste disorder was studied in both acute and late phases [51] in a small sample size. Taste ability was measured by the taste threshold for the four basic tastes using a filter-paper disk method in patients before, during, and after radiotherapy. The subjects were divided into two groups. In group A, the radiation fields included most of the tongue ($n = 100$), and in group B, the radiation fields did not include the tip of the tongue ($n = 18$). In group A, there was a significant impairment of the threshold of all four basic tastes at 3 weeks after starting radiotherapy (RT), and this impairment remained at 8 weeks ($p < 0.05$). This was not seen in group B. In group A, there was no significant difference in the patterns of taste sensitivity change between the high-dose (>20 Gy) and low-dose (≤20 Gy) groups. In the late phase, recovery of taste loss was seen in both groups even 4 months after completing RT. Researchers concluded that unless the anterior part of the tongue was irradiated, taste loss was not observed during RT. When the anterior part of the tongue was irradiated, a difference by radiation dose was not observed in the taste-loss pattern. Additionally, radiation-induced taste dysfunction appears to be a temporal effect [51].

Previous studies have reported the alteration of the four basic tastes in patients with head and neck cancer during radiotherapy. However, only a few studies have been conducted on the effects of irradiation on the function of umami taste, a novel and basic taste recently recognized. In a prospective study, 52 patients undergoing radical head and neck irradiation were assessed for taste loss. Taste ability was measured by the taste threshold for umami quality using the whole-mouth taste method in patients before, during, and immediately after radiotherapy. Umami taste declined on the third week after the start of radiotherapy and improved on the 8 week. Yamashita [52] and Shi [52] investigated the recognition threshold of umami and the four basic tastes at different irradiation dose intervals during radiotherapy for head and neck cancer in 30 patients with malignant neoplasm of head and neck. Objective taste thresholds were examined by use of a whole-mouth method at pre-radiotherapy with irradiation doses at 15, 30, 45, and 60 Gy, respectively. Subjective taste loss and some distresses were recorded simultaneously. Sweet, sour, salty, and bitter tastes showed temporarily and slightly increased thresholds during the treatment, but no statistical difference was found between the threshold at preradiotherapy and that at 15, 30, 45, and 60 Gy in any taste quality (all $p > 0.05$). Significantly impaired threshold of umami taste was revealed at 30 Gy ($p < 0.05$) and remained throughout the following treatment (at 45 and 60 Gy, both $p < 0.01$). Subjective taste impairment, appetite loss, and satisfaction with the current state tended to deteriorate significantly during the irradiation. Mean body weight of the patients experienced a continuous loss, decreasing from an average of 60.4 kg before treatment to 57.3 kg at 60 Gy ($p < 0.01$). Scores of satisfaction with current state showed a significant correlation with umami taste thresholds ($p = 0.035$). They concluded that the clinical impairment pattern of umami taste is different from that of the other four basic tastes in HNC patients during radiotherapy. Impaired umami taste acuity plays an important role in impacting the quality of life of the patients irradiated to the head and neck. Taste alterations, whether caused by chemotherapy or a side effect of the chemotherapy, lead to food aversions, compromising nutritional intake. Poor oral hygiene, infection of the oral cavity, and dentures have been associated to worsen chemotherapy-induced taste alterations [6, 53].

Based on these studies, it is clear that patients who received radiation therapy for head and neck cancers and had high-dose chemotherapy experienced a loss of taste and smell during and after treatment. Six months to 1 year after RT, taste acuity recovers to its previous level in many patients, but some patients show incomplete or no recovery even several years later [25]. With the implementation of new radiation techniques, such as conformal and intensity-modulated RT in head and neck irradiation, the late radiation effects can probably be reduced, but the remaining sequelae are still bothersome to the patients [45, 54].

12.3.3   Other Causes of Taste and Smell Alterations in Cancer

Bernhardson et al. [5] found that taste changes to be more prevalent among women and younger patients. Several differential diagnoses are associated with clinical presentation of dysgeusia. Taste alteration may be the result of mucositis, nausea, xerostomia, oral infections, zinc deficiency, or depression [21, 55, 56]. Medications such as antidepressants, antihypertensives, and antiemetics may be responsible for taste changes, and use of such medications needs to be assessed during clinical evaluation [14, 33, 57]. Dysfunction of the olfactory sense could also lead to taste changes, and diagnoses such as sinusitis and nasal polyps should be considered. Surgery of the oral and nasal cavity can also compromise taste and smell. Tumors obstructing airflow in the nasal cavity can also alter smell since up to 80% of the taste of a meal is related to how it smells [58–62].

12.4   Current Treatment Strategies

The treatment of dysgeusia has vexed clinicians for decades. This is partially due to incomplete understanding of its pathophysiology, but also because this diagnosis has been understudied. Current principles of management have relied on early detection and management that involves alteration and enhancement of nutritional intake tailored to the individual patient. In a recent meta-analysis of dysgeusia induced by cancer therapies, Hovan et al. [17] examined the prevalence and management of dysgeusia as an oral side effect of cancer treatment. A total of 30 papers were reviewed; the results of 26 of these papers were included in the present systematic review. Results of these studies indicated that both pharmacological and nonpharmacological approaches to the management of taste and smell alterations have been examined.

12.4.1 Assessment

Assessment of gustatory sensitivity in a clinical setting is the prerequisite for correct diagnosis and adequate treatment of taste dysfunction. Although quantitative, objective methods for detection or recognition of threshold values of the five basic tastes have been used in laboratory settings (e.g., gustometers) [61, 62], patient-reported qualitative assessments have been found to have a relatively better utility value in clinical settings. Quantitative assessment of gustatory function in a clinical context using impregnated "taste strips." More recent studies using "taste strips," [39] which is a rapid, lateralized, gustatory bedside identification test based on impregnated filter papers. The investigation involved 537 participants reporting a normal sense of smell and taste (318 female, 219 male, mean age 44 years, age range 18–87 years). The taste test was based on spoon-shaped filter paper strips ("taste strips") impregnated with the four (sweet, sour, salty, and bitter) taste qualities in four different concentrations. The strips were placed on the left or right side of the anterior third of the extended tongue, resulting in a total of 32 trials. With their tongue still extended, patients had to identify the taste from a list of four descriptors, i.e., sweet, sour, salty, and bitter (multiple forced choice). To obtain an impression of overall gustatory function, the number of correctly identified tastes was summed up for a "taste score." Result of these studies indicated that taste function decreased significantly with age. Women exhibited significantly higher taste scores than men, which was true for all age groups. The taste score at the 10(th) percentile was selected as a cutoff value to distinguish normogeusia from hypogeusia. Results from a small series of patients with ageusia confirmed the clinical usefulness of the proposed normative values based on over 500 subjects tested. Using this assessment technique, which may have clinical utility in cancer patient populations, Mueller et al. [65] administered this to 69 subjects. Each subject received 18 taste strips (four concentrations of each taste quality plus two blanks) in a pseudorandomized sequence. Results from this new procedure correlated significantly with the results of the well-established extensive three-drop technique (r69=0.67). Repeated measures indicated good reproducibility of the results for the taste strips (r69=0.68). These data suggest the usefulness of this new technique in routine clinical practice. Major advantages are long shelf life, convenience of administration, short time needed for testing (approximately 8 min), and the possibility to test each side of the tongue separately [65]. In a prospective study of ovarian and breast cancer patients by Steinbach et al. [7], olfactory function was tested using Sniffin' Sticks (Burghart, Wedel, Germany) and gustatory function was tested using taste strips before, during, and immediately and 3 months after chemotherapy. Results indicated that olfactory and gustatory function significantly decreased during chemotherapy and recovered almost completely 3 months after chemotherapy. Scores of odor thresholds were affected more than those of discrimination or identification. The olfactory function of older patients was affected more than that of younger patients. There was no difference in the olfactory function during chemotherapy with respect to the chemotherapeutic agent or initial diagnosis (breast or ovarian cancer). Regarding taste, scores of salty taste were affected more than scores of sweet, sour, or bitter taste. The gustatory function did not differ significantly during chemotherapy with respect to age or diagnosis but did differ with respect to the chemotherapeutic agent. Taxane-based chemotherapy caused the most severe disorders. These initial studies inform clinicians of the validity of utilizing these techniques that can be applied to efficiently identify those subjects who experience this symptom cluster and provide an opportunity to intervene to treat these symptoms.

12.4.2 Pharmacological

With regard to pharmacological approaches, several studies have evaluated the use of zinc sulfate in mitigating taste alterations. Two pilot studies found that zinc supplementation increased recovery in taste acuity, but a larger phase III trial found that zinc supplementation had no effect on taste alteration [26, 54]. Anecdotal observations and pilot studies have suggested zinc may mitigate these symptoms. In a multi-institutional, double-blind, placebo-controlled trial, Haylard et al. (2007) [22] attempted to provide definitive evidence of zinc's palliative efficacy. A total of 169 evaluable patients were randomly assigned to zinc sulfate 45 mg orally three times daily versus placebo throughout RT and for 1 month after. All patients were scheduled to receive >2,000 cGy of external beam RT to >30% of the oral cavity, were able to take oral medication, and had no oral thrush at study entry. Changes in taste were assessed using the previously validated Wickham questionnaire. Results indicated that overall, 61 zinc-treated (73%) and 71 placebo-exposed (84%) patients described taste alterations during the first 2 months ($p=0.16$). The median interval to taste alterations was 2.3 versus 1.6 weeks in the zinc-treated and placebo-exposed patients, respectively ($p=0.09$). The reported taste alterations included the absence of any taste (16%), bitter taste (8%), salty taste (5%), sour taste (4%), sweet taste (5%), and the presence of a metallic taste (10%), as well as other descriptions provided by a write-in response (81%). Zinc sulfate did not favorably affect the interval to taste recovery in this study, indicating that zinc, as prescribed in this trial, did not prevent taste alterations in cancer patients who were undergoing RT to the oral pharynx. This treatment should be used with caution until further research confirms its efficacy because excessive zinc supplementation can negatively impact the immune system [55].

The amino acid glutamine has also been investigated as a treatment for dysgeusia [56–58]. Strasser et al. (2008) [58] investigated glutamine's role in reducing taste alterations because research supports the use of glutamine in improving mucositis and recovery time in patients receiving high-dose chemotherapy. Taste alteration (dysgeusia), an underrecognized toxicity associated with taxane-based chemotherapy (TaxCh), lacks standard treatment. Jacobson et al. and SD et al. [59] investigated prevention of dysgeusia with oral glutamine in patients undergoing first-time taxane-based chemotherapy; adult patients were randomized to receive either 30 g/day glutamine or placebo (maltodextrin) from day 1 of TaxCh. Dysgeusia was measured daily with a visual analogue scale (VAS). On each chemotherapy cycle, objective (sour, sweet, salty, bitter) and subjective (four-category scale) taste and toxicity (National Cancer Institute Common Toxicity Criteria, v.3) were assessed. Stomatitis and zinc deficiency were treated. For primary outcomes, repeated dysgeusia scores were analyzed with a linear mixed model. Repeated data on each objective or subjective taste item were analyzed with a generalized estimating equation. Of 52 patients randomized, 41 completed treatment (median study duration, 74 days). At baseline, the glutamine ($n = 21$) and placebo ($n = 20$) groups were comparable for age (64 years), gender (32% men), tumor types, chemotherapy (docetaxel, 44%; paclitaxel, 56%), schedule (weekly, 78%; triweekly, 22%), treatment intention (15% adjuvant), dysgeusia (VAS, 11/100), and taste recognition (88%). Twenty-four patients had peripheral neuropathy grades 1–2; none had grade 3. Glutamine and placebo were not different for maximal dysgeusia and increase from baseline, with an insignificant linear time effect. Separate subgroup analyses for patients with baseline dysgeusia ≤11 or >11 did not alter the results. Objective or subjective taste tests were not different, nor were adverse events. Compared with placebo, oral glutamine did not prevent or decrease subjective taste disturbances or altered taste perception associated with TaxCh. The role of glutamine in supportive care of taxane-associated dysgeusia seems limited. Based on these studies, there is limited evidence supporting the use of zinc sulfate or glutamine for treatment of these symptoms, and more research needs to occur before pharmacological recommendations can be made.

12.4.3 Nonpharmacological

Nonpharmacological management strategies and patient education have been the mainstay of treatment for dysgeusia. Many of the suggested recommendations deal with nutritional counseling including food preparation techniques to ameliorate symptoms [1, 60, 61]. Most studies suggest strategies to improve flavors as additional spices and flavoring may compensate for this diminished chemosensory function, enhancing patient compliance and quality of life [5, 23], and suggest psychological strategies for dealing with chemosensory changes such as dysgeusia. Patients in this study stated giving up expectations of food and drink and using taste memory helped them with taste changes. Remembering how things tasted and using these memories in meal situations was found to be helpful when dysgeusia occurred. Having someone else prepare the meal was also found to be effective at reducing food aversion. Both chemotherapy and radiation therapy alter the pleasure produced by taste and smell through the formation of conditioned aversions. i.e., foods consumed in proximity with the nausea of therapy come to be unpleasant. The impact of conditioned aversions can be diminished by providing a scapegoat food just before therapy. Alterations in foods may be beneficial to the cancer patient.

Increasing the concentrations of flavor ingredients can compensate for sensory losses, and providing pureed foods that retain the cognitive integrity of a meal can benefit the patient who has chewing or swallowing problems [62]. Stress of the patient may be further alleviated to know that dysgeusia is a transient condition lasting approximately 3–6 months after completion of chemotherapy and/or radiation therapy [5, 23]. Patients must be counseled regarding these critical timelines which may be helpful to some patients in minimizing the symptoms of dysgeusia.

12.5   Guidelines for Management

Currently, no guidelines exist for the pharmacological management of dysgeusia. These suggestions, though useful, do not resolve the recurring incidence of taste and odor abnormalities among cancer patients.

The following guidelines are considered best practice standards. Improved management of these symptoms may require a *multimodal approach by multidisciplinary teams*. Systematic screening of symptoms, current and past treatments, other medications, infections, oral care, and additional symptoms of cancer treatments must be taken into account prior to providing modification of food preparation and nutritional intake recommendations. The modifications in nutritional intake and behaviors appear to be the only effective management approach at this time.

12.5.1 Education of Patient and Family About These Symptoms

Taste and smell alterations not only affect the QOL of patients undergoing cancer treatment, but have the potential to prolong morbidity and decrease response to therapy. Taste and smell alteration varies with each patient, and specific suggestions for management of symptoms must be tailored on an individual basis. Modification of food preparation appears to be only the effective management approach at this time. Since alterations in taste and smell are rarely brought up by the healthcare provider, a conversation about dysgeusia needs to take place before the initiation of chemotherapy or radiation therapy. Stress of the patient may be further alleviated to know that dysgeusia is a transient condition lasting approximately 3–6 months after completion of chemotherapy and/or radiation therapy. Patients must be counseled regarding these critical timelines which may be helpful to some patients in minimizing the symptoms. The patient can therefore prepare for the psychological and physical manifestations of taste alteration.

12.5.2 Referral to Dentist

Since poor oral hygiene, infection of the oral cavity, and dentures have been associated with chemotherapy-induced taste alterations, a visit to the dentist and frequent periodical check with dental hygienist to ensure that dental care is maintained is recommended. Patients should be examined for any dental problems that may affect the taste or smell of food. Frequent oral hygiene such as regularly rinsing the mouth and brushing the teeth is a good suggestion. Routine dental visits are also helpful and may help in identifying any new infections. Practicing good oral hygiene, including frequent tooth brushing and use of mouthwash must be emphasized.

12.5.3 Treatment of Infections

Patients should be checked prior to start of treatment and periodically thereafter to monitor for mucositis, nausea, xerostomia, oral infections, and any dysfunction of the olfactory sense which could also lead to taste changes, and diagnoses such as sinusitis and nasal polyps should be included.

12.5.4 Screening for Alterations in Taste and Smell

Assessment of gustatory sensitivity in a clinical setting is the prerequisite for correct diagnosis and adequate treatment of taste dysfunction. A variety of approaches to the assessment of taste and smell alterations have evolved in the literature including self-reported tools that continue to generate a description of the development, duration, and recovery of distorted chemosensory perception in cancer patients. Quantitative assessment of gustatory function in a clinical context using impregnated "taste strips" or "Sniffin' Strips" has been validated by several groups and has been found to be used in 8–10 min by the patient at bedside. The taste from a list of four to now five descriptors, i.e., sweet, sour, salty, bitter, and umami (multiple forced choice), can be assessed serially using these strips objectively.

12.5.5 Current Treatment

Patients should be screened for history of recent treatments for cancer as well as the current treatments that the patient is receiving. Surgery of the oral and nasal cavity can also compromise taste and smell. Tumors obstructing airflow in the nasal cavity can also alter smell since up to 80% of the taste of a meal is related to how it smells. Similarly, specific cytotoxic regimens and radiation therapy, including dose and region of therapy, must be taken into consideration.

12.5.6 Other Causes Must Be Examined

Taste changes are more prevalent among women and younger patients. Several differential diagnoses are associated with clinical presentation of dysgeusia. Patients should also be screened for other contributing factors such as mucositis, nausea, xerostomia, oral infections, zinc deficiency, or depression.

Dysfunction of the olfactory sense could also lead to taste changes, and diagnoses such as sinusitis and nasal polyps should be considered.

Medications such as antidepressants, antihypertensives, and antiemetics may be responsible for taste changes, and use of such medications needs to be assessed during clinical evaluation.

12.5.7 Nutrition Guidelines

Nutritional assessment must be performed within 24 h of admission of the patient by a Registered Dietitian.
1. Assess current nutritional status and estimate caloric, protein, and multivitamin/mineral needs.
2. Provide adequate nutrition by including education material on "calorie" and "protein" boosters and nutritional supplements to ensure intake of proteins 0.8 g–1.0 g/kg/day and dense caloric supplements up to 400 cal/day containing 1.5 kcal/mL (Ensure Plus or alternate). The choice of nutritional supplements will be based in the personal choice of the patient. Supplement diet if inadequate with smoothies, instant breakfast powders, Scandishake®, Ensure Plus®, Boost Plus®, and Resource®.
3. Include a standard multivitamin/mineral supplementation to prevent any further deficits and meet increased needs.
4. Assess adequacy of intake and provide an appetite stimulant (megestrol acetate 800 mg/day or alternate) if patient has cancer anorexia to ensure adequate intake and prevent further weight loss.
5. Provide each patient with nutritional guidelines to ensure adequate intake of calories and proteins and a list of suggested high-caloric and high-protein nutritional supplements to choose from, taking into consideration taste alterations, early satiety, nausea, and vomiting that are common symptoms observed in this patient population.
6. Other tips to enhance nutritional intake:
   - Studies of taste sensitivity in malignant disease have shown variable results indicating that different people may have different experiences. Research has shown that overall sweet tastes may be perceived very weakly, while metallic and bitter tastes come to the fore and seem very intense.
   - Patients should avoid being in a room where food is prepared or where these odors can be detected.
   - Cancer patients often prefer cold foods; foods that require less cooking, such as breakfast foods; and foods that require minimum cooking.
   - Recommend use of plastic utensils if there is a need to minimize metallic taste and avoid the use of metallic silverware.
   - Additional sweeteners can be used to reduce bitter taste or acid taste.
   - Increasing the honey or sugar in foods may decrease bitter or acid tastes.

- To improve flavor, suggest flavoring food with herbs such as basil, oregano, rosemary, tarragon, or mint and other flavorings such as vinegar, mustard, and catsup. Use fresh herbs and lemon for more robust flavors.
- Garlic, onions, citrus, and ripe berries, if tolerated, can significantly increase food flavors.
- Marinating and cooking foods using tart or sweet flavors help foods to taste better. Suggestions include cooking in sweet juices or with fruits and using marinades made with fruits, dressings, or wine. Examples would include sweet-and-sour pork, chicken with mustard, or marinating and basting beef in Italian dressing.
- If foods taste "off," recommend clearing taste buds before eating by rinsing or drinking water, tea, ginger ale, or fruit juices mixed with club soda, lemon ice, or lemon sorbet.
- Season foods with tart flavors such as a lemon wedge, citrus fruits, and vinegar, which all help to stimulate saliva flow and taste (avoid if patient has mucositis or esophagitis).
- Hard candies, lemon drops, mints, or chewing gum is recommended. Use sialogogues (agents that stimulate salivary secretion), such as sugar-free gums or sour-tasting drops.
- Use smell, texture, and eye appeal to help stimulate the desire to eat. The smell of fresh bread baking may help stimulate appetite, and visual appeal is essential.
- Increase garnishes on foods.
- Fresh fruits and vegetables may be more appealing than canned or frozen ones.
- Experiment with different food textures as crunchy, creamy, and crispy foods.
- When shopping, recommend choosing foods that are beautiful, fresh, and full flavored.
- Include other protein sources in the diet such as poultry, fish, milk, eggs, bean group, tofu, peanut butter, and other nut butters if patient is unable to tolerate meats during this time.
- Marinating meat, poultry, or fish in yogurts, sweet fruit juices, sweet wine, Italian dressing, or sweet-and-sour sauce or honey may reduce odors.
- Since eating is a social event, patients no longer derive enjoyment from the experience because of taste alteration. Patients report avoiding eating around friends and family and isolate themselves during profound episodes of dysgeusia. Make patients and families aware of this, including understanding of patient's needs as well as providing encouragement.
- Reduce consumption of bitter- or metallic-tasting foods such as coffee and chocolate.
- Fruit intake can be enhanced by freezing fruits such as melon balls, grapes, or oranges.
- Recommend drinking more water with meals to help with swallowing or to rinse away bad taste. Recommend rinsing with cool black or green tea, lightly

salted water, or baking soda and water to "clear" taste buds before eating. Fruit sorbets such as lemon or lime sorbets can also help.

• When drinking liquids, recommend use of a cup with a lid or cover to further reduce odors.

• Use liquid nutrition products to fill in the nutrition gaps if nutritional intake is not adequate.

• If patient has nausea and vomiting, recommend that they avoid their favorite foods.

12.5.8 Pharmacotherapy

Use saliva substitutes and lubricating solutions containing mucin and carboxymethyl cellulose. Concomitant medications such as antidepressants, antihypertensives, and antiemetics may be responsible for taste changes, and use of such medications needs to be assessed during clinical evaluation (Comeau, Epstein, and Migas 2001).

12.5.9 Markers and Instruments for Patient Monitoring and Assessment of Response to Treatment by the Interdisciplinary Medical Team

1. *Anthropometric measurements* such as participant's height, weight, and body mass index can be performed at admission and at regular intervals established by the medical team.
2. *Body composition by DXA scan*: DXA should be used to assess both total lean body mass (LBM), fat mass (FM), and total bone mineral density (BMD). Total bone mineral density (BMD) is a valid indirect measure of skeletal muscle and patient activity. Total LBM is sometimes called total fat-free mass (FFM), depending upon specific DXA manufacturer. DXA instruments use an X-ray source that generates or is split into two energies to measure bone mineral mass and soft tissue from which fat and fat-free mass are estimated. The exam is quick (1–2 min), precise (0.5–1%), and noninvasive. DXA scanners have the precision required to detect changes in muscle mass as small as 5%. Radiation exposure from DXA scans is minimal. The National Council of Radiation Protection and Measurements (NCRP) has recommended that the annual effective dose limit for infrequent exposure of the general population is 5,000 μSv and that an annual effective dose of 10 μSv be considered a negligible individual dose. The effective dose of a dual-energy X-ray absorptiometry whole-body scan on an adult is 2.1 μSv. Studies have shown that quality assurance is an important issue in the use of DXA scans to determine body composition including lean body mass and bone mineral density. DXA instrument manufacturer and model should remain consistent, and their calibration should be monitored throughout treatment. Use of a standardized scan acquisition protocol and appropriate and unchanging scan acquisition and analysis software is essential to achieve consist results.

3. *Dietary intake* must be assessed at baseline and periodical intervals by conducting random weekly, 2 weekdays + 1 weekend day, 24-h dietary recalls (gold standard for collecting dietary data) using a five-step multipass procedure (which has been found to assess mean energy intake within 10% of actual intake) and using the frequently updated University of Minnesota Nutrition Data System for Research (NDS-R) version database for analysis of nutrient composition. Food portion visuals can be provided to patients to estimate portion sizes of foods while monitoring intake..

4. *Symptom log* may be completed daily and collected from patients on a monthly basis. Based on these symptoms, all anticipated and unanticipated, grades of constitutional, dermatological, gastrointestinal (GI), metabolic, and pain symptoms can be continuously monitored including those symptoms affecting nutritional intake and utilization.

5. *CMP and CBC*: Monthly CMP and CBC should be monitored to assess electrolytes and organ function.

6. *Functional markers (Karnofsky performance score)*: Evaluation of patients' functional status and barriers to obtaining adequate nutrients are also necessary. A physical exam combined with personal interview should include the evaluation of functional status such as the ability to chew and swallow, dental or oral problems causing odynophagia or dysphagia, signs of muscle wasting or anasarca, presence of edema, presence of skin or mouth lesion, and ability to perform instrumental activities of daily living (IADLs) such as cooking shopping, and self-feeding. It is critical to assess activities of daily living, physical activity, exercise, and sleep and ability to work and perform other functional roles. Limitations in the activities of daily living have been identified secondary to and as a cause of weight loss in cancer patients. Cancer and other chronic diseases pose difficulties specifically for the cancer patient receiving treatment and the elderly in carrying out activities of daily living. A loss of postural and locomotive muscle mass has been observed within 7 days of inactivity. The Karnofsky Performance Scale Index allows patients to be classified as to their functional impairment. This has been used to compare effectiveness of different therapies and to assess the prognosis in individual patients and has been validated in cancer patient populations.

7. *Godin Leisure-Time Exercise Questionnaire* weekly to monitor physical activity.

8. *Handgrip strength dynamometry assessment*: A validated tool commonly used to assess handgrip strength is the Jamar dynamometer, which is a fast, reliable, and an easy-to-perform device commonly used by our team to measure improvements in functional strength. The Jamar dynamometer has a lower % coefficient of variation and is thus a more precise device than other handgrip dynamometers.

9. *Biochemical markers of protein status (serum albumin and transferrin)*: Assessment of protein status is critical in the identification and treatment of abnormalities in protein metabolism. There is substantial evidence of the correlation between serum hepatic proteins and inflammation, making these the most relevant biomarkers in cancer patient populations. Serum transferrin, prealbumin, and albumin have been observed as intermediate endpoint biomarkers and independently associated with clinical outcomes. Measurements of body

composition combined with more objective and sensitive measure of protein nutriture are ideal for the biochemical assessment of intravascular and visceral protein stores. We have thus included the three major valid intermediate endpoint biomarkers (IEBs) that represent intravascular and visceral protein pools – transferrin, prealbumin and albumin – as the biochemical indicators of protein status. Although transferrin levels are affected by iron status, serum transferrin, either singly or as part of a multiparameter index, is the strongest predictor of cancer patient morbidity and mortality.

10. *Immune and inflammatory markers*: A range of metabolic responses triggered by inflammatory and immunological responses in cancer patients. Cytokines can be measured in a panel including IL-1, IL-4, IL-6, IL-8, IL-10, GM-CSF, IFN-κ, TNF-α, and CRP (Bio-Rad-Bio-Plex). All of these biomarkers have been shown to increase with disease, aging, and cytotoxic agents. Though we realize these intermediate endpoint biomarkers of cytokines cannot be reliably interpreted, as over 70% of the subjects as observed in our studies were on active treatment with cytotoxic agents, these variables are important to determine as they may provide useful information and contribute to the better understanding of the mechanistic process.

11. *Quality of life* should be measured at baseline and monthly using the Rand Short Form (SF)-36 (Medical Outcomes Study SF36) [66]. The SF-36 has been used extensively with general, high-risk, and cancer populations and has available norms for mail and telephone versions and comparisons between group and individual scores. Scores are calculated and transformed to a 0–100 scale, with higher scores indicating increased health status. Reliability of the SF-36 scales was measured by Cronbach α coefficient and the results ranged from 0.78 in general health perceptions to 0.91 in the physical functioning domain.

12. *Assessment for alterations in taste and smell*: Assessment of gustatory sensitivity in a clinical setting is the prerequisite for correct diagnosis, adequate treatment, and evaluation of taste dysfunction. A variety of approaches to the assessment of taste and smell alterations have evolved in the literature including self-reported tools that continue to generate a description of the development, duration, and recovery of distorted chemosensory perception in cancer patients. Quantitative assessment of gustatory function in a clinical context using impregnated "taste strips" or "Sniffin' Strips" has been validated by several groups. The duration of these tests range between 8 to 10 minutes and can be completed at patient's bedside. The taste from a list of four to now five descriptors, i.e., sweet, sour, salty, bitter, and umami (multiple forced choice), can be assessed serially using these strips objectively. This ongoing assessment will inform the interdisciplinary team as to the effectiveness of the intervention.

12.5.10 Follow-up

Patients must be seen by the multidisciplinary team on a regularly scheduled basis to monitor progress and to review compliance to intervention including diet intake adequacy, symptom logs, change in concomitant medications, and any other issues related to treatment. Reassessment/reevaluation for monitoring and evaluation of nutritional therapy must include monitoring of clinical, functional, dietary, and behavioral outcomes that were identified by the comprehensive nutritional assessment

12.6   Future Directions

As with all symptoms of cancer treatment and interventional approaches to prevent and/or ameliorate these symptoms, alteration in smell and taste continue to perplex the medical teams treating cancer patients as well as frustrate patients and families. In general, there is no cure for chemotherapy-induced dysgeusia, only strategies to help manage the disorder. There is a paucity of high-level evidence on potentially useful interventions and a continued need for new and innovative research, incorporating quality-of-life measurements in patients experiencing these symptoms.

Summary for the Clinician

Current principles of management have relied on early detection and management that involves alteration and enhancement of nutritional intake tailored to the individual patient.

Results of research over the past decade indicate that both pharmacological and nonpharmacological approaches to the management of taste and smell alterations have been examined.

Assessment of gustatory sensitivity in a clinical setting is the prerequisite for correct diagnosis and adequate treatment of taste dysfunction.

Although quantitative, objective methods for detection or recognition of threshold values of the five basic tastes have been used in laboratory settings, patient-reported qualitative assessments have been found to have a relatively better utility value in clinical settings.

Since alterations in taste and smell are rarely brought up by the healthcare provider, a conversation about these symptoms needs to take place before the initiation of chemotherapy or radiation therapy.

Improved management of these symptoms may require a *multimodal approach by multidisciplinary teams*.

With regard to pharmacological approaches, several studies have evaluated the use of zinc sulfate in mitigating taste alterations and the amino acid glutamine as a treatment for dysgeusia. Based on these studies, there is limited evidence supporting the use of zinc sulfate or glutamine for treatment of these symptoms, and more research needs to occur before pharmacological recommendations can be made.

Nonpharmacological management strategies and patient education have been the mainstay of treatment for dysgeusia.

Taste and smell alteration varies with each patient, and specific suggestions for symptom management must be tailored on an individual basis.

Systematic screening of symptoms, current and past treatments, other medications, infections, oral care, and additional symptoms of cancer treatments must be taken into account prior to providing modification of food preparation and nutritional intake recommendations. The modifications in nutritional intake and behaviors appear to be the only effective management approach at this time.

There is a paucity of high-level evidence on potentially useful interventions and a continued need for new and innovative research, incorporating quality-of-life measurements in patients experiencing these symptoms.

References

1. Hong JH, Omur-Ozbek P, Stanek BT, Dietrich AM, Duncan SE, Lee YW, Lesser G (2009) Taste and odor abnormalities in cancer patients. J Support Oncol 7(2):58–65
2. American Institute for Cancer Research (2010) Nutrition of the cancer patient. [Brochure], Washington, DC. Retrieved from http://www.aicr.org/site/DocServer/Nutrition_of_Patient. pdf,docID=1567
3. Leopold DA, Holbrook EH. Disorders of taste and smell. Available at. http://www.emedicine. com/ent/topic333.htm. Accessed 11 Feb 2009
4. Leopold D (2002) Distortion of olfactory perception: diagnosis and treatment. Chem Senses 27:611–615 [2200340]
5. Bernhardson BM, Tishelman C, Rutqvist LE (2008) Self-reported taste and smell changes during cancer chemotherapy. Support Care Cancer 16(3):275–283, Epub 2007 Aug 21
6. Camp-Sorrell D (2005) Chemotherapy toxicities and management. In: Yarbro C, Frogge M, Goodman M (eds) Cancer nursing. Jones and Bartlett Publishers, Sudbury, pp 412–457
7. Steinbach S, Hundt W, Zahnert T, Berktold S, Böhner C, Gottschalk N, Hamann M, Kriner M, Heinrich P, Schmalfeldt B, Harbeck N (2010) Gustatory and olfactory function in breast cancer patients. Support Care Cancer 18(6):707–713, Epub 2009 Jun 3
8. Halyard MY, Jatoi A, Sloan JA, Bearden JD 3rd, Vora SA, Atherton PJ, Perez EA, Soori G, Zalduendo AC, Zhu A, Stella PJ, Loprinzi CL (2007) Does zinc sulfate prevent therapy-induced taste alterations in head and neck cancer patients? Results of phase III double-blind, placebo-controlled trial from the North Central Cancer Treatment Group (N01C4). Int J Radiat Oncol Biol Phys 67(5):1318–1322
9. Capra S, Ferguson M, Ried K (2001) Cancer: impact of nutrition intervention outcome – nutrition issues for patients. Nutrition 17(9):769–772, Review
10. Sarhill N, Mahmoud F, Walsh D, Nelson KA, Komurcu S, Davis M, LeGrand S, Abdullah O, Rybicki L (2003) Evaluation of nutritional status in advanced metastatic cancer. Support Care Cancer 11(10):652–659, Epub 2003 Aug 15
11. Brisbois TD, de Kock IH, Watanabe SM, Baracos VE, Wismer WV (2011) Characterization of chemosensory alterations in advanced cancer reveals specific chemosensory phenotypes impacting dietary intake and quality of life. J Pain Symptom Manage 41(4):673–683, Epub 2011 Jan 28

12. Rehwaldt M, Wickman R, Purl S, Tariman J, Blendowski C, Shott S, Lappe M (2009) Self-care strategies to cope with taste changes after chemotherapy. Oncol Nurs Forum 36:E 47–E 56. doi:doi: 10.1188/09.ONF.E47-E56

13. Bernhardson B-M, Tishelman C, Rutqvist LE (2007) Chemosensory changes experienced by patients undergoing cancer chemotherapy: a qualitative interview study. J Pain Symptom Manage 34:403–411. doi:10.1016/j.jpainsymman.2006.12.010

14. Comeau TB, Epstein JB, Migas C (2001) Taste and smell dysfunction in patients receiving chemotherapy: a review of current knowledge. Support Care Cancer 9:575–580. doi:10.1007/s005200100279

15. Bernhardson BM, Tishelman C, Rutqvist LE (2009) Olfactory changes among patients receiving chemotherapy. Eur J Oncol Nurs 13(1):9–15, Epub 2008 Nov 22

16. Bartoshuk LM (1990) Chemosensory alterations and cancer therapies. NCI Monogr 9:179–184

17. Hovan AJ, Williams PM, Stevenson-Moore P, Wahlin YB, Ohrn KE, Elting LS, Spijkervet FK, Brennan MT, Dysgeusia Section, Oral Care Study Group, Multinational Association of Supportive Care in Cancer (MASCC)/International Society of Oral Oncology (ISOO) (2010) A systematic review of dysgeusia induced by cancer therapies. Support Care Cancer 18(8):1081–1087, Epub 2010 May 22

18. Wickham RS, Rehwaldt M, Kefer C, Shott S, Abbas K, Glynn-Tucker E, Potter C, Blendowski C (1999) Taste changes experienced by patients receiving chemotherapy. Oncol Nurs Forum 26(4):697–706

19. Ravasco P (2005) Aspects of taste and compliance in patients with cancer. Eur J Oncol Nurs 9(Suppl 2):S84–S91, Review

20. Berteretche MV, Dalix AM, Cesar d'Ornano AM, Bellisle F, Khayat D, Faurion A (2004) Decreased taste sensitivity in cancer patients under chemotherapy. Support Care Cancer 12:571–576. doi:doi: 10.1007/s00520–004–0589-2

21. Strasser F, Demmer R, Böhme C, Schmitz SF, Thuerlimann B, Cerny T, Gillessen S (2008) Prevention of docetaxel- or paclitaxel-associated taste alterations in cancer patients with oral glutamine: a randomized, placebo-controlled, double-blind study. Oncologist 13(3):337–346

22. Ravasco P (2011) Nutritional support in head and neck cancer: how and why? Anticancer Drugs 22(7):639–646

23. Steinbach S, Hummel T, Böhner C, Berktold S, Hundt W, Kriner M, Heinrich P, Sommer H, Hanusch C, Prechtl A, Schmidt B, Bauerfeind I, Seck K, Jacobs VR, Schmalfeldt B, Harbeck N (2009) Qualitative and quantitative assessment of taste and smell changes in patients undergoing chemotherapy for breast cancer or gynecologic malignancies. J Clin Oncol 27(11):1899–1905, Epub 2009 Mar 16

24. Dirix P, Nuyts S, Vander Poorten V, Delaere P, Van den Bogaert W (2008) The influence of xerostomia after radiotherapy on quality of life: results of a questionnaire in head and neck cancer. Support Care Cancer 16(2):171–179, Epub 2007 Jul 6

25. Ruo Redda MG, Allis S (2006) Radiotherapy-induced taste impairment. Cancer Treat Rev 32(7):541–547, Epub 2006 Aug 2

26. Ripamonti C, Zecca E, Brunelli C, Fulfaro F, Villa S, Balzarini A, Conno F (1998) A randomized, controlled clinical trial to evaluate the effects of zinc sulfate on cancer patients with taste alterations caused by head and neck irradiation. Cancer 82:1938–1945

27. Murphy C, Schubert CR, Cruickshanks KJ, Klein BE, Klein R, Nondahl DM (2002) Prevalence of olfactory impairment in older adults. JAMA 288:2307–2312

28. Sandow PL, Hejrat-Yazdi M, Heft MW (2006) Taste loss and recovery following radiation therapy. J Dent Res 85:608–611 [16798859]

29. Yamashita H, Nakagawa K, Nakagawa N et al (2006) Relation between acute and late irradiation impairment of four basic tastes and irradiated tongue volume in patients with head-and-neck cancer. Int J Radiat Oncol Biol Phys 66:1422–1429 [17084561]

30. Yamashita H, Nakagawa K, Tago M et al (2006) Taste dysfunction in patients receiving radiotherapy. Head Neck 28:508–516 [16619275]

31. Halyard MY (2009) Taste and smell alterations in cancer patients – real problems with few solutions. J Support Oncol 7(2):68–69
32. McDaniel RW, Rhodes VA (1998) Development of a preparatory sensory information videotape for women receiving chemotherapy for breast cancer. Cancer Nurs 21:143–148
33. Epstein JB, Phillips N, Parry J et al (2002) Quality of life, taste, olfactory and oral function following high-dose chemotherapy and allogeneic hematopoietic cell transplantation. Bone Marrow Transplant 30:785–792
34. Muller A, Landis BN, Platzbecker U, Holthoff V, Frasnelli J, Hummel T (2006) Severe chemotherapy-induced parosmia. Am J Rhinol 20:485–486
35. Hoffman H, Ishii EK, Macturk RH (1998) Age-related changes in the prevalence of smell/taste problems among the United States adult population. Ann N Y Acad Sci 855:716–722 [9929676]
36. Zabernigg A, Gamper EM, Giesinger JM, Rumpold G, Kemmler G, Gattringer K, Sperner-Unterweger B, Holzner B (2010) Taste alterations in cancer patients receiving chemotherapy: a neglected side effect? Oncologist 15(8):913–920, Epub 2010 Jul 8
37. Sánchez-Lara K, Sosa-Sánchez R, Green-Renner D, Rodríguez C, Laviano A, Motola-Kuba D, Arrieta O (2010) Influence of taste disorders on dietary behaviors in cancer patients under chemotherapy. Nutr J 9:15
38. Watters AL, Epstein JB, Agulnik M (2011) Oral complications of targeted cancer therapies: a narrative literature review. Oral Oncol 47(6):441–448, Epub 2011 Apr 22
39. Landis BN, Scheibe M, Weber C, Berger R, Brämerson A, Bende M, Nordin S, Hummel T (2010) Chemosensory interaction: acquired olfactory impairment is associated with decreased taste function. J Neurol 257(8):1303–1308, Epub 2010 Mar 11
40. Landis BN, Welge-Luessen A, Brämerson A, Bende M, Mueller CA, Nordin S, Hummel T (2009) "Taste strips" – a rapid, lateralized, gustatory bedside identification test based on impregnated filter papers. J Neurol 256(2):242–248, Epub 2009 Feb 7
41. Sugawara S, Takimoto N, Iida A, Mori K, Sugiura M, Yamamura K, Adachi M (2009) Incidence of taste disorder associated with cancer patients undergoing chemotherapy on an ambulatory basis. Gan To Kagaku Ryoho 36(11):1871–1876
42. Jensen SB, Pedersen AM, Vissink A, Andersen E, Brown CG, Davies AN, Brennan MT (2010) A systematic review of salivary gland hypofunction and xerostomia induced by cancer therapies: prevalence, severity and impact on quality of life. Support Care Cancer. doi:10.1007/s00520-010-0827-8
43. Epstein JB, Barasch A (2010) Taste disorders in cancer patients: pathogenesis and approach to assessment and management. Oral Oncol 46:77–81. doi:10.1016/j.oraloncology.2009.11.008
44. Perry M (2008) The chemotherapy source book. Lippincott Williams & Wilkins, Philadelphia
45. Roeder F, Zwicker F, Saleh-Ebrahimi L, Timke C, Thieke C, Bischof M, Debus J, Huber PE (2011) Intensity modulated or fractionated stereotactic reirradiation in patients with recurrent nasopharyngeal cancer. Radiat Oncol 6:22
46. Johnson FM (2001) Alteration in taste sensation: a case presentation of a patient with end-stage pancreatic cancer. Cancer Nurs 24:149–155
47. Mattes RD, Arnold C, Boraas M (1987) Learned food aversion among cancer chemotherapy patients. Cancer 60:2576–2580
48. DeWys WD, Walters K (1975) Abnormalities of taste sensation in cancer patients. Cancer 36:1888–1896
49. Mirza N, Machtay M, Devine PA, Troxel A, Abboud SK, Doty RL (2008) Gustatory impairment in patients undergoing head and neck irradiation. Laryngoscope 118(1):24–31
50. Yamashita H, Nakagawa K, Tago M, Nakamura N, Shiraishi K, Eda M, Nakata H, Nagamatsu N, Yokoyama R, Onimura M, Ohtomo K (2006) Taste dysfunction in patients receiving radiotherapy. Head Neck 28(6):508–516
51. Yamashita H, Nakagawa K, Nakamura N, Abe K, Asakage T, Ohmoto M, Okada S, Matsumoto I, Hosoi Y, Sasano N, Yamakawa S, Ohtomo K (2006) Relation between acute and late irradiation impairment of four basic tastes and irradiated tongue volume in patients with head-and-neck cancer. Int J Radiat Oncol Biol Phys 66(5):1422–1429, Epub 2006 Nov 2

52. Shi HB, Masuda M, Umezaki T, Kuratomi Y, Kumamoto Y, Yamamoto T, Komiyama S (2004) Irradiation impairment of umami taste in patients with head and neck cancer. Auris Nasus Larynx 31(4):401–406

53. Sadler GR, Stoudt A, Fullerton JT, Oberle-Edwards LK, Nguyen Q, Epstein JB (2003) Managing the oral sequelae of cancer therapy. Medsurg Nurs 12(1):28–36

54. Lee N, Puri DR, Blanco AI, Chao KS (2007) Intensity-modulated radiation therapy in head and neck cancers: an update. Head Neck 29(4):387–400

55. Smeets MA, Veldhuizen MG, Galle S, Gouweloos J, de Haan AM, Vernooij J, Visscher F, Kroeze JH (2009) Sense of smell disorder and health-related quality of life. Rehabil Psychol 54(4):404–412

56. Cunningham RS (2004) The anorexia-cachexia syndrome. In: Yarbro C, Frogge M, Goodman M (eds) Cancer symptom management. Jones and Bartlett Publishers, Sudbury, pp 137–167

57. Doty RL, Bromley SM (2004) Effects of drugs on olfaction and taste. Otolaryngol Clin North Am 37(6):1229–1254

58. Windfuhr JP, Sack F, Sesterhenn AM, Landis BN, Chen YS (2010) Post-tonsillectomy taste disorders. Eur Arch Otorhinolaryngol 267(2):289–293, Epub 2009 Aug 23

59. Bonfils P, Jankowski R, Faulcon P (2001) Smell dysfunction in nasal and paranasal sinus disease: a review of the literature (II). Ann Otolaryngol Chir Cervicofac 118(3):143–155

60. Briner HR, Simmen D, Jones N (2003) Impaired sense of smell in patients with nasal surgery. Clin Otolaryngol Allied Sci 28(5):417–419

61. Ovesen L, Sørensen M, Hannibal J, Allingstrup L (1991) Electrical taste detection thresholds and chemical smell detection threshold in patients with cancer. Cancer 68:2260–2265 [1913462]

62. Berteretche MV, Dalix AM, d'Ornano AM, Bellisle F, Khayat D, Faurion A (2004) Decreased taste sensitivity in cancer patients under chemotherapy. Support Care Cancer 12:571–576

63. Marín Caro MM, Laviano A, Pichard C (2007) Impact of nutrition on quality of life during cancer. Curr Opin Clin Nutr Metab Care 10(4):480–487, Review

64. Yamashita H, Nakagawa K, Hosoi Y, Kurokawa A, Fukuda Y, Matsumoto I, Misaka T, Abe K (2009) Umami taste dysfunction in patients receiving radiotherapy for head and neck cancer. Oral Oncol 45(3):e19–e23, Epub 2008 Jul 11

65. Mueller C, Kallert S, Renner B, Stiassny K, Temmel AF, Hummel T, Kobal G (2003) Quantitative assessment of gustatory function in a clinical context using impregnated "taste strips". Rhinology 41(1):2–6

66. Garratt AM, Ruta DA, Abdalla MI, Buckingham JK, Russell IT (1993) The SF36 health survey questionnaire: an outcome measure suitable for routine use within the NHS? BMJ 306(6890):1440–1444

Index